Springer Series in Statistics

Advisors:
P. Bickel, P. Diggle, S. Fienberg, K. Krickeberg,
I. Olkin, N. Wermuth, S. Zeger

T0135269

Springer

New York
Berlin
Heidelberg
Barcelona
Hong Kong
London
Milan
Paris
Singapore
Tokyo

Springer Series in Statistics

Andersen/Borgan/Gill/Keiding: Statistical Models Based on Counting Processes.
Atkinson/Riani: Robust Diagnotstic Regression Analysis.
Berger: Statistical Decision Theory and Bayesian Analysis, 2nd edition.
Bolfarine/Zacks: Prediction Theory for Finite Populations.
Borg/Groenen: Modern Multidimensional Scaling: Theory and Applications
Brockwell/Davis: Time Series: Theory and Methods, 2nd edition.
Chan/Tong: Chaos: A Statistical Perspective.
Chen/Shao/Ibrahim: Monte Carlo Methods in Bayesian Computation.
David/Edwards: Annotated Readings in the History of Statistics.
Devroye/Lugosi: Combinatorial Methods in Density Estimation.
Efromovich: Nonparametric Curve Estimation: Methods, Theory, and Applications.
Eggermont/LaRiccia: Maximum Penalized Likelihood Estimation, Volume I:
    Density Estimation.
Fahrmeir/Tutz: Multivariate Statistical Modelling Based on Generalized Linear
    Models, 2nd edition.
Farebrother: Fitting Linear Relationships: A History of the Calculus of Observations
    1750-1900.
Federer: Statistical Design and Analysis for Intercropping Experiments, Volume I:
    Two Crops.
Federer: Statistical Design and Analysis for Intercropping Experiments, Volume II:
    Three or More Crops.
Fienberg/Hoaglin/Kruskal/Tanur (Eds.): A Statistical Model: Frederick Mosteller's
    Contributions to Statistics, Science and Public Policy.
Fisher/Sen: The Collected Works of Wassily Hoeffding.
Glaz/Naus/Wallenstein: Scan Statistics.
Good: Permutation Tests: A Practical Guide to Resampling Methods for Testing
    Hypotheses, 2nd edition.
Gouriéroux: ARCH Models and Financial Applications.
Grandell: Aspects of Risk Theory.
Haberman: Advanced Statistics, Volume I: Description of Populations.
Hall: The Bootstrap and Edgeworth Expansion.
Härdle: Smoothing Techniques: With Implementation in S.
Harrell: Regression Modeling Strategies: With Applications to Linear Models,
    Logistic Regression, and Survival Analysis
Hart: Nonparametric Smoothing and Lack-of-Fit Tests.
Hartigan: Bayes Theory.
Hastie/Tibshirani/Friedman: The Elements of Statistical Learning: Data Mining,
    Inference, and Prediction
Hedayat/Sloane/Stufken: Orthogonal Arrays: Theory and Applications.
Heyde: Quasi-Likelihood and its Application: A General Approach to Optimal
    Parameter Estimation.
Huet/Bouvier/Gruet/Jolivet: Statistical Tools for Nonlinear Regression: A Practical
    Guide with S-PLUS Examples.
Ibrahim/Chen/Sinha: Bayesian Survival Analysis.
Kolen/Brennan: Test Equating: Methods and Practices.

(continued after index)

Joseph Glaz
Joseph Naus
Sylvan Wallenstein

Scan Statistics

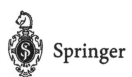

Springer

Joseph Glaz
Department of Statistics
The College of Liberal Arts and Sciences
University of Connecticut
Storrs, CT 06269
USA

Joseph Naus
Department of Statistics
Rutgers, The State University of
  New Jersey
Piscataway, NJ 08854
USA

Sylvan Wallenstein
Department of Biomathematical Sciences
Mount Sinai School of Medicine
New York, NY 10029
USA

Library of Congress Cataloging-in-Publication Data
Glaz, Josesph.
    Scan statistics / Joseph Glaz, Joseph Naus, Sylvan Wallenstein.
      p. cm. — (Springer series in statistics)
    Includes bibliographical references and index.
     ISBN 978-1-4419-3167-2
    1. Order statistics.   I. Naus, Joseph   II. Wallenstein, Sylvan.   III. Title.   IV. Series.
QA278.7 .G57 2001
519.5—dc21   00-053197

Printed on acid-free paper.

Photocomposed pages prepared by TeXniques, Inc., Cambridge, MA.

Printed in the United States of America.

9 8 7 6 5 4 3 2 1

Springer-Verlag   New York Berlin Heidelberg
A member of BertelsmannSpringer Science+Business Media GmbH

To our parents and wives

Preface

This book summarizes research on scan statistics. These statistics arise naturally in the scanning of time and space looking for clusters of events.

The first part of the book concentrates on applications of the different types of scan statistics. This part summarizes useful formulae for approximate and exact probabilities and moments of scan statistics, and references available tables and computer programs. Applications of a wide variety of scan statistics to fields ranging from epidemiology, quality control, reliability, molecular biology, astronomy, photographic science, telecommunications, mineral exploration, stress engineering, visual perception, sports statistics, military science, meteorology, and other fields are illustrated. This part of the book is designed for researchers in many applied fields, and is written from the point of view of methodology and applications of the scan statistics.

The second part of the book is designed for mathematical statisticians and probabilists who are interested in doing further research into the scan statistic. This part of the book brings together and reviews the mathematical approaches used to develop exact and approximate results for the scan statistics. It is hoped that bringing this material together will be an aid and impetus for further development in this field.

The authors thank Martin Gilchrist and John Kimmel (Editors, Springer-Verlag) for inviting us to write this book and for providing continual support and encouragement. We also thank the people at the production office of Springer, including, Production Editor Tony Orrantia, the copy editor, Brian Howe, and the typesetter, TEXniques, for producing this attractive volume. We thank our colleagues for ideas and inspiration, and our institutions for their support during the course of writing this book.

Joe Glaz thanks his parents, David and Emi Glaz, for their loving support and encouragement throughout the years. He thanks his wife, Sarah, for her continuous loving support and encouragement and for the wise advice in all his professional activities. He thanks his son, Ron, for his loving support and encouragement and for the fun we have observing clusters of wins by the Yankees and the UConn Huskies.

Joe Naus thanks his wife, Sarah, for 40 years of patient listening about scan statistics. Sarah, clearly a *woman of valor*, brings love to all around her and has developed an impressive cluster of friends who share her birthday. He thanks his parents, Maximillian and Charlotte Naus, his wife Sarah and his children, Alisa and Eric, Laura, Julie and Patrick, and Mark for their love, encouragement, and for the joy they bring to his life.

Sylvan Wallenstein thanks his wife, Helene, for her love and for her encouragement in writing this book and in all his professional efforts. He thanks his children Josh and Rachel, Elana, and Tami in listening to hours of talk on the scan statistic over the dinner table and on vacations. He thanks his parents Morris and Dina Wallenstein for the examples they have set.

Contents

Preface   **vii**

I Methods and Applications   **1**

1 Introduction   **3**
   1.1   The Discrete Scan Statistic   5
   1.2   Scan Statistics in Two Dimensions   6
   1.3   Power of the Scan Statistic   7
   1.4   Clusters and Intuition   8

2 Retrospective Scanning of Events Over Time   **11**
   2.1   Conditional Case: Uniform Distribution of Events   11
         2.1.1   Approximate Results for $P(k; N, w)$ 12
   2.2   The Scan Statistic on the Circle   18
   2.3   The Ratchet Scan Statistic   20
   2.4   Moments of Scan Statistics   21
         2.4.1   Exact Values for Moments of the Scan Statistic S_w   21
         2.4.2   The Expectation and Variance of the W_k, the Size of the
                 Smallest Interval   22

3 Prospective Scanning of Events Over Time   **25**
   3.1   Poisson Distribution of Events   25
         3.1.1   The Poisson Process   27

3.2   Approximate Formula for $P^*(k; \lambda T, w/T)$ 28

3.3   Handling Trends or Seasonality in Data   35

      3.3.1   The Disjoint Week Procedure   36

      3.3.2   Continuous 7-Day Scan   37

      3.3.3   Comparison of Disjoint Week with 7 Day Scan for
           a 52 Week Year   37

3.4   Moments of Scan Statistics   37

      3.4.1   The Expectation and Variance of W_k, the Size of
           the Smallest Interval   38

      3.4.2   The Expected Waiting Time until a Cluster   38

3.5   The Distribution of the Number of Clusters in $[0, T)$ 39

      3.5.1   The Distribution of the Number of Nonoverlapping Clusters   40

      3.5.2   The Distribution of the Number of Overlapping Clusters .   40

3.6   The Scan Statistic on the Circle   41

4   Success Scans in a Sequence of Trials   **43**

4.1   Binomial Distribution of Events: Discrete Time, Unconditional Case   43

4.2   A Null Model for the Unconditional Case: The Bernoulli Process .   44

      4.2.1   Approximations for $P'(k \mid m; N; p)$ with Applications . .   45

      4.2.2   The Length of the Longest Quota   54

4.3   The Charge Problem   54

4.4   Binomial Distributed Events: Discrete Time, Conditional Case . .   56

4.5   Related Statistics   58

4.6   Longest Run of any Letter in a Sequence of r Letters   58

4.7   Moments of Scan Statistics   59

      4.7.1   The Expectation and Variance of S'_m, the Size of
           the Largest Cluster   59

      4.7.2   The Expectation and Variance of W'_k, the Size of
           the Smallest Interval   59

      4.7.3   The Expected Waiting Time until a Cluster   60

5   Higher-Dimensional Scans   **61**

5.1   Introduction   61

5.2   The Conditional Problem   63

      5.2.1   Effect of the Shape of the Scanning Rectangle   65

5.3   The Unconditional Problem   75

5.4   Clustering on the Lattice   76

6   Scan Statistics in DNA and Protein Sequence Analysis   **81**

6.1   Introduction   81

6.2   Scanning for Clusters of Patterns   82

6.3   Matching in DNA Sequences   85

6.4   Matching in Multiple Random Letter Sequences   91

6.5   Sequencing Fragments to Reconstruct a Genome   94

6.6   Using Double Scans for More Effective Searches for Homologies   95

6.7   Correlated Descendant Sequences Scan Statistics   95

II Scan Distribution Theory and its Developments   97

7 Approaches Used for Derivations and Approximations   99
  7.1 Introduction 99
  7.2 Order Statistics and a Direct Integration Approach 99
  7.3 Combinatorial Approach 101
     7.3.1 The Karlin–McGregor Theorem 103
  7.4 Bonferroni-Type Inequalities 104
  7.5 The Q_2/Q_3 Approximation for Scan Statistics 107
  7.6 Poisson and Compound Poisson Approximations 108

8 Scanning N Uniform Distributed Points: Exact Results   113
  8.1 Introduction 113
  8.2 The Direct Integration Approach 114
  8.3 The Combinatorial Approach 115
  8.4 The Derivation of $P(k; N, w)$ for $k > (N + 1)/2, w \le 1/2$ 117
     8.4.1 Finding $P(B_1)$ 117
     8.4.2 Finding $P(B_1 \cap B_2)$ for $k > N/2$ 119
  8.5 A General Formula for $P(k; N, 1/L)$ for Integer L 119
  8.6 Simplifying Theorem 8.1 for the Special Case $P(k; N, 1/3)$ . . . 122
  8.7 General Formula for $P(k; N, w)$ 123
  8.8 Simplifying the General Formula 126
     8.8.1 Finding $P(\mathcal{A})$ 127
     8.8.2 Finding $P(B)$ 127
  8.9 Generating the Piecewise Polynomials from the General Formulas 131
  8.10 The Approach of Huffer and Lin 133
  8.11 The Expectation and Variance of W_k, the Size of
       the Smallest Interval 136
  8.12 The Scan Statistic on the Circle 137
     8.12.1 Derivation of Exact Results 138
     8.12.2 Relation of Scan Statistic on Circle and
            Coverage Problems 140

9 Scanning N Uniform Distributed Points: Bounds   141
  9.1 Bounds Based on the Scanning Process Representation 141
  9.2 Bounds Based on Spacings 147
  9.3 Method of Moments Bounds Using Linear Programming 154
  9.4 Bounds for $E(S_w)$ 156
  9.5 Bounds for the Distribution of a Scan Statistic on a Circle 158

10 Approximations for the Conditional Case   161
  10.1 Spacings 162
  10.2 Approximations Involving Probabilities 164
  10.3 Declumping Techniques 165
  10.4 The Method of Moments Based on Two Moments 166

      10.4.1 Two-Moment "Markov-Chain" Approximation (MC2) . . 167
      10.4.2 Two-Moment Compound Poisson Approximations 168
      10.4.3 Two-Parameter Compound Poisson Geometric (CPG2) . . 169
      10.4.4 Glaz's et al. Compound Poisson Approximation 169
      10.4.5 Other Methods of Moments Approximations 170
  10.5 Cell Occupancy Approximations: Introduction 170
      10.5.1 Conditional Probabilities 171
      10.5.2 Unconditional Probabilities 171
      10.5.3 Joint Unconditional Probabilities 173
  10.6 Markov-Type Approximation (Naus, 1982) 174
  10.7 Very Simple Approximations based on Multiples of $b(k; N, w)$ . . 175
      10.7.1 Derivation of Wallenstein–Neff Approximations 176
      10.7.2 Related Approximations 177
  10.8 Approximations Based on Bounds 178
      10.8.1 Approximation Based on Two-Way Intersections 178
      10.8.2 Approximation Based on Three-Way Intersections 179
  10.9 Other Methods 179
  10.10 Comparisons 180
  10.11 Circular Case 182

11 Scanning Points in a Poisson Process   **185**
  11.1 Poisson Distribution of Events 185
      11.1.1 The Poisson Process 185
  11.2 Exact Results for $P^*(k; \lambda T, w/T)$ 186
  11.3 Bounds for the Distribution of the Scan Statistic 189
  11.4 Approximations for the Distribution of the Scan Statistics 196
      11.4.1 Alm's Approximation 197
      11.4.2 Moments of Scan Statistics 199

12 The Generalized Birthday Problem   **201**
  12.1 Binomial Distribution of Events: Discrete Time,
      Unconditional Case 201
  12.2 The Conditional Case: Exact Results 201
  12.3 Bounds for the Conditional Scan Statistic 205
  12.4 Approximations for the Conditional Scan Statistic 212
      12.4.1 Approximations for i.i.d. 0–1 Bernoulli Trials 212
            12.4.1.1 Product-Type Approximations 212
            12.4.1.2 Poisson Approximations 214
            12.4.1.3 Compound Poisson Approximations 215
            12.4.1.4 Approximations for the Expected Size and
                     Standard Derivation of the Scan Statistic 217
      12.4.2 Scan Statistics for Binomial and Poisson Distributions
            Conditional on the Total Number of Events 218
            12.4.2.1 Poisson Model 218
            12.4.2.2 Binomial Model 218

13 Scan Statistics for a Sequence of Discrete I.I.D. Variates   **221**

13.1   Binomial Distribution of Events. Discrete Time, Unconditional
Case. The Bernoulli Process 221

13.2   Exact Results for the Distribution of the Scan Statistics 222

13.2.1   The Distribution of the Length of the Longest Success
Run: $P'(k \mid k; N, p)$ 222

13.2.2   Exact Results for $P'(k \mid m; N, p)$ 223

13.3   Bounds for S_m' for i.i.d. Integer Valued Random Variables 225

13.4   Approximations for $P'(k \mid m; N, p)$ 231

13.4.1   The Special Case $k = m$: The Length of the Longest Run . 232

13.4.2   Erdös–Rényi Laws 233

13.4.3   Approximating the Discrete Problem by the Continuous . 235

13.5   The Charge Problem 236

13.5.1   Exact Results 236

13.5.2   Saperstein's Recursion for $G_{k,m}(2m)$ 236

13.5.3   The Case $2m < N \leq 3m$ 239

13.5.4   Approximate Results 239

13.5.5   Asymptotic Approximations 239

13.6   Longest Run of Any Letter in a Sequence of r Letters 240

13.7   Moments of Scan Statistics 241

13.7.1   The Expected Waiting Time till a Quota 241

14 Power   **243**

14.1   Introduction 243

14.1.1   Step Function Alternatives 244

14.2   Very Simple Approximations 246

14.2.1   Conditional Case 246

14.2.2   Unconditional Case 247

14.2.3   Discrete 247

14.3   Exact Results 247

14.4   Markovian Approximations for a Pulse of Width w 249

14.4.1   Approximation Applied in the General Context 249

14.4.2   Power when the Width of the Pulse and
Window are Identical 251

14.4.3   A Further Simplification 251

14.5   Intermediate Calculations: Exact Power when $w/T = 1/2$ or $1/3$. 252

14.5.1   One-Way Probabilities 252

14.5.1.1   Continuous Case 252

14.5.2   Joint Probabilities 254

14.5.2.1   Continuous Case 254

14.6   Simple, Somewhat ad hoc Approximation for Power 256

14.6.1   A Very Simple Approximation to Power:
Unconditional Case 256

14.6.2   Conditional Continuous Case 257

14.6.3   Power for a Pulse Starting at $b < w$ 257

14.6.4 Accuracy of Approximations 257
14.7 Power for Other Alternatives 258
14.8 Practical Implementation of Power: Conditional Case 258

15 Testing for Clustering **261**
15.1 Introduction 261
15.2 Weinstock's Approach 262
15.3 An Optimal Test Statistic 263
  15.3.1 Derivation of Approximate Significance Level 265
15.4 A Reasonable, but Nonoptimal Statistic 267
  15.4.1 Proof of Approximation 267
15.5 Practical Implementation: Estimating $f_0(t)$ 269
  15.5.1 Linearly Changing Density 270
15.6 Exact Distribution of a Statistic 270

16 Two-Dimensional Scan Statistics **273**
16.1 A Discrete Scan Statistic 273
  16.1.1 Approximations and Inequalities for $P(S'_{m_1,m_2} = m_1 m_2)$
         for i.i.d. Bernoulli Trials 275
  16.1.2 A Product-Type Approximation 277
  16.1.3 A Bonferroni-Type Inequality 279
  16.1.4 Poisson-Type Approximations 281
  16.1.5 A Compound Poisson Approximation 282
  16.1.6 A Markov Chain Embedding Method for the
         Bernoulli Model 283
  16.1.7 Approximations for the Expected Size and
         Standard Deviation 286
  16.1.8 A Multiple Scan Statistic 287
16.2 A Conditional Discrete Scan Statistic 287
  16.2.1 Product-Type Approximations 288
  16.2.2 Poisson Approximations 290
  16.2.3 A Compound Poisson Approximation 291
  16.2.4 Bonferroni-Type Inequalities 292
  16.2.5 Approximations and Inequalities for the Expected Size
         and Standard Deviation 293
  16.2.6 Simulation Algorithms 295
         16.2.6.1 Binomial Model 295
         16.2.6.2 Poisson Model 296
16.3 A Scan Statistic for a Two-Dimensional Poisson Process 297
16.4 A Scan Statistic for N Points 299

17 Number of Clusters: Ordered Spacings **301**
17.1 Notation and Introduction 301
17.2 Local Declumping which Mimics the Global One 303
17.3 A Markovian Method of Declumping 304

17.4 Compound Poisson Approach 305
17.5 The Dandekar-Modified Binomial 307
17.6 Another Approach Based on the Q_2/Q_3 Approximation 308
17.7 Summary of Results and Comparison of Procedures 309
    17.7.1 Overlapping Clusters 309
    17.7.2 Nonoverlapping Clusters 309
17.8 Exploratory Approach when r Cannot be Specified 309
    17.8.1 Calculations with Fixed r 310
    17.8.2 Calculations with Multiple Values of r Compared with
               Experimental Results 311
    17.8.3 Further Discussion of Example 312

18 Extensions of the Scan Statistic   **313**
18.1 The Double Scan Statistic 313
18.2 Clustering of Two Types of Letter Patterns 317
18.3 The Skip–Scan Statistic 320
18.4 Unusually Small Scans 322
18.5 The Ratchet Scan 326
    18.5.1 Definition of Ratchet Scan and Exact Distribution 326
    18.5.2 Approximate Distributions 327
    18.5.3 Equal Size Intervals, Combinatorial-Type Bounds 327
    18.5.4 Multivariate Normal Asymptotic for Circular Ratchet Scan
               when $L = 12$ 329
18.6 Unknown Value of w 330
    18.6.1 Other Statistics 332

References   **333**

Index   **367**

Part I

Methods and Applications

What is a plague? A city that sends forth five hundred men and three dead went forth from it within three days this one after this one, then this is a plague; less than this, this is not a plague.

Mishna (3rd century codification of Jewish Law)
Tractate Ta'anit, Chapter 3, Mishna 4
Translation by Nahman Kahana and Leonard Oschry in the Kehati Mishna

1
Introduction

In many fields, decision-makers give great weight to clusters of events. Public Health investigators look for common causal factors to explain clusters of cancer cases or birth defects. Molecular biologists look for palindrome clusters in DNA for clues to the origin of replication of viruses. Telecommunications engineers design capacity to accommodate clusters of calls being simultaneously dialed to a switchboard. Quality control experts investigate clusters of defectives. The probabilities of different types of clusters under various conditions are tools of the physical, natural, and social sciences.

This book summarizes research on scan statistics. These statistics arise naturally in the scanning of time and space, looking for clusters of events. The following are two examples of scan statistics. Given N points distributed over a time period $(0, T)$, S_w is the largest number of events in a window of fixed length w of time. This maximum cluster, S_w, is called the *scan statistic*, from the viewpoint that one scans the time period $(0, T)$ with a window of size w, and observes a large number of points (see Figure 1.1). W_k is the shortest period of time containing a fixed number k of events. A special case, W_N, is the sample range. The interval W_{r+1} is called the *minimum r-th-order gap*, or *r-scan statistic*. The distributions of the statistics S_w and W_k are related. If the shortest window that contains k points is longer than w, then there is no window of length w that contains k or more points, $P(W_k > w) = P(S_w < k)$.

The following example clarifies the meaning of the scan statistic. Over a five year period, 1991 to 1995, there were 19 cases of a particular type of cancer reported in a city. In reviewing the data, the epidemiologist notes that there is a 1 year period (from April 4, 1993, through April 13, 1994), that contains eight cases. This is illustrated in Figure 1.1. The researcher asks the following question:

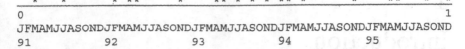

Figure 1.1. Scanning the unit time interval with a window of length $w = .2$. The *'s represent times of occurrence of $N = 19$ events, $S_{.2} = 8$.

Given 19 cases over 5 years, how unusual is it to have a 1 year period containing as many as eight cases?

We might try to answer the researcher's question as follows. Each of the 19 cases could either fall in the period (April 14, 1993 to April 13, 1994) or not fall in it, independently of the other cases. The probability of as many as eight cases falling in this interval is found by computing the binomial probability for $N = 19$, $p = 1/5$, and summing terms for $k \geq 8$. This calculation does not answer the question posed; the researcher wants to know how unusual it is to get any 1 year period (not a specific year) containing as many as eight cases.

We might try to get around this problem by dividing the five years up into five disjoint 1 year periods, and using the distribution of the maximum number of cases falling in any 1 year. However, this too does not answer the researcher's question, since the specific year observed overlaps two of the disjoint years. The researcher is not limiting the question to calendar years. The researcher is in effect scanning the 5 year period with a window of length 1 year, and focusing on the scan statistic S_w, the maximum number of points in the scanning window. Application 2.4 of Chapter 2 shows how to compute $P(S_{.2} \geq 8 \mid N = 19)$, the answer to the researcher's question for this example.

Epidemiologists and public health officials focus on unusual clusters of disease cases. The following recent research shows the range of epidemiologic applications that use scan statistics to test for unusual clustering: Anderson and Titterington (1997), laryngeal cancer; Morris, Alberman, and Mutton (1998), Down's Syndrome; Hourani, Warrack, and Cohen (1997), suicide; Ward and Carpenter (2000), blowfly strike in sheep; Moreno, Ardanaz, Olivera, Castilla, and de Pedro-Cuesta (1994), Sudden Infant Death Syndrome; Hjalmers, Kulldorf, Gustafsson, and Nagarwalla (1996), childhood leukemia; Doheer, Carpenter, Wilson, and Gardner (1999), equine *C. pseudoturberculosis*; Ekbom, Zack, Adami, and Helmick (1991), inflammatory bowel disease; Jiang, Cheng, Link, and de Pedro-Cuesta (1997), Guillain–Barre syndrome; Velandia, Fridkin, Cardenas, Boshell, Ramirez, Bland, Iglesias, and Jarvis (1995), HIV in dialysis patients; Calzolari, Volpato, Bianchi, Cianciulli, Tenconi, Clementi, Calabro, Lungarotti, Mastroiacovo, Botto, Spagnolo, and Milan (1993), *Omphalocele* and *Gastroschisis*; Singer, Case, Carpenter, Walker, and Hirsh (1998), resistant *Pasturella* in cattle; Kulldorff, Feurer, Miller, and Freedman (1997), brain cancer and (1998), breast cancer.

Scan statistic clusters of many types grab attention, demand explanation, and spark action. Two recent articles illustrate this:

> *USA Today* (February 23, 1996, front page): Headline, "Another F-14 crash prompts *stand-down.*" On February 22, the U.S. Navy suspended all operations of the F-14 jet after the third crash in 25 days. The three crashes in less than a month was about seven times the expected rate based on the 5 year period. (Here, $S_{25} = 3$; $W_3 = 25$.)

> *Home News* (August 11, 1995): In a 10 month period, 11 residents died at a Tennessee State Institution for individuals with serious physical and mental handicaps. The number dying was about twice what was expected, and a U.S. District judge was angry, "Find the cause for the increase and correct it!" Until then, the judge ordered the State of Tennessee to pay a fine of $5000 a day, and the mental health commissioner to spend one in four weekends at the state institution.

The decision-makers in these two cases took action because of scan statistic clusters that were intuitively very unusual. However, intuition can mislead. This book gives tools to measure the unusualness of scan statistic clusters. Chapter 3 analyzes the above examples in detail using these tools. The results may surprise you.

1.1 The Discrete Scan Statistic

The scan statistics above were defined over a continuous time interval $[0, T)$. They can be similarly defined over a sequence of T trials (the discrete case). A special case of the discrete scan statistic is the length of the longest *success* run in a sequence of Bernoulli trials. The distribution of the length of the longest run of successes in a sequence of N Bernoulli trials is a classical problem in probability theory, with a generating function approach, going back to 1738 by Abraham de Moivre, explicit expressions by Simpson in 1740, and Laplace's recursion relation solution in 1812 (see Hald (1990, pp. 417–423)). The problem and its generalizations, asymptotic results, and Erdös–Rényi laws, continue to challenge and stimulate.

The maximum number of successes within any m contiguous trials within the N trials, denoted S'_m, is a *discrete scan statistic*. For the special case where $S'_m = m$, a success run of length m has occurred within the N trials. For the general case where $S'_m = k$, a *quota* of at least k successes within m consecutive trials has occurred. Chapter 4 describes a variety of applications of the discrete scan statistic; Chapte 12 reviews exact and asymptotic distributional results.

An important application of discrete scan statistics arises in matching DNA or protein sequences. Scientists in fields ranging from evolution to medicine compare sequences from several biological sources. These can be viewed as sequences of letters from an alphabet. The scientist look for similarity between different sequences to suggest commonality of functions, or genetic material that is preserved. Unusually large matches between viral DNA and host DNA provides clues to understanding and treating diseases.

Researchers with newly sequenced segments search the databank looking for similarities. Computer algorithms have been developed to scan two long sequences, searching for subsequences or fragments that match perfectly or almost perfectly. In the process of comparing two long sequences, one would expect to find, purely by chance, some matching subsequences. To search efficiently, the researcher seeks to determine, for various chance models, what is an unusually large match. Chapter 6 details how scan statistics are used for this purpose.

1.2   Scan Statistics in Two Dimensions

Astronomy provides some of the earliest and also the most recent uses of the scan statistic in one and two dimensions.

In 1734, Daniel Bernoulli studied the inclinations of the planes of orbits of the planets and sought to test whether the observed clustering was unusual. He did this calculation under a variety of randomness models; for a detailed review see Gower (1987), which provided all of the historical information and quotes used in this example.

There were six planets known at the time: Mercury, Venus, Earth, Mars, Saturn, and Jupiter. Bernoulli's stated approach was to "... look for the two planetary orbits between which there is the greatest angle in inclination; after which I will calculate what probability there is that all the other orbits will be included by chance within the limits of these two." Since the angles of inclination may be thought of as points on the circumference of a circle, Bernoulli was dealing with the sample range on the circle W_6.

Sir Ronald A. Fisher (1959) deals with quantitative inference. He starts Chapter 3 explaining the concept of a test of significance. His illustrative example involved a scan statistic test in two dimensions. In an earlier chapter, Fisher notes that this example was used by George Boole (1854) in *The Laws of Thought* to discuss the probability of causes, and inverse probability. The example went back to 1767 when the Reverend Michell, scanning the heavens, noted the visual closeness of six stars in the Pleiades. Michell calculated the probability of such a cluster of stars all within a small visual circle within the celestial sphere. In Fishers' words:

> The example chosen by Boole of Michell's calculation with respect to the Pleiades will serve as an illustration. ... Michell [1767] supposed that there were, in all, 1500 stars of the required magnitude and sought to calculate the probability, on the hypothesis that they are individually distributed at random, that any one of them should have five neighbors within a distance of a minutes arc from them. ...

Fisher states that he finds Michell's calculations "obscure," and then goes on to bound the probability as less than 1 in 33,000. (We will return to this example and detail the calculations in Chapter 5.) Fisher then explains the essential idea of a simple test of significance:

> The probability... is amply low enough to exclude at a high level of significance any theory involving a random distribution. The force with which such a conclusion is supported is logically that of the simple disjunction: Either an exceptionally rare chance has occurred, or the theory of random distributions is not true.

Astronomers use scan statistics to search the heavens for clustered galaxies, particles, signals, or radiation sources. Orford (2000) reviews approaches for analyzing cosmic ray data in one and two dimensions, with extensive discussion of the scan statistic. He discusses methods to analyze unusual burst of high-energy arrival direction data from space. He notes the importance of these analyses for satellite gamma-rays and X-rays and for very high-energy cosmic rays not deflected by the magnetic field of our Galaxy. He compares several methods for analyzing large bursts, or clusters, including fixed grid and scan methods. He notes:

> Simple methods rely on a grid placed on the events and counts in the grid cells taken as independent Poisson-distributed events. If the cells are fixed absolutely, there is no problem in ascribing suitable Poisson probability to the largest number detected in any cell. If there is freedom to incrementally move the cell containing the largest count, a larger number is generally found... simple application of Poissonian probabilities is inappropriate.

Orford goes on to discuss alternative methods of spatial analysis looking for unusually large bursts. He concludes that the two-dimensional scan statistic

> is a preferred general statistic for those cases where events are located randomly on a plane, within fixed bounds, and where there is no a priori expectation such as a known source with known instrumental spread function.

1.3   Power of the Scan Statistic

Orford also considers the one-dimensional problem of determining whether a high count on a detector is due to variability in background or due to a "real outburst of events." One approach is to bin the time-tagged data by superimposing a time grid. The practical problem with binning is that the researcher often uses the freedom in placing the grid to maximize the cluster. As a result, more bursts are claimed "significant" than is justified, resulting in a skepticism that requires five sigmas to be convinced.

The test based on the scan statistic uses a significance level that takes into account the sliding of the grid to maximize a cluster. The scan test uses a more realistic significance level than the fixed grid test in cases where such sliding occurs. The scan test is also more powerful than a test that looks at the maximum within a fixed grid. For cases where one is searching for a "real" localized burst within a prescribed sized window, superimposed on random (uniform or Poisson) background variability, the standard scan statistic is a generalized likelihood ratio test. Chapter 14 discusses the power of the scan statistic.

Orford concludes for the one-dimensional case:

> In summary, of possible methods suggested for searching for bursts using classical statistics, the scan statistic is recommended, both for time-tagged data and for time-binned data.

Hoh and Ott (2000) apply scan statistic approaches to screen a genome for susceptibility to a complex trait. They note that

> Our result of a genome-wide significance level of $P = .038$ for autism data is remarkable—for complex traits, it has been difficult to find global significance levels smaller than .05.

Their paper concludes that

> The increased power provided by scan statistics has the effect that smaller number of observations (or families) may yield as strong a result as do conventional statistics based on larger numbers of observations.

1.4   Clusters and Intuition

Unusual clusters and coincidences have startling effects in many areas of life. Arthur Koestler, wrote in *The Roots of Coincidence* (1972) about Kammerer and Jung who kept log-books of coincidences. Kammerer wrote a book on the idea that coincidences come in series. Koestler notes Kammerer defines coincidence as

> a lawful recurrence of the same or similar things and events—a recurrence, or clustering, in time or space, whereby the individual members in sequence—as far as can be ascertained by careful analysis—are not connected by the same active cause.

Koestler quotes Jung "I have often come up against the phenomena in question and could convince myself how much these inner experiences meant to my patients." Mactavish (1998) studies the phenomena of the coincidence of psychic and physical events, and notes the "extraordinary quality" of the experience and its impact on a person's development.

Such apparently unusual clusters defy intuition. In part this is due to the fact that people tend to underestimate the probability of a cluster occurring at random. The classical birthday problem illustrates this. People in small groups are surprised to find a pair of individuals who share a birthday. (See Chapter 4, Application 4.7, for a generalized birthday scan statistic.) Some individual's reaction to such clusters and coincidence is to reject randomness, even in randomized environments; this is even true for individuals with much experience in these environments. Gamblers commonly believe in lucky days, or being on a hot streak.

Recently, a book hit the bestseller list simultaneously in several countries. *The Bible Code* by Drosnin (1997) scans the text of the *Bible* with a two-dimensional approach, and finds what appears to intuition to be unusual clustering of related words, a hidden code. In Chapter 18 we look at some of these clusters.

2

Retrospective Scanning
of Events Over Time

2.1   Conditional Case: Uniform Distribution
of Events

Researchers studying events occurring over a period of time may observe what
appears to be a large cluster of events all occurring within a short period of time.
The researchers ask whether the cluster is unusual in the sense that it is unlikely
to have arisen by chance if events were distributed independently and completely
at random over time. The relative frequency of large clusters that occur purely by
chance is one tool to answer such questions.

   In this chapter we focus on two statistics that describe large clusters given a
particular randomness model. The randomness model assumes that the times of
events are distributed independently of each other, and are equally likely to occur
anywhere in the time period. The two related statistics are the largest number of
events in a fixed period of time, and the shortest period of time containing a fixed
number of events.

   Given N points independently drawn from the uniform distribution on $[0, 1)$, let
S_w denote the largest number of points to be found in any subinterval of $[0, 1)$ of
length w. The maximum cluster S_w is called the *scan statistic*, from the viewpoint
that one scans time with a window of size w, and observes a large number of
points. Let W_k be the size of the smallest subinterval of $[0, 1)$ that contains k
points. The interval W_{r+1} is called the *minimum rth-order gap*. The distributions
of the statistics S_w and W_k are related, $P(S_w \geq k) = P(W_k \leq w)$. We denote the
common probability, $P(k; N, w)$, and let $Q(k; N, w) = 1 - P(k; N, w)$.

In certain applications the researcher may want highly accurate estimates of $P(k; N, w)$, while in other applications reasonable approximations may suffice. This section gives a simple approximation for $P(k; N, w)$ valid when $P(k; N, w)$ is small. A web site gives more accurate approximations and exact bounds for $P(k; N, w)$ for $N \leq 100$, $w \geq .01$; this approximation is exact for $k > N/3$. The web site address is

http//c3.biomath.msmm.edu/scan.html.

Chapter 10 reviews the more accurate but complex approximations; Chapter 8 gives exact results for a variety of cases, and references tables of values; and Chapter 9 bounds the probabilities. Section 2.4 gives results on the moments of the distributions of S_w and W_k. We illustrate the results with a variety of applications.

2.1.1 Approximate Results for $P(k; N, w)$

Wallenstein and Neff (1987) give the following easy to compute approximation for $P(k; N, w)$, as a simple sum of binomial and cumulative binomial probabilities. Let

$$b(k; N, w) = \binom{N}{k} w^k (1 - w)^{N-k}, \tag{2.1}$$

$$G_b(k; N, w) = \sum_{i=k}^{N} b(i; N, w). \tag{2.2}$$

Then, approximately,

$$P(k; N, w) \approx (N - k + 1)b(k - 1; N, w) - (N - k - 1)b(k; N, w)$$
$$+ 2G_b(k + 1; N, w)$$
$$= (kw^{-1} - N - 1)b(k; N, w) + 2G_b(k; N, w). \tag{2.3}$$

We have found (2.3) to be accurate for values of $P(k; N, w) < .10$, and even for larger values. Chapter 8 notes that (2.3) is exact for $k > N/2$, $w \leq .5$, and gives exact results for other cases.

Application 2.1 (Parasuicide Clustering). Smeeton and Wilkinson (1988) note that some individuals have a pattern of a "burst" of repeated attempts at suicide within a short period, followed by longer periods between clusters. Their goal was to identify those patients with such a pattern, from other individuals with a random pattern of frequent attempts. This would allow helping the former group at appropriate times. They use the scan statistic to help identify the clustered group. They illustrate the approach with data for all patients admitted to the Edinburgh Regional Poisoning Treatment Centre during a 2 year period. The Centre records incidents to the exact day. The review period was 2 years. The scanning interval was 3 months, or three twenty-fourths of the review period.

The distribution of S_w depends on the ratio of the sizes of the scanning window and review period. This ratio is the same whether we take the unit of time to be 1 month with scan window of 3 months and review period of 24 months, or whether the unit of time is 24 months and the scanning window is three-twenty fourths of a 24 month period, and the review period is one (24 month) unit. The formulas (2.1) to (2.3) always take the length of the review period as the unit of time. Taking 24 months as the unit of time, the scanning window's length is $w = 3/24 = .125$.

Only patients that had at least five suicide attempts during the 2 years were included ($N \geq 5$). There were 31 such patients, and a separate scan test was carried out for each patient's suicide attempts. The critical values for the scan statistic were based on (2.3), and a significance level of .05. The critical values for the scan statistic $S_{.125}$ were 4 (for $N = 5, 6$); 5 (for $N = 7, 8$); 6 (for $N = 9, 10, 11$); and 7 (for $N = 12, 13, 14$). The reader can check these using (2.3). For examples, $P(7; 14, .125) \approx .03$, while $P(6; 12, .125) \approx .06$, both by (2.3) and by the exact tables in Neff and Naus (1980).

Based on using this test for differentiating chronic from clustered parasuicide patients, eight of the 31 patients were identified as having clustered patterns. The authors note that the chronic and clustered pattern groups had one important difference. Of the 20–29 year olds, 56% had clustered patterns, as compared to 10% for ages other than 20–29.

Application 2.2 (Cluster of HIV in Dialysis Patients). There had been anecdotes of unusual clustering of HIV among dialysis patients in developing countries. Velandra, Fridkin, Cardenas, et al. (1995) investigated a cluster of HIV among patients at a dialysis center in Columbia, South America. They did a retrospective study of these dialysis patients from January, 1988, through December, 1993. There were 13 definite HIV seropositive patients during this 72 month period, and among these there were a cluster of eight during the last 6 months of 1992. They used the scan statistic to test for significance, and found the cluster highly unusual at the $p < .0002$ level. (They used an epidemiologic software statistics package: epi.info version 5.01 b.) Here, the cluster size $k = 8$, total number of points $N = 13$, and window size $w = 6/72 = .0833$. Since $k > N/2$, (2.3) is exact, and $P(8; 13, .0833) = .00016 < .0002$. This cluster was unlikely to have occurred by chance. Finding unsual clusters helps to focus further investigation. The investigators focused on procedures at the Centre. They found that during the cluster period patients' access needles were processed incorrectly prior to reuse. A key step was to place the used needles in a soaking pan with a sterilizing chemical (benzalkonium chloride), at a recommended 1% solution. In fact, only a .16% solution was used.

Application 2.3 (Developability in Photographic Series). Silberstein (1945, p. 319), Berg (1945, p. 340), and Mack (1948, p. 784) derive approximation formula for $P(k; N, w)$ for the case of sufficiently rare clusters. These authors were motivated by a photographic theory problem, the developability of silver specks. Under certain conditions, when a developer puts layers of silver on a glass, silver atoms randomly fall on a smooth surface. Silver specks form from clusters, or "aggregates" of silver atoms, where k points form an aggregate if "they are

all contained within a subinterval, w, of $[0, 1)$, no matter how placed in $[0, 1)$."
Additional layers of silver deposit on sufficiently large aggregates and make them
visible. Silberstein states that

> the rigorous determination of the probability of any given number of
> aggregates among N points is exceedingly complicated and becomes
> to all purposes impracticable when N exceeds a few units.

Silberstein makes two exceptions, namely the probability of no aggregate of two
or more points, $Q(2; N, w)$, and the probabiity that all N points form a single
aggregate $P(N; N, w)$.

Exact formulas for the two special cases, $P(2; N, w)$ and $P(N; N, w)$, appear
in various probability texts and had been known for many years. An exact formula
for $P(N; N, w)$, the cumulative distribution function (c.d.f.) of W_N, the sample
range of the N points, is derived in Burnside (1928, p. 22):

$$P(N; N, w) = Nw^{N-1} - (N - 1)w^N, \qquad 0 \le w \le 1. \qquad (2.4)$$

An exact formula for $P(2; N, w)$ the cumulative distributions function of W_2, the
smallest distance between any of the N points, is derived in Parzen (1960, p. 304),
by a direct integration approach

$$P(2; N, w) = 1 - (1 - [N - 1]w)^N, \qquad 0 \le w \le 1/(N - 1)$$
$$= 1, \qquad\qquad\qquad 1/(N - 1) \le w \le 1. \qquad (2.5)$$

Silberstein (1945, p. 322) notes that $P(k; N, w)$ is a polynomial in w of order
N. Mack (1948, p. 783) notes that $P(k; N, w)$ is piecewise polynomial, that is,
that the polynomial expressions may change for different ranges of w.

Application 2.4 (Cluster of Cancer Cases). Epidemiologists and public health
officials focus on unusual clusters of cancer cases. A 1998 motion picture film, *A
Civil Action*, starring John Travolta highlights the public's interest in such cases.
The scan statistic has been used to test for unusual clustering of different types of
cancer cases.

Over a 5 year period, 1991 to 1995, there were 19 cases of a particular type of
cancer reported in a city. In reviewing the data, the epidemiologist notes that there
is a 1 year period (from April 14, 1993, through April 13, 1994) that contains eight
cases. The researcher asks the following question: Given 19 cases over 5 years,
how unusual is it to get a 1 year period containing as many as eight cases?

We might try to answer the researcher's question as follows. Each of the 19
cases could either fall in the period (April 14, 1993, to April 13, 1994) or not
fall in it, independently of the other cases. The probability of as many as eight
cases falling in this interval is given by computing the binomial probabilities for
$N = 19$, $p = 1/5$, and summing terms for $k \ge 8$. This gives the value .023, which
indicates that the observed cluster is somewhat unusual. But this calculation does

not answer the question posed; the researcher wants to know how unusual it is to get any 1 year period (not a specific year) containing as many as eight cases.

We might try to get around this problem by dividing the 5 years up into five disjoint 1 year periods, and using the distribution of the maximum number of cases falling in any 1 year. However, this too does not answer the researcher's question, since the specific year observed overlaps two of the disjoint years. The researcher is not limiting the question to calendar years. Ederer, Myers, and Mantel (1964) in a study of leukemia clusters, note this difficulty:

> The reader will recognize that a 5 year period in fact contains a continuum of overlapping periods 1 year in length. However, the distribution of the maximum number of cases in 1 year under the null hypothesis cannot be readily determined unless the number of periods is restricted in some way.

$P(k; 19, 1/5)$ is the distribution of the maximum number of cases in a year, under the null hypothesis model for the unrestricted continuum of 1 year periods. The null model used was that the 19 cases were distributed independently and completely at random over the 5 year period. The answer to the researcher's question is given by a scan statistic probability. Here the cluster size is $k = 8$; the total number of cases over the whole 5 year period is $N = 19$; and the window size w is one year out of five, or $w = 1/5$. The answer is given by the probability, $P(8; 19, 1/5)$. From (2.3):

$$P(8; 19, .2) = 12b(7; 19, .2) - 10b(8; 19, .2) + 2G_b(9; 19, .2)$$
$$= 12(.04432) - 10(.016621) + 2(.0066577) = .379.$$

This tells our researcher that the observed cluster is not unusual.

How accurate is (2.3) for this example? Very! The exact tabled result from Neff and Naus (1980) is .376. For this example where k is close to $N/2$, we would expect (2.3) to be very accurate, since it is exact for $k > N/2$.

Application 2.5 (Clustering of Inflammatory Bowel Disease). Ekbom, Zack, Adami, and Helmick (1991) investigate the clustering by birth date (and mother's residence) in a cohort group of 2175 patients in an Uppsala health care region in Sweden. These patients had been diagnosed with inflammatory bowel disease, 845 with Crohn's disease, and 1330 with ulcerative colitis. Previous research had suggested possible common causes or events including perinatal and other infections and month of birth/seasonality might have contributed to precipating these diseases. This paper gives an excellent example of various methodological and practical issues involved in such studies. The authors applied four tests for clustering, the first being the scan statistic adjusted to account for variations in monthly number of births. The basic adjusting approach, due to Weinstock (1981), is to stretch the time period studied so that the length of any subinterval is proportional to the expected number of events (in this case, proportional to the number of births) in the subinterval.

For the present study, the authors chose 15 and 30 day scanning intervals for the overall Uppsala region, and 30 day scanning intervals for individual counties in the region. In the overall region, the scan statistic for a 15 day interval was six cases, and for a 30 day interval was nine cases of Crohn's disease; neither of these are more than expected.

For one of the counties, Vasternorrland County, the scan statistic for the 30 day period was four Crohn's disease cases, out of 80 cases for the entire 34 years of the study period (12,419 days). This the authors found to be borderline significant ($p = .07$).

Based on previous studies' evidence of increased rates of inflammatory bowel disease after World War II, the authors also focused on this period. In Vasternorrland County after 1944 there were 194 cases of inflammatory bowel disease. Of these, the 30 day scan statistic was eight cases. That is, given 194 cases in 4748 days (the 13 years 1945 to 1957), there was a cluster of eight cases in 30 days. The authors found this to be statistically significant ($p = .036$). To illustrate the simple formula, if there had been no adjustment for varying number of births over time, the significance level would have been

$$P(k = 8; N = 194, w/T = 30/4748) = P(8; 194, .00632).$$

From (2.3):

$$P(8; 194, .00632) = 187b(7; 194, .00632) - 185b(8; 194, .00632)$$
$$+ 2G_b(9, 194; .00632) = .036.$$

In computing this, we used the exact binomial probabilities; the same result follows using the normal approximation to compute the cumulative G_b. (Using the Poisson approximation for the individual binomial terms would give an answer of .038.)

Application 2.6 (Representativeness of Samples). For a given population, how big a sample should one take so that it is likely that the sample will be representative? Kruskal and Mosteller (1979) consider many interpretations that are given to be *representative*. One of the interpretations is closely related to scan statistics.

A researcher may be sampling individuals from a large population and measuring their ages. For the sample to be representative the researcher would like, with high (95%) probability that for every age interval that contains 1% of the population, that the percent of the sample that falls in that age interval will be no more than 2%. What is the smallest sample the researcher can take? We will show below that the answer is $n = 1850$.

If the researcher was only interested in the representativeness of the sample for one particular 1% age interval in the population, a sample of about 400 would be adequate. But here the researcher requires that an infinite number of possible overlapping age intervals (each containing 1% of the population) will each contain between 0 to 2% of the sample.

Formally, let $Z_1, Z_2, \ldots, Z_n$ be independently and identically distributed (i.i.d.) continuous random variables with known common c.d.f. $F(z) = P(Z_i \leq z)$. Then it is known that the random variables $F(Z_1)$, $F(Z_2), \ldots,$ $F(Z_n)$, are independently and identically distributed uniform random variables on the interval $[0, 1)$. Because of this transformation, and because F is known, we can, without loss of generality, let $X_i = F(Z_i)$ and just consider the case where the X_i's are indepently and identically distributed uniform $[0, 1)$ variates.

One interpretation of the "representativeness" of a sample, is for a given w to see if the proportion of the sample in any window of length w within $[0, 1)$ is never far from the population proportion. Let $Y_t(w)$ denote the number of X_i's in the interval $(t, t + w)$. Kruskal and Mosteller describe this interpretation with the question: "For given α and β, how large must n be so that

$$P \left(\max_{0 \leq t \leq 1-w} |n^{-1} Y_t(w) - w| \leq \beta \right) \geq 1 - \alpha?" \tag{2.6}$$

In general (2.6) could also be stated as

$$P \left(\left\{ \max_{0 \leq t \leq 1-w} Y_t(w) \leq n(w + \beta) \right\} \right.$$

$$\text{and} \quad \left. \left\{ \min_{0 \leq t \leq 1-w} Y_t(w) \geq n(w - \beta) \right\} \right) \geq 1 - \alpha. \tag{2.7}$$

Note that $\max_{0 \leq t \leq 1-w} Y_t(w)$ is the scan statistic S_w, and $\min_{0 \leq t \leq 1-w} Y_t(w)$ is the related scan statistic, the minimum number of points in a scanning interval. For the uniform case the distribution of the maximum scan is discussed in this chapter; the distribution of the minimum scan is discussed in Chapter 18.

Kruskal and Mosteller (1979) give the example where $w = .1$, $\beta = .3$, and $1 - \alpha = .95$. For this example, the researcher asks what sample size n will give at least a 95% chance that any interval containing .10 of the population will have a sample relative frequency that will not be further than .30 away from .10. For this example, Kruskal and Mosteller use the results in Neff and Naus (1980) for the scan statistic of this chapter. Inequality (2.6) becomes

$$P \left(\left\{ \max_{0 \leq t \leq .9} Y_t(.1) \leq .4n \right\} \text{ and } \left\{ \min_{0 \leq t \leq .9} Y_t(.1) \geq 0 \right\} \right) \geq .95.$$

The researcher seeks the sample size n, such that

$$P(S_{.10} \leq .4n) \geq .95 \tag{2.8}$$

or, for $[x]$ denoting the largest integer in x:

$$P([.4n] + 1; n, .1) \leq .05. \tag{2.9}$$

From the tables in Neff and Naus (1980), Kruskal and Mosteller (1979) find that the smallest sample size satisfying (2.9) is $n = 13$. They note that $n = 14$ does not satisfy (2.9), but that $n \geq 15$ works. $P(5; 10, .1) = .06$; $P(5; 11, .1) = .10$; $P(5; 12, .1) = .15$; $P(6; 13, .1) = .04$; $P(6; 14, .1) = .06$; $P(7; 15, .1) = .016$; $P(7; 16, .1) = .024$; $P(7; 17, .1) = .037$; $P(8; 18, .1) = .010$; $P(8; 19, .1) = .015$.

We can use (2.3) to look at some special cases:

Case 1: $w = .01$, $\beta = .01$, and $1 - \alpha = .95$.

We seek that for every interval corresponding to .01 of the population, the sample will be within $\pm.01$ of the population proportion with probability .95. The smallest sample is $n = 1850$, since $P(38; 1850, .01) = .0446$, and $P(37; 1849, .01) > P(37, 1800, .01) = .054$. Because of the discreteness of k, it is not true that any sample size greater than 1850 will work. For example, $P(39, 1949, .01) = .06$, so 1949 does not work. For this case the following sample sizes work: $n = 1850$ to 1859, 1900 and 1929, 1950 to 1998, and 2000, or greater.

Case 2: $w = .05$, $\beta = .05$, and $1 - \alpha = .95$.

For every interval corresponding to .05 of the population, the sample will be within $\pm.05$ of the population proportion. The sample sizes that work are $n = 260$, 270 to 273, 280 to 287, and ≥ 290. So the smallest sample size is $n = 260$.

Case 3: $w = .10$, $\beta = .10$, and $1 - \alpha = .95$.

For every interval corresponding to .10 of the population, the sample will be within $\pm.10$ of the population proportion. The sample sizes that work are $n = 105, 111, 112$, and 115, or higher.

Cunui Zhang (personal communication) points out that the sample sizes necessary to get the sample simultaneously representative over the whole range of the distribution are approximately $\log_e(1/w)$ times what is necessary to gain representativeness within just one interval corresponding to w of the population. The approximation follows from large deviation theory. That is, the required sample size is approximately $\{4w(1 - w)/\beta^2\} \log_e(1/w)$. For the three cases: $w = .01$, .05, .10 the large deviation approximation gives sample sizes 1824, 228, 83 as compared to the more accurate 1850, 260, and 105.

Application 2.7 (Breakdowns Due to Closeness of Flaws). Newell (1958) notes how several flaws all within a given distance in a crystal can cause breaks. On a somewhat larger scale, Shepherd, Creasey, and Fisher (1981) apply the scan statistic to clustering of discontinuities in coal mines. Chapter 4 deals with discrete variations on these applications, where the reliability of systems may be compromised by several failures of close components.

2.2   The Scan Statistic on the Circle

Do angles of inclinations of planetary orbits cluster? Do accidents or birthdays cluster on certain adjacent days of the year? Do the directions of flights of birds or insects cluster? In these cases researchers study clusters on the circle.

Given N points independently drawn completely at random from the circumference of the unit circle, let S_w^c denote the largest number of points to be found in any subarc of length w. Let W_k be the size of the smallest subarc that contains k points. We denote the common probability

$$P(S_w^c \geq k) = P(W_k \leq w) = P_c(k; N, w)$$

and let

$$Q_c(k; N, w) = 1 - P_c(k; N, w).$$

Wallenstein, Weinberg, and Gould (1989) give the simple approximation for small probabilities

$$P_c(k; N, w) \approx b(k; N, w)(k - Nw)/\{w(1 - w)\}, \tag{2.10}$$

where $b(k; N, w)$ is the binomial probability defined in (2.1).

Application 2.8 (Seasonal Clustering of Adolescent Suicide). Quetelet (1835) is credited by Kevan (1980) to first note seasonal variation in suicide. Kevan's overall evaluation of more than 75 studies indicates a peak in suicide in late Spring or early Summer. Barraclough and White (1978) evaluate data from England and Wales for the period 1968 to 1972 where the highest suicide rate months were March, April, May, and July. The explanation for seasonality of suicide remains unclear, with both climatic and socioeconomic factors hypothesized as the underlying cause.

Wallenstein, Weinberg, and Gould (1989) review data on seasonality of adult and teenage suicide. They investigate possible seasonal clustering of adolescent (age 15 to 19) suicide in the United States for the two calendar years 1978, 1979. They used data from the Vital Statistics Mortality Detail tapes from the National Center for Health Statistics. Neither the data for 1978 to 1979, nor the more complete data for 1978 to 1985 shows a strong secular trend that would require adjustment prior to use of the scan statistic.

There were 3474 adolescent suicides over the 2 year period. The data for each day of the 2 years are pooled, (e.g., the suicides on January 1, 1978, are combined with those on January 1, 1979). The combined data is viewed as a circle with days from January 1 through December 31. A window of length 91 days (3 months) was selected a priori as the choice for seasonal effects. Taking the year as a unit circle, the length of the scanning window is $w = 91/365 = .249$. The maximum number of suicides in the scanning window was 966, and was for the period from January 1 through April 1. Substituting $w = .249$, $k = 966$, and $N = 3474$ into (2.10) gives

$$P_c(966; 3474, .249) \approx (8.5 \times 10^{-6})(966 - 865)/\{.249(.751)\} = .0045.$$

The observed seasonal pattern of clustering of suicides among adolescents is statistically significant. This cluster pattern is different than that of adults.

2.3   The Ratchet Scan Statistic

In Application 2.8, the exact dates of suicide were available, and a continuous scan
with a window of 91 days was a reasonable approach. In many cases, especially
with applications utilizing vital statistics data, the original raw data is difficult to
obtain, and only monthly totals are available. Wallenstein, Weinberg, and Gould
(1989) introduce the concept of a *ratchet scan statistic* to handle such cases.

View the unit interval (line or circle) as divided into L disjoint subintervals.
Given that N events occur in the unit interval, let $n_1, n_2, \ldots, n_L$ denote the number of events in the L intervals. Given the N events are distributed completely at
random, $(n_1, n_2, \ldots, n_L)$ have a joint multinomial distribution. For a given m, let
$w = m/L$, and

$$
\begin{aligned}
Y_i &= (n_i + \cdots + n_{i+m-1}), & i &= 1, 2, \ldots, L - m + 1, \\
&= (n_i + \cdots + n_L + n_1 + \cdots + n_{m+i-1-L}), & i &= L - m + 2, \ldots, L,
\end{aligned}
$$

and define the linear and circulat ratchet scan statistics, respectively, by R_w and
R_w^c where

$$
R_w = \max_{1 \le i \le L-m+1} \{Y_i\} \tag{2.11}
$$

and

$$
R_w^c = \max_{1 \le i \le L} \{Y_i\}. \tag{2.12}
$$

Wallenstein, Weinberg, and Gould (1989) derive results for a circular ratchet
scan statistic, for $L = 12$, and given that the N events are distributed completely at
random over the year. They give tables of exact upper tail probabilities, $P(R_w^c \ge k)$ for $L = 12$, $m = 2, 3$, and $N = 8(1)25(5)35$, and upper tail approximations
for other m and N. (The notation $N = a(b)c$, means that values are tabled for
$N = a, a + b, a + 2b, \ldots, c$; thus, $N = 2(1)10(5)20$ means that values are
tabled for $N = 2, 3, 4, 5, 6, 7, 8, 9, 10, 15, 20$.)

The approximation for the case $L = 12$, first transforms the circular scan statistic to another scale by computing

$$
R = (R_w^c - 1 - Nw)/\{Nw(1 - w)\}^{.5}. \tag{2.13}
$$

Use R to read the approximate upper-tail p-value, $P(R_w^c \ge k)$, from Figure 1
in Wallenstein, Weinberg, and Gould (1989). Application 2.9 illustrates this approach.

Application 2.9 (Seasonal Clustering of Adolescent Suicide). In Application 2.8
the exact dates of the 3474 suicides were known. In many applications using vital
statistics, only the monthly totals may be available. For the 3474 suicides, the 2
year totals for each of the 12 months were as follows:

334	291	332	284	311	257	282	261	275	289	290	268
Jan.	Feb.	Mar.	Apr.	May	Jun.	Jul.	Aug.	Sep.	Oct.	Nov.	Dec.

Taking a 3 month circular ratchet scan, we look for the maximum of

$$(334 + 291 + 332), (291 + 332 + 284), \ldots, (289 + 290 + 268),$$
$$(290 + 268 + 334), (268 + 334 + 291)$$
$$= \max\{957, 907, 927, \ldots, 847, 892, 893\} = 957.$$

Substitute $R_w^c = 957$, $m = 3$, $L = 12$, $w = 3/12$, $N = 3474$ into (2.13) to find $R = 3.92$. Entering Figure 1 in Wallenstein, Weinberg, and Gould (1989) with $R = 3.92$, the p-value is less than .005. (See Chapter 18 for an alternative method.)

Krauth (1992a,b) gives bounds for upper tail probabilities for the linear and circular ratchet scan statistic. Krauth (1999) gives an excellent summary and surveys results for the ratchet scan statistic, including more general distributions of the N points. These statistics are discussed further in Chapter 18.

2.4   Moments of Scan Statistics

2.4.1   Exact Values for Moments of the Scan Statistic S_w

Denote S_w by $S_w(N)$ to indicate dependence of the moments on N and w. There are very few analytic formula for the moments of $S_w(N)$ in the literature. Naus (1966a) gives means and variances for $N \leq 10$, $w = .1(.1).9$, although simulations are used for $w < .5$, $N \geq 6$. Wallenstein, Gould, and Kleinman (1989) tabulate means and variances of $S_w(N)$ for $N = 2(1)40$, 40(5)70, 85, 100, 125, 150, 200(100)500, 1000; and $w - 1/T$, $T = 3(1)6, 8, 12$. The values for $N < 19$ are computed from the exact values in Neff and Naus (1980); the other values by simulation. Unpublished tables were produced for $T = 15, 18, 26, 52, 104$, and an even finer grid on N. For $20 \leq N \leq 40$, estimates were based on 20,000 simulations; while for $N > 40$ from 7500 to 20,000 simulations were performed.

The mean was believed to be accurate to three significant digits, and the variance to two or three places. Interpolation was used occasionally in Neff and Naus's tables but since the tabulation in that book were produced on a fine grid the values are essentially exact.

In order to enable investigators to obtain means for N, in the range $100 < N < 1000$, Wallenstein, Gould, and Kleinman (1989) fit the model

$$E\{S_w(N)\} = wN + b_w N^{.5} \tag{2.14}$$

and

$$\text{Var}\{S_w(N)\} = a_w N + c_w N^{.5}. \tag{2.15}$$

Table 2.1. Coefficient to use in approximating mean and variance of $S_w(N)$.

$L = 1/w$	2	3	4	6	8	12	24	52	104
b :	.8551	.8530	.8157	.7724	.7009				
a :	.0811	.0608	.0391	.0291	.0177				
c :	.0387	.0780	.1128	.1044	.1125				
d :	.113	.095	.083	.068	.061	.050	.055	.054	.055
f :	1.0	.976	.958	.931	.907	.876	.728	.627	.527

In an unpublished manuscript, they fit

$$\text{Var}\{S_w(N)\} = d_w N^{f_w}. \tag{2.16}$$

Table 2.1 gives the coefficients they obtained.

Application 2.10 (Testing for Copy-Cat Suicides). Some well-publicized clusters of adolescent suicides have raised the question of whether one suicide leads to another. If so, one would expect many sporadic small clusters, at different times and places. We select C counties, and for the ith county compute the scan statistic, $S_{w,i}$ for $i = 1, 2, \ldots, C$. In the spirit of the Ederer–Myers–Mantel approach, we pool information for the C counties by computing the pooled scan statistic

$$S_{w,\text{(pooled)}} = \sum \{S_{w,i} - E(S_{w,i})\} / \left(\sum \text{Var}(S_{w,i}) \right)^{.5}. \tag{2.17}$$

The statistic has approximately a standard normal distribution for C moderate to large. Wallenstein, Weinberg, and Gould (1989) used this statistic computed from data on 21 counties in the United States with large ($> 100{,}000$) adolescent populations, for the years 1981 to 1984, with a scan window of 365 days. Approximations (2.14) and (2.15) were used to compute the expectations and variances for the individual counties. The observed value of the pool scan statistic was 1.69, and the one-tailed p-value was .044.

2.4.2 The Expectation and Variance of the W_k, the Size of the Smallest Interval

Naus (1966a, p. 1198) proves for $(N + 1)/2 < k \le N$, that

$$E(W_k) = \{k - 2(N - k + 1)b\}/(N + 1), \tag{2.18}$$

where

$$b = b(N - k + 1; 2(N - k + 1), .5),$$

and

$$\text{Var}(W_k) = (N - k + 1)\{(N + k + 1) + 2(2k - N - 1)b$$
$$- 4(N + 2)(N - k + 1)b^2\}/(N + 1)^2(N + 2). \tag{2.19}$$

Neff and Naus (1980) generate tables for the expectation and variance of W_k for $\{k = 3, 4, 5; N = k(1)19\}; \{k = 6; N = 6(1)17\}; \{k = 7; N = 7(1)20\}; \{k = 8; N = 8(1)23\}; \{k = 9; N = 9(1)25\}.$

3
Prospective Scanning of Events Over Time

3.1 Poisson Distribution of Events

Chapter 2 deals with the scan statistic given that a fixed number N of events have occurred at random in a time period. This conditional (on N) case is called retrospective because in typical applications the researcher scans and makes inferences about N events that have occurred.

The present chapter deals with the distribution of the scan statistic given that the events occur from a Poisson process. The number of points in the time period is not viewed as a fixed number N that has already occurred, but rather as a random variable with a known probability distribution. In this chapter the distribution of the total number of points is a Poisson variate with an average of λ points per unit time. The typical application is prospective. The researcher seeks to use the scan statistic to monitor future data or to design a system to prevent overloading capacity.

The Poisson process has been used to model many phenomena dealing with the occurrence of events in time or space. Applications include telephone traffic, physical particles registered by counters, arrival of customers for service, locations or times of cancer cases. The distribution of scan statistics under the Poisson process is a tool for researchers working in many areas, as shown in the many applications in this chapter. We begin with two applications to highlight the motivation behind a prospective use of the scan statistic. We then present useful formula for carrying out the test. This is followed by additional applications. The first application contrasts a retrospective and a prospective use of the scan statistic.

Application 3.1 (Carbon Monoxide Poisoning). Over an 8 year period, there were 19 isolated cases of carbon monoxide poisoning reported in a county. A public health official is on the look out for unusual clusters of such poisonings and asks how likely is it (given no change in the underlying process, and assuming a Poisson process) that in the next 8 years there would be a cluster of 8 or more cases in a 1 year period.

One might think that the probability of the cluster (8 cases in a year) is about the same whether there are exactly 19 cases over 8 years, or an average of 19 cases over 8 years. The former case, the conditional (on N) version of the problem is considered in Chapter 2. The latter case, the prospective (or unconditional) version, is described here. The scan probabilities in the conditional and unconditional cases are denoted P and P^*, respectively. (A formal definition of P^* is given later in this section.) In the present example, the unconditional and conditional probabilities can lead to different practical conclusions. For the conditional case, $P(8; 19, 1/8) = .04811$, while for the unconditional case, $P^*(8; 19, 1/8) = .09293$. Researchers who choose a .05 level of significance would not want to use P^* to approximate P for this example. The next application illustrates a case where a prospective use of the scan statistic is particularly appropriate. This involves designing a system to have capacity to handle heavy loads. Application 3.11 below illustrates an application designing surveillance or monitoring systems to detect changes that occur in disease clusters.

Application 3.2 (Designing Telephone Systems to Avoid Overloads). A telephone traffic engineer designs a system with capacity to handle clusters during peak load periods. The engineer assumes that dialing of calls occurs at random times in the hour and that the dialing time for a call is 15 seconds. During a peak hour there are, on average, 4800 calls dialed, or about 20 calls being dialed in a typical 15 second period. The engineer asks how likely is it that at some point in a peak hour there will be more than 40 phone calls all being dialed simultaneously (dialing time starting within the same 15 second period). The engineer uses the Poisson distribution to calculate that the probability that a particular 15 second period has more than 40 calls is .000025. This is highly unlikely. It is also irrelevant to the engineer's original question about any 15 second period, rather than a particular 15 second period.

In fact, there are an infinite number of overlapping intervals of 15 seconds each in an hour, although the numbers of calls in them are correlated in a complex way. Feller (1958, p. 397) observed in reference to compound events such as these (his example was "seven calls within a minute on a certain day") that they involve complicated sample spaces, and went on to say "We cannot deal here with such complicated sample spaces and must defer the study of the more delicate aspects of the theory."

The engineer might try to approximate the probability by using the fact that in 1 hour there are 240 disjoint intervals of 15 seconds each. The probability that at least one of these disjoint 240 intervals contains more than 40 calls is

$1 - (1 - .000025)^{240} = .006$. This *disjoint* approximation is poor. Here $k = 41$, $\lambda = 20$, $w = 1$, $T = 240$, where the time unit is 15 seconds. Applying (3.3) we find that the correct scan probability $P^*(k; \lambda T, w/T) = P^*(41; 4800, 1/240)$ is about .066.

Chapter 2 dealt with two related scan statistics for the case of a fixed number N of points independently drawn from the uniform distribution. In Chapter 2 the time units are chosen so that $T = 1$. In this section we define the two scan statistics of Chapter 2 for general T, and relate them to a third scan statistic.

Let $Y_t(w)$ denote the number of points (X's) in the interval $(t, t + w)$. The scan statistic $S_w = \max_{0 \le t \le T - w} \{Y_t(w)\}$, denotes the largest number of points to be found in any subinterval of $[0, T)$ of length w. Let $X_{(1)} \le X_{(2)} \le \ldots$, denote the ordered values of the X's. The statistic W_k, the size of the smallest subinterval of $[0, T)$ that contains k points, equals

$$\min_{0 \le w \le T} \{w : S_w \ge k\} = \min_{1 \le i} \{X_{(i+k-1)} - X_{(i)}\}.$$

The distributions of the scan statistics S_w and W_k are related, $P(S_w \ge k) = P(W_k \le w)$. For the case where the N points are uniformly distributed on $[0, T)$, the common probabilities $P(S_w \ge k) = P(W_k \le w)$ are denoted $P(k; N, w/T)$. The maximum cluster S_w is called the *scan statistic*, and the smallest interval W_{r+1} is called the *r-scan statistic*.

3.1.1 The Poisson Process

In certain applications, the researcher is not interested in the distribution of scan statistics given a fixed total number N of events in $[0, T)$. Instead, the total number of events in $[0, T)$ is a random variable. Events are viewed as occurring at random times according to some process. The Poisson process is one completely-at-random chance model that corresponds to a random number of points (events) and a uniform distribution of points over time. In this process, let λ denote the (expected) average number of events in any unit interval. The number of events $Y_t(w)$ in any interval $[t, t + w)$ is Poisson distributed with mean λw. That is,

$$P(Y_t(w) = k) = e^{-\lambda w}(\lambda w)^k / k!, \qquad k = 0, 1, 2, \ldots.$$

The number of events in any disjoint (nonoverlapping) intervals are independently distributed. There are various other ways to characterize the Poisson process. For the Poisson process the arrival times between points are independent exponential random variates. Conditional on there being a total of N points from the Poisson process in $[0, T)$, these N points are uniformly distributed over $[0, T)$.

Given events occurring at random over time, let $T_{k,w}$ denote the waiting time until we first observe at least k events in an interval of length w. Formally, $T_{k,w} = X_{(i+k-1)}$ for the smallest i such that $X_{(i+k-1)} - X_{(i)} \le w$. The three scan statistics S_w, W_k, and $T_{k,w}$ are related by $P(S_w \ge k) = P(W_k \le w) = P(T_{k,w} \le T)$.

For the Poisson process, with mean λ *per unit time*, we denote these common probabilities by $P^*(k; \lambda T, w/T) = 1 - Q^*(k; \lambda T, w/T)$.

The distribution of $T_{k,w}$ under the Poisson model is of importance in the classical theory of visual perception described in Application 3.5 below. In other applications, the researcher is interested in the maximum cluster statistic S_w or the smallest kth-order gap W_k. Section 3.2 gives a highly accurate approximate formula for $P^*(k; \lambda T, w/T)$, as well as some rougher but even simpler to compute approximations. Section 3.2 also gives a series of applications of these formulas.

For some applications the researcher may need exact results, or at least bounds on the probability as a supplement to the approximation. Chapter 11 gives exact formulas for $P^*(k; \lambda T, w/T)$. In cases where one needs accurate but not necessarily exact results, the approximations of Section 3.2 can be supplemented by bounds on the probability. Chapter 11 gives tight bounds for the probability.

3.2 Approximate Formula for $P^*(k; \lambda T, w/T)$

In this section we list a variety of approximations and illustrate their application. Details on the development of these approximations, and further comparisons are given in Chapter 11.

Newell (1963) and Ikeda (1965) derive the asymptotic formula

$$P^*(k; \lambda T, w/T) \approx 1 - \exp\{-\lambda^k w^{k-1} T/(k-1)!\}. \tag{3.1}$$

This formula gives useful rough approximations for certain purposes when P^* is sufficiently small. The asymptotic convergence of this formula is very slow. In the following let L denote T/w and let $\psi = \lambda w$ denote the expected number of points in an interval of length w (the width of the scanning window).

Conover, Bement, and Iman (1979) give an alternative approximation

$$P^*(k; \psi L, 1/L) \approx 1 - 1.5 F_p(k-1; \psi) \exp\{-\psi(L-1) $$
$$\cdot \left(1 - (F_p(k-2; \psi)/F_p(k-1; \psi))\right)\} $$
$$+ .5 \exp\{-\psi L(1 - F_p(k-2; \psi))\}, \tag{3.2}$$

where

$$p(j; \psi) = \exp\{-\psi\}\psi^j/j!, \qquad F_p(k; \psi) = \sum_{i=0}^{k} p(i; \psi).$$

Approximation (3.2) is intended for cases where $k \leq 7$, and is most accurate for P^* small. For the case of $L = T/w$ large, and $P^*(k; \psi L, 1/L)$ small, the following approximation is sometimes useful:

$$P^*(k; \psi L, 1/L) \approx 1 - \exp\{-\delta\}, \tag{3.3}$$

where

$$\delta = (k-1)(L-1)p(k; \psi).$$

Naus (1982) gives the highly accurate approximation

$$P^*(k; \psi L, 1/L) \approx 1 - Q_2^*(Q_3^*/Q_2^*)^{L-2}, \tag{3.4}$$

where $Q_2^* = Q^*(k; 2\psi, 1/2)$ and $Q_3^* = Q^*(k; 3\psi, 1/3)$, are given in readily computable forms in (3.5) and (3.6). In addition, tables of Q_2^* and Q_3^* are given in Neff and Naus (1980). Approximation (3.4) is accurate even when $L = T/w$ is not an integer.

Let $F_p(i; \psi) = 0$ for $i < 0$. The following are exact probabilities for

$$Q_2^* = 1 - P^*(k; 2\psi, 1/2) \qquad \text{and} \qquad Q_3^* = 1 - P^*(k; 3\psi, 1/3),$$

$$\begin{aligned} Q^*(k; 2\psi, 1/2) &= (F_p(k-1; \psi))^2 - (k-1)p(k; \psi)p(k-2; \psi) \\ &\quad - (k-1-\psi)p(k; \psi)F_p(k-3; \psi), \end{aligned} \tag{3.5}$$

and

$$Q^*(k; 3\psi, 1/3) = (F_p(k-1; \psi))^3 - A_1 + A_2 + A_3 - A_4, \tag{3.6}$$

where

$$A_1 = 2p(k; \psi)F_p(k-1; \psi)\{(k-1)F_p(k-2; \psi) - \psi F_p(k-3; \psi)\},$$

$$\begin{aligned} A_2 &= .5(p(k; \psi))^2\{(k-1)(k-2)F_p(k-3; \psi) \\ &\quad - 2(k-2)\psi F_p(k-4; \psi) + \psi^2 F_p(k-5; \psi)\}, \end{aligned}$$

$$A_3 = \sum_{r=1}^{k-1} p(2k-r; \psi)(F_p(r-1; \psi))^2,$$

$$A_4 = \sum_{r=2}^{k-1} p(2k-r; \psi)p(r; \psi)\{(r-1)F_p(r-2; \psi) - \psi F_p(r-3; \psi)\}.$$

Alm (1983) develops the approximation

$$P^*(k; \lambda T, w/T) \tag{3.7}$$
$$\approx 1 - F_p(k-1; \lambda w) \exp\{-[(k-w\lambda)/k]\lambda(T-w)p(k-1; \lambda w)\}.$$

Alm gives further simplifications of (3.7) for cases where λT is large, and a further simplification if, in addition, w/T is small. Alm provides some tables and quantiles for the (3.7) for the case $T = 3600$, $\{w = 1, 2, 5, \text{ and } \lambda = 1(1)70\}$, and for $\{w = 1, \lambda = 10(5)50\}$.

We compare the five approximations for $P^*(k; \psi L, 1/L)$ with the exact values from Neff and Naus (1980) for several examples in Table 3.1.

In many fields decision-makers give great weight to a cluster that they perceive to be significant. The next two applications illustrate how a cluster will spark action.

Application 3.3 (Clusters of Plane Crashes). On the front page of the February 23, 1996, issue of *USA Today* is a news item headlined "Another F-14 crash prompts

Table 3.1. Approximations and exact values for $P^*(k; \psi L, 1/L)$.

Application	Exact value	Naus (3.4)	(3.3)	Alm (3.7)	CBI (3.2)	Newell–Ikeda (3.1)
$P^*(4; 10, .1)$	.374	.374	.339	.351	.386	.811
$P^*(5; 12, .25)$	.765	.765	.702	.555	.816	1.000–
$P^*(5; 8, 1/6)$	.896	.896	.867	.703	.945	1.000–
$P^*(41; 4800, 1/240)$	—	.066	.121	.061	.076	1.000–
$P^*(11; 33, 1/6)$	—	.381	.510	.342	.431	1.000–
$P^*(6; 342, 1/674.51)$	—	.051	.051	.051	.053	.091

Of all the approximations listed, our experience is that (3.4) is highly accurate for the widest range of values. Note that (3.3) is simple to compute with a calculator, while (3.4) is easily computed on a PC with a program.

stand-down." Over the past 5 years 32 of the Navy's 369 F-14 figher jets crashed. On February 22, 1996, the Navy suspended all operations of the F-14 after the third crash in 25 days. The first crash was on January 29, 1996, and the third on February 22. The three crashes in less than a month were about seven times the expected rate based on the 5 year period. Was there some new common cause that was increasing the chance of crashes? This is certainly worth exploring.

There are two questions that, if answered, could be useful to decision-makers. The first question is retrospective. The cluster of three crashes in 25 days certainly appears unusual given the overall accident rate. But how unusual is it? The second question is prospective. Suppose the Navy does not find any new cause of increase in accidents, and the overall regular rate of accidents (prior to this cluster) continues. If the Navy suspends all operations on this plane whenever three crash in a 25 day period, how often will they be suspending operations?

We will answer the second question using the methods of this chapter. The reader can use the methods of Chapter 2 to answer the first question.

The Table 3.2 shows the probabilities of getting a cluster of three crashes in 25 days somewhere within an i year period, where $i = 1, 2, 3, 4, 5$. The results are given for two different rates; the first uses a rate of .438 crashes per 25 days period (based on 32 per 5 years); the second uses a rate of .403 crashes per 25 days (based on 29 per 59 months). This table indicates, given the overall crash rate, that a cluster of three crashes in 25 days, somewhere in the five year period, is not particularly unusual. In fact, if there is no reduction in the overall crash rate, then such a cluster is more likely than not to occur somewhere in a 3 year or greater period, and is not particularly unusual even in a 1 year period.

Application 3.4 (Cluster of Deaths in a State Healthcare Facility). Epidemiologists and public health officials are often called upon to find explanations of clusters of cancer cases, suicides, accidents, or other causes of illness or death. These *cluster busters* will look for common causal factors. In cases where they find no such factors, and in screening situations where they are deciding which

Table 3.2. Probability of a 25 day period in K years having 3 crashes.

K	Average rate per 25 day period	
	.438	.403
1 year	.29	.24
2 years	.50	.43
3 years	.65	.57
4 years	.75	.68
5 years	.83	.76

clusters to choose to investigate, the epidemiologists seek to distinguish unusual from chance clusters. Intuition on such clusters is often misleading.

The following article from the August 11, 1995, issue of *The Home News* (p. A7, New Brunswick, NJ) illustrates this. The article describes how in a 10 month period, 11 residents died at a Tennessee State institution. The article notes that the number dying was approximately double the expected rate for a 400-bed institution housing individuals with such serious physical and mental handicaps.

A doubling of the expected rate of deaths calls out for explanation. Were some deaths due to lack of supervision in feeding patients, as some witnesses suggested? In any case, the number dying was about twice what was expected, and an angry U.S. District judge was tired and frustrated about the "pass-the-buck job" being done. The judge fined the State of Tennessee $5000 a day, and ordered Tennessee's mental health commissioner to spend one in four weekends at the state institution.

We find that the observed 11 cases in a 10 month period could have easily happened due to chance variations over a 3 to 5 year review period. Among institutions that have, on the average, 5.5 deaths in a 10 month period, purely by chance, we would expect that over a 5 year review period, that 38% of them have some 10 month period with 11 or more deaths. Here $k = 11$, $\psi = 5.5$, $w/T = 10/60 = 1/6 = 1/L$. Applying (3.4), $P^*(11; 33, 1/6) \approx .38$. (This is the next to last example in Table 3.1). Even for a 3 year review period, 23% of institutions would have such a cluster.

This application illustrates the use of the unconditional on N (total number of deaths) formula in a retrospective setting. The judge is reacting to what has already happened; however, insight can be added by considering what might have happened under similar situations at other institutions with a similar background rate.

Application 3.5 (Visual Perception). In studies of visual perception, photons are assumed to arrive at a receptor in the retina according to a Poisson process. Researchers observe that under conditions of low illumination the retinal neurones do not discharge for each photon. Instead there appears to be a triggering effect from several photons leading to patterns of neuron discharge spikes. A classical theory of perception is that if k or more photons arrive within an *integration time* w, an impulse triggers the neurones to discharge. Researchers seek to compare the observed patterns of times between neuronal spikes with what would be expected under the classical chance model. Leslie (1969, p. 379) noted that the distribution of waiting time till discharge under the classical model is intractable. Van de Grind, Koenderink, Heyde, Landman, and Bowman (1971) stated that an analytic solution was lacking, and used a Monte Carlo approach to simulate the distribution. The present chapter gives the distribution of the waiting times till k or more photons arrive within an integration time w for the above model.

Application 3.6 (Adequacy of Number of Spare Parts). Goodwin and Giese (1965) study whether the number of spare parts is adequate to provide reliability for a complex system. They assume that when a part fails, it is immediately replaced by a spare part if available. The failed part is repaired and is kept as a spare until needed. The repair time is a constant w. The number of parts that fail in a given time is assumed to have a Poisson distribution. Given $k - 1$ spares, if at any time in $[0, T)$ there are k or more failures within a time w then the system goes down. They give an approximation, their approximation (21), for the probability that the system does not fail, $Q^*(k; \lambda T, w/T)$. (In their notation $p_\tau = Q^*(N + 1; \lambda \tau, r/\tau)$.) For enough spares, such that there is a very small probability of the system going down, their approximation appears reasonable. For large probability of the system going down, their approximation is not accurate. For example, for $\lambda = 3$, $w = 1$, $T = L = 6$, and 4 spares (our $k = 5$), the probability that the system is up is $Q^*(5; 18, 1/6) = .104$, their equation (21) gives .0370.

Application 3.7 (Cluster of Police Deaths in the Line of Duty). *The Newark Star Ledger* (Nov. 26, 1997, p. 15) comments on the multiple tragedies. "The recent string of police deaths—three in 5 weeks—is unusual. In the previous 10 years, ten New Jersey officers were killed in the line of duty."

Given an average of one death per 52 weeks, three deaths in 5 weeks is more than 31 times the expected number. In any particular 5 week period it would be very unusual to get three or more cases; the chance probability is .00014. However, this in itself is misleading. Note that even one death in 5 weeks would be more than ten times the expected number, yet it would not be surprising to find some 5 week period in 1 year where there is one death. What strikes us as unusual is three deaths within some 5 week period within some larger period of time.

Given an average rate of one death per year, the probability that somewhere in a 10 year period there would be a 5 week period with three or more deaths is $P^*(3; 10, 5/520) = .04$. From the retrospective perspective of Chapter 2, given ten deaths over a 10 year period, the probability of three or more deaths in some 5 week period within the 10 year period is from the tables in Neff and Naus (1980), $P(3; 10, 5/520) = .03$. Here the two views give similar results.

Application 3.8 (Reliability of Pipeline Networks). Laszlo and Mihalyko (1992) describe the application of the scan statistic to the following example of overflow in a pipeline network servicing a factory. A large factory has 100 sections. Each section has a storage unit that has a tank that collects water to be discharged, and has its own pump. When a tank is full the pump will work for 1 hour to empty the water from the tank into the main drain that is linked to all the tanks. The starting times for the pumps to start (or, equivalently, for the tanks to be full) are independent from pump to pump, and random according to a Poisson process. Experience indicates that individual tanks fill, on average, in 20 hours. Now suppose that the principal drain pipe is sized to handle the discharge of up to 22 pumps, but will overflow if more than 22 pumps are pumping simultaneously. Is this an adequate sizing of the main drain if the goal is that the chance of overflow in a 10 year period is less than .001?

   To view the problem in terms of the scan statistic, slide a window of 1 hour over the 10 year ($3652.5 \times 24 = 87,660$ hours) period. If 23 or more pumps start pumping within the same hour the main drain pipe will overflow. The number of pumps working in any given hour is assumed to be a Poisson distributed random variable with expectation $\lambda = 100 * (1/20) = 5$. To apply (3.4) for $P^*(k; \psi L, 1/L)$ for this example, k is the critical overflow amount, $k = 23$. The average number within a 1 hour window is $\psi = \lambda = 5$. The total time period is 87,660 window lengths; $L = 87,660$. From (3.4), $P^*(23; 5 * 87,660, 1/87,660) = .005$. Laszlo and Mihalyko's asymptotic results give the same answer for this case. The pipeline should be sized bigger to handle at least 24 simultaneous pumps to meet the goal that the chance of overflow in a 10 year period is less than .001. This follows from $P^*(24; 5 * 87,660, 1/87,660) = .00106$ and $P^*(25; 5 * 87,660, 1/87,660) = .00021$.

Application 3.9 (Cluster of Cases of Guillian–Barre Syndrome). Jiang, Cheng, Link, and de Pedro-Cuesta (1997) apply the scan statistic to analyze the temporal clustering of Guillain–Barre syndrome in Sweden during the period 1978 to 1993. They carried out a systematic search over time for all cases in the whole population of 12 counties, using the scan test. They used both a 1 month and a 3 month moving window. They found a significant cluster of 23 cases in the 3 month period from July to September, 1983, for individuals younger than 40 years. This was much higher than the average expected rate for that period of 9.17 cases. They found the observed significance level to be .042. Assuming the cases followed a Poisson distribution with constant rate of 9.17 cases in a 3 month period, the probability, that somewhere in the 15 year period (i.e., 60 3 month periods) there would be a cluster as large as 23, is given by $P^*(k = 23; \psi L = 9.17L; 1/L = 1/60) \approx .044$, from (3.4).

Application 3.10 (Open-Loop Window Flow Control). Berger and Whitt (1993) describe window flow control schemes that can be used to control the flow of information packets into a network. They contrast the benefits of the closed and open-loop window control mechanisms. In both schemes a sender of information packets (the source) tries to keep track of the flow of information packets into a network, and will stop sending when there is evidence that the flow may be overloading the system. In the closed-loop mechanism, the receiver provides feedback to the sender about the information received. When a certain amount of sent information has not been acknowledged, the sender will stop sending. Berger and Whitt note that given the large amounts of information sent over high-speed networks and over long distances, the closed-loop feedback mechanism can lead to delays in recognizing important changes in the state of the network. The open-loop control mechanism avoids the feedback and delays by basing the control mechanism on the maximum number of information packets in a sliding time window of fixed prespecified length. Berger and Whitt note that the maximum number of points in a sliding window is the scan statistic, and derive asymptotic results using strong approximations for a variety of probability input models. (They also look at disjoint windows which they call the "jumping window" and also some "leaky bucket" models.) Their asymptotic results are designed to give reasonable approximations for scanning window length w, small relative to the total time T, but both w and T large. (More precisely, they assume that T is much larger than w, which in turn is greater than $\log T$.) For large w and very large T they compare their asymptotic approximations with simulations and demonstrate that the asymptotic results provide good approximations for the mean (i.e., expected) size of the maximum sliding window content. They also approximate the standard deviation.

They note and document that for smaller values of w and T, one should use the more accurate (3.4) for the Poisson case. For example, in Berger and Whitt (1993, Table 2), the smallest window length is for $w = 20$, $T = 1,000,000$ and a Poisson process with an average of one observation per unit of time. For this case, their asymptotic approximation for the mean is 42, and for the standard deviation it is 1.2. This compares with two small simulations which gave 44 and 45 for the mean and 1.8 and .9 for the standard deviation. For this example, (3.4) can be used to compute $Q^*(k; \psi L, 1/L) = 1 - P^*(k; \psi L, 1/L)$ with $\psi = 20$, $L = 1,000,000/20 = 50,000$, and a range of k-values. Table 3.3 gives the needed range of k that causes Q^* to take values between ε and $1 - \varepsilon$, where ε is small.

From Table 3.3, the maximum window size has mean 44.84 and standard deviation 1.60, consistent with the simulations. (The mean can be computed as $\sum_k P^*(k; 20(50,000); 1/50,000) = 52 - 7.1572 = 44.84$.) For the case $w = 20$, $T = 1,000,000$, the asymptotic results of 42 and 1.2 appear too small. For the case of $w = 200$ and $T = 1,000,000$ the simulations and asymptotic results are close.

3.3   Handling Trends or Seasonality in Data

Application 3.11 (Monitoring Systems for Disease Clusters). Farrington, Andrews, Beale, and Catchpole (1996) describe a monitoring system to scan au-

Table 3.3. $Q^*(k; 20(50,000); 1/50,000)$ for $k = 41(1)52$ for Poisson input.

k	$Q^*(k; 20(50,000); 1/50,000)$
41	6.6E−7
42	8.2642E−4
43	.0317
44	.1946
45	.4682
46	.7098
47	.8594
48	.9365
49	.9726
50	.9885
51	.9952
52	.9999
Sum	7.1572

tomatically weekly reports to provide an early warning of outbreaks of infectious diseases. This early detection allows interventions such as removing contaminated food, or the different treatment of water supplies, or vaccination, or other prophylactic treatments. They focus on a prospective view:

> In the prospective context the aim is to detect clustering of events at one extremity of the data series, typically in the most recent time interval.... The primary purpose... is to identify outbreaks sufficiently early to allow time for intervention.

At the Communicable Disease Surveillance Centre in London (CDSC), reports come in each week on 200 to 350 distinct organisms. The week's data is gathered and processed over the weekend. They need one general automatic approach that would apply to all organisms. The most important requirements for their routine monitoring are

> timeliness, sensitivity and specificity, together with readily interpretable outputs. Timeliness and sensitivity are required to ensure that outbreaks are detected in time for interventions to take place.

The specificity is required to avoid high false positive detection which would result in a waste of investigative time and effort.

They use a (log-linear) regression model to calculate expected values for the number of cases for each organism for a given week (taking into account seasonality and trends). Thresholds are based on counts for similar periods in previous years, and are determined empirically. They chose the threshold to keep the number of detections to a workable level and not to focus on a few cases of very rare diseases. In their approach they are dividing up time into nonoverlapping periods, and (adjusting for nonuniformities over time) they look at unusually large values in a given calendar week. This is reasonable, in part, from the fact that the data is summarized on a weekly basis. There is an important reason to base the decision rule on a small time period. One wants to investigate unusual clusters before it is obvious that there is an epidemic. If the natural development of the epidemic is such that it will become obvious after time t, then one would want to use a decision time interval smaller than t.

They describe an incident where eight isolated cases of *Salmonella agona* were reported in the week beginning October 31, 1994. Again in December, and in January, excessive numbers of cases were reported. Because the time series of weekly reports did not appear that unusual, and were not limited to some clearly defined group, the excesses were assumed to be false positives, and they did not follow up with further investigation. In February, 1995, another cluster of cases of this somewhat unusual type of salmonella was reported. It turned out that the source of infection was contamination in a popular snack that was distributed worldwide. Standard surveillance methods led to an investigation, and "it soon became apparent that the outbreak was not limited to Britain." In this example, their approach had detected the cluster and gave an earlier warning than previous approaches.

The CDSC data is not presently summarized as it comes in, but is rather analyzed for disjoint (nonoverlapping) weeks. In this context, it would not be appropriate to use the scan statistic. However, when one can monitor continuously, the scan statistic, appropriately applied, offers advantages over the disjoint week procedure. In a monitoring system that continuously updates reports, one could look at the number of cases during the past 7 day period. This is scanning with overlapping 1 week periods. If the number of cases in this scanning window is at any point unusually high (relative to the expected number for a 7 day period), one would tag the occurrence as unusual. We describe below ways to set the thresholds within the window. The clustering of *Salmonella agona* provides a useful comparison of the disjoint and continuous scan approaches. It is possible to use the scan statistic to incorporate the threshold rates (based on the CDSC regression model or some other way). See Chapter 15 for a full discussion.

3.3.1 The Disjoint Week Procedure

Farrington, Andrews, Beale, and Catchpole (1996) in Figure 6 plot weekly counts for the *Salmonella agona*. There is seasonal variability over time. The CDSC chose the critical number in a specific week to have a false positive rate of .005. For this purpose of illustration, assume that during the week of interest, the background number of cases, is a Poisson variate with a mean of two. Then the critical number to warn of a possible problem would be seven cases. This is because $1 - F_p(6; \psi = 2) \approx .005$.

Requiring a critical value of seven or more cases within a disjoint week (where the background expected rate is two) will lead to a false positive rate of .005 for that organism for that week. Over the course of a 52 week year, the false positive chance, that at least 1 week will be over its threshold, is given by $1-(1-.005)^{52} =$ .23. Given that all organisms are monitored using a weekly false positive rate of .005, then one would expect (due purely to natural variability about background) that about 23% of all organisms would lead to a false positive warning at least once a year.

To put this seemingly high 23% in perspective, Farrington, Andrews, Beale, and Catchpole note that about 20 organisms are flagged each week out of some 200 to 350 reported. Their experience using this system indicates that about 40% of the cases flagged as being unusual were of health interest; the remaining 60% were either due to chance, or batching, or other aspects of the reporting. Routine monitoring has to consider many clusters; this is why an automated system was needed.

3.3.2 Continuous 7-Day Scan

For an organism with a background weekly expectation of two cases, the comparable critical value of the continuous scan statistic is eight cases in any 7 day period. This is computed by finding the value of k for which $P^*(k; \psi L; 1/L) = .23$, where $\psi = 2$, $L = 52$ and $w = 1$, $P^*(8; 104; 1/52) \approx .23$.

3.3.3 Comparison of Disjoint Week with 7 Day Scan for a 52 Week Year

The critical value of the disjoint test and the scan test are each chosen relative to the expected backgrounds for the year. The critical values for both tests can vary from week to week based on the background rates. For the disjoint test this can be done by setting the critical value for a specific week to yield a weekly .005 rate; this results in a false alarm rate of .23 for the year. Chapter 15 shows how to set overall rates for the scan test given variability in background rates.

3.4 Moments of Scan Statistics

Recall that S_w denotes the largest number of points to be found in any subinterval of $[0, T)$ of length w; W_k denotes the size of the smallest subinterval of $[0, T)$ that contains k points; and $T_{k,w}$ denotes the waiting time until we first observe at least k points in an interval of length w. The distribution of all three variables are directly related to $P^*(k; \lambda T, w/T)$. Chapter 2 described results for the first two moments of S_w and W_k for the conditional on N case.

3.4.1 The Expectation and Variance of W_k, the Size of the Smallest Interval

The continuous random variable W_k has cumulative distribution function $P(W_k \leq w/T) = P^*(k; \lambda T, w/T)$. The sth moment of W_k can be evaluated by integrating over the appropriate densities. Alternatively, one can average the conditional moments (about the origin) over the distribution of N.

3.4.2 The Expected Waiting Time until a Cluster

For the Poisson process, Solev'ev (1966), Glaz (1979), Naus (1982), and Samuel-Cahn (1983) give various approximations for the expectation of $T_{k,w}$, the waiting time until a cluster of k points within a window w first occurs. Samuel-Cahn (1983) gives approximations and bounds for the expectation and variance of the waiting time until a cluster, and bounds for the expectation for general point processes with i.i.d. interarrival times between the points. Details are given for the Poisson, Bernoulli, and compound Poisson processes. We now discuss Samuel-Cahn's results for the Poisson case. Let $\delta_{k,w}$ denote the total number of points observed until first getting a cluster of k points within an interval of length w. For the Poisson process with mean λ per unit time, the expected waiting times between points is $1/\lambda$. Samuel-Cahn applies Wald's lemma, to find for the Poisson case

$$E(T_{k,w}) = E(\delta_{k,w})/\lambda, \tag{3.8}$$

and derives a series of approximations for $E(\delta_{k,w})$. The simplest of these is

$$E(\delta_{k,w}) \approx k + \left\{ (F_p(k-2; \lambda w))^2 / P(\delta_{k,w} = k+1) \right\}, \tag{3.9}$$

where

$$P(\delta_{k,w} = k+1) = \sum_{i=0}^{k-2} (-1)^{k-2-i} p(i; \lambda w) + (-1)^{k-1} \exp\{-2\lambda w\}, \tag{3.10}$$

and where $p(i; \lambda w)$ and $F_p(k-2; \lambda w)$ are Poisson probability functions defined in (3.2).

Naus (1982, Sect. 2.2) also gives an approximation for the expected waiting time until a cluster for the Poisson case. Let $\psi = \lambda w$ denote the expected number of points in a window of w units in length. Let Q_2^* denote $Q^*(k; 2\psi, 1/2)$, and let Q_3^* denote $Q^*(k; 3\psi, 1/3)$, where exact expressions for these quantities are given in (3.5) and (3.6). Naus (1982, Eq. (2.12)) gives the approximation

$$E(T_{k,1}) \approx 2 + \left\{ Q_2^* / \log_e(Q_2^*/Q_3^*) \right\}. \tag{3.11}$$

Approximation (3.11) follows from writing $E(T_{k,1}) = \int_0^\infty P(T_{k,1} > T)dT$ and using (3.4) to approximate $P(T_{k,1} > T)$ by $Q_2^*(Q_3^*/Q_2^*)^{T-2}$.

The following example, based on simulations and calculations in Samuel-Cahn and Naus, compare the approximations. Let $w = 1$, $\lambda = 1$. The following are the approximations for $E(T_{k,w})$, the expected waiting time until a *k-in-w cluster*. In parentheses are a second stage approximation by Samuel-Cahn, given by (2.9) and (4.3) of her paper. For these examples, the approximations are fairly similar:

	Samuel-Cahn (1983)	Naus (1982)	10,000 simulations
For $k = 3$	7.0 (6.6)	6.8	6.6
For $k = 5$	80.7 (81.8)	80.8	81.1

Note that one can use the tight bounds for $P(T_{k,1} > T)$ for the Poisson case, in Janson (1984) to construct bounds on the expectation of $T_{k,1}$.

3.5　The Distribution of the Number of Clusters in $[0, T)$

The previous section dealt with probabilities of getting somewhere in $[0, T)$ at least one cluster of k points in a scanning window of length w. Results were given for the distribution and moments of variables associated with the largest cluster, the largest number of points in any window w, the length of the smallest interval containing k points, and the waiting time till getting at least one cluster of k points in a scanning window w.

The present section deals with the distribution and moments of the numbers of clusters of k points within a scanning window w. In dealing with the number of clusters, we face a new difficulty. How should clusters be counted? The following example illustrates this question.

Let $k = 4$, $w = 1$, and $T = 10$. Suppose 12 points are observed, and their values are .1, .2, .3, .4, .5, 4.6, 7.7, 7.9, 8.3, 8.4, 8.6, 8.8. There are five cases of four points within a window of size 1.0: (.1, .2, .3, .4), (.2, .3, .4, .5), (7.7, 7.9, 8.3, 8.4), (7.9, 8.3, 8.4, 8.6), (8.3, 8.4, 8.6, 8.8). Each of these cases *starts with a different point*, and we could count this as five clusters. This is the counting method in Glaz and Naus (1983). They derive moments and distributional results for this method that count overlapping clusters as distinct if they start with a different point. It is also closely related to the counting in the r-scan method of Dembo and Karlin (1992). We describe below the exact and approximate distributional results for these methods of counting overlapping clusters.

There are alternative ways of counting overlapping clusters. One might only count overlapping clusters as separate clusters, *as long as one point within the window of size 1 is different*. This will only count four clusters. The case of (.1, .2, .3, .4, .5) is special in that any window of length 1 that contains (.1, .2, .3, .4), must also contain .5.

Many of the clusters counted under either of the above methods involve overlapping sets of points. For the above example, counting only clusters with disjoint sets gives two nonoverlapping clusters. We now describe approximate distributional results for nonoverlapping clusters.

3.5.1 The Distribution of the Number of Nonoverlapping Clusters

Let $\eta_k(T)$ denote the number of nonoverlapping (k points in unit time) clusters occurring in $[0, T)$. For the case where clusters are relatively rare, the distribution of $\eta_k(T)$ will be approximately Poisson distributed with parameter $\delta = E\{\eta_k(T)\}$. For a discussion of Poisson approximation and the declumping involved with dealing with nonoverlapping clusters, see Aldous (1989), and Barbour, Holst, and Janson (1992). In the present problem we can approximate $E\{\eta_k(T)\}$ in several ways:

Method 1. $Q^*(k; \lambda T, w/T)$ gives the probability of no clusters. Given the Poisson approximation, $Q^*(k; \lambda T, w/T) = Q^*(k; \psi L, 1/L) \approx \exp\{-\delta\}$, where $T = L/w$. Solving for δ gives

$$E\{\eta_k(T)\} = \delta \approx -\log_e\{Q^*(k; \psi L, 1/L)\} \approx -\log_e\{Q_2^*\{Q_3^*/Q_2^*\}^{L-2}\}. \tag{3.12}$$

Method 2. For the case where clusters are relatively rare, the result for the expected waiting time till a cluster provides an approximation for the expected number of nonoverlapping clusters occur in $[0, T)$:

$$E\{\eta_k(T)\} = \delta = T/E(T_{k,1}) \approx T/(2 + \{Q_2^*/\log_e(Q_2^*/Q_3^*)\}). \tag{3.13}$$

For example, let $w = 1$, $k = 3$, $\lambda = \psi = 1$, $L = T = 100$. From (3.5) and (3.6), $Q_2^* = .77817792$ and $Q_3^* = .66251375$. The expected waiting time until three points in $w = 1$ is from (3.11) approximately 6.8. The expected number of nonoverlapping clusters in $[0, 100)$ is from Method 2, (3.13) approximately $100/6.8 = 14.7$. From Method 1, the expected number of nonoverlapping clusters is approximately 15.8.

The distribution of the number of nonoverlapping clusters (for the case of rare clusters) is approximately Poisson, with

$$P(\eta_k(T) = r) = p(r; \delta). \tag{3.14}$$

3.5.2 The Distribution of the Number of Overlapping Clusters

First condition on there being a total of N points. Let $X_{(1)} \leq X_{(2)} \leq \cdots \leq X_{(N)}$ denote the ordered values of the X's. Define the indicator variables, Z_i by

$$Z_i = \begin{cases} 1 & \text{if } X_{(i+k-1)} - X_{(i)} \leq w, \\ 0 & \text{otherwise.} \end{cases} \tag{3.15}$$

Glaz and Naus (1983) define the number of overlapping clusters by

$$\zeta(k, w, N) = \sum_{i=1}^{N-k+1} Z_i, \qquad (3.16)$$

and find

$$E(\zeta(k, w, N)) = (N - k + 1)P(Z_i = 1)$$
$$= (N - k + 1)G_b(k - 1; N, w) \qquad (3.17)$$

and

$$\mathrm{Var}(\zeta(k, w, N)) = E\big(\zeta(k, w, N)\big)(1 - E(\zeta(k, w, N)))$$
$$+ 2 \sum_{t=0}^{N-k-1} (N - k - t)P\{(Z_1 = 1) \cap (Z_{t+2} = 1)\}, \qquad (3.18)$$

and give a formula for $P\{(Z_1 = 1) \cap (Z_{t+2} = 1)\}$ for $w \leq .5$. Glaz and Naus (1983) give tables for $E(\zeta(k, w, N))$ and $\mathrm{Var}(\zeta(k, w, N))$ for $n = 5(1)10$, $k = 2(1)N$, $w = .1(.1).5$. For the case where N is a random variable with a Poisson distribution with mean λT, one can average the expressions in (3.17) and (3.18) over the distribution of N. See Chapter 17 for further details.

3.6 The Scan Statistic on the Circle

Chapter 2 notes that for certain applications it is reasonable to view the points as being randomly distributed over a circle rather than a line. In that chapter, a fixed number N of points were independently drawn from the uniform distribution on the unit circle. In the present chapter, the total number of points is a Poisson random variable, with expectation λ per unit length. Define S_w to be the maximum number of the points in any arc of length w on the unit circle. Define W_k as the size of the smallest subarc of the unit circle that contains k points. For the unit circle $T = 1$, $w/T = w = 1/L$, and $\psi = \lambda w = \lambda/L$. We denote the common probability

$$P(S_w \geq k) = P(W_k \leq w) = P_c^*(k; \lambda T, w/T) = P_c^*(k; \lambda, w),$$

and let $Q_c^*(k; \lambda, w) = 1 - P_c^*(k; \lambda, w)$. The conditional on N results of Wallenstein (1971) for $P_c(k; N, w)$ can be averaged over the Poisson distribution of N to find $P_c^*(k; \lambda, w)$. For the case $w \leq .2$, Naus (1982, Eq. (5.2)) gives a highly accurate approximation for $P_c^*(k; \lambda, w)$ that uses as input the quantities $Q^*(k; r\psi, 1/r)$ for $r = 2, 3, 4$. The formula for $r = 2, 3$ are given by (3.5) and (3.6). The values for $r = 4$ are tabled in Neff and Naus (1980), or can be derived from (11.6) for $L = 4$. The approximation in Naus (1982) is heuristically shown to be

$$Q_c^*(k; \psi L, 1/L) \approx Q^*(k; 4\psi, 1/4)\{Q^*(k; 3\psi, 1/3)\}^{L-2}/\{Q^*(k; 2\psi, 1/2)\}^{L-1}. \qquad (3.19)$$

As a further step, we can approximate $Q^*(k; 4\psi, 1/4)$ in (3.19) from the $r = 2, 3$ terms, and find the simpler approximation

$$Q_c^*(k; \psi L, 1/L) \approx \{Q^*(k; 3\psi, 1/3)/Q^*(k; 2\psi, 1/2)\}^L. \qquad (3.20)$$

For the example, $k = 5$, $L = 6$, $\psi = 1$, $Q^*(5; 3, 1/3) = .971277358$, $Q^*(5; 2, 1/2) = .983483383$, and $Q^*(5; 4, 1/4) = .959220621$. Approximations (3.19) and (3.20) give $Q_c^*(5; 6, 1/6) \approx .9278$, and this is within .0001 of the exact result from averaging over the conditional values in Wallenstein (1971). See Barbour, Holst, and Janson (1992, pages 156 and following) for discussion of the scan statistic on the circle and line for the Poisson process.

4
Success Scans in a Sequence of Trials

4.1 Binomial Distribution of Events: Discrete Time, Unconditional Case

Many researchers deal with data that can be viewed as a series of trials, each with two possible outcomes. We will arbitrarily label the two alternative possible outcomes of a trial as *success* and *failure*. In a quality control chart, consecutive points may be in or out of a warning zone. After a period of learning, a subject may correctly or incorrectly perform a series of cognitive tasks. A sports team wins and loses games over a season. In a stream of items sampled from an assembly line some are defective, some acceptable.

Sometimes the researcher seeks to determine whether there have been changes in the underlying process that generates the outcome. Given that there is no change, a simple (null) model for the underlying process assumes independent trials with constant probability of success on each trial. Several statistical criteria have been developed to test for specific types of changes in an underlying process. One such type of change is where the probability of success increases at some point in the process. Given $N = Lm$ trials, L an integer, one criterion commonly used divides the N trials into L disjoint sets each of m consecutive trials, and observes the number of successes within each set. If the number of successes in any of the sets is too large this suggests a change in the underlying process. To determine what is *too large* relative to the null model, note that under the null model the number of successes in m trials is a binomial random variable. However, the researcher is looking at the number of successes in L sets of m trials, and needs an experiment-wide level of significance. The distribution of the maximum of L independently and identically distrituted (i.i.d.) binomial variates is used.

Another naturally and commonly used criterion is based on all the sets of m contiguous trials (disjoint or overlapping) within the N trials. At each trial the researcher counts the number of successes in the last m trials. If at any trial this number is too big, this suggests a change in the underlying process. The maximum number within any m contiguous trials within the N trials, denoted S'_m, is called the *scan statistic*. For the special case where $S'_m = m$, a *success-run* of length m has occurred within the N trials. For the general case where $S'_m = k$, a *quota* of at least k successes within m consecutive trials has occurred (terminology (Goldman and Bender, 1962)).

In some applications the researcher conditions on a known observed value of the total number of successes in the N trials. We call this the *conditional* or *retrospective* case. In other applications the total number of successes in N trials is treated as a random variable; we call this the *unconditional* or in other applications the *prospective* case. Section 4.2 deals with a simple model for the unconditional case. Section 4.3 considers generalizations to trials with more than two outcomes. Section 4.4 gives a simple model for the conditional case.

4.2   A Null Model for the Unconditional Case: The Bernoulli Process

Let $X_1, X_2, \ldots, X_N$ be a sequence of i.i.d. discrete random variables, where $P(X_i = 1) = p = 1 - P(X_i = 0)$. We refer to the X's as a sequence of Bernoulli trials, and the process as a Bernoulli process. For m an integer, and $i = 1, 2, \ldots, N - m + 1$, define the random variables

$$Y_i = \sum_{j=i}^{i+m-1} X_j.$$

The Y's define a moving sum of m of the X's. The scan statistic, S'_m is defined as the maximum of the moving sums, that is, the maximum number of ones in any m consecutive trials

$$S'_m = \max_{1 \le i \le N-m+1} \{Y_i\}.$$

A related statistic is W'_k, the smallest number of consecutive trials that contain k ones. That is,

$$W'_k = \min_{k \le m \le N} \{m : \text{such that, } S'_m = k\}.$$

Given a Bernoulli process on $(1, \infty)$, let $T_{k,m}$ denote the waiting time until we first observe at least k ones in an interval of length m. Formally, $T_{k,m}$ is the smallest i (greater than or equal to m) such that $Y_{i-m+1} \ge k$. The three statistics, S'_m, W'_k, and $T_{k,m}$, are related by

$$P(S'_m \geq k) = P(W'_k \leq m) = P(T_{k,m} \leq N). \tag{4.1}$$

We denote these common probabilities for the Bernoulli process by $P'(k \mid m; N, p)$. These three statistics have similar counterparts in the continuous time Poisson process considered in Chapter 3.

A fourth statistic defined for the discrete-time process considered in the present chapter is the length of the longest number of consecutive trials, V_r, that have at most r zeros. For the special case $r = 0$, V_r is the length of the longest run of ones. For a sequence of N trials, the statistic V_r is probabilistically related to the scan statistic S'_m by the relation

$$P(V_r \geq k + r) = P(S'_{k+r} \geq k) = P'(k \mid k + r; N; p). \tag{4.2}$$

Note: In the matching in molecular biology examples in Chapter 6, researchers sometimes focus on the length of the longest, almost perfectly, matching sequence, and this is directly measured by V_r. For the special case $r = 0$, the researcher is looking at the length of the longest perfectly matching sequence, and this is directly related to the length of the longest run of ones.

4.2.1 Approximations for $P'(k \mid m; N; p)$ with Applications

Let $Q'(k \mid m; N; p) = 1 - P'(k \mid m; N; p)$, and abbreviate $Q'(k \mid m; Lm; p)$ by Q'_L. Naus (1982) provides the following highly accurate approximation for Q'_L in terms of Q'_2 and Q'_3:

$$Q'_L \approx Q'_2 \{Q'_3 / Q'_2\}^{((N/m)-2)}. \tag{4.3}$$

Equations (4.4) and (4.5) give exact results for Q'_2 and Q'_3. Let

$$b(k; m, p) = \binom{m}{k} p^k (1 - p)^{m-k},$$

and

$$F_b(r; s, p) = \sum_{i=0}^{r} b(i; s, p), \qquad r = 0, 1, \ldots, s,$$

$$= 0, \qquad r < 0.$$

For $2 < k < N, 0 < p < 1$, let

$$Q'_2 = \left(F_p(k - 1; m, p)\right)^2 - (k - 1)b(k; m, p)F_b(k - 2; m, p)$$
$$+ mpb(k; m, p)F_b(k - 3; m - 1, p), \tag{4.4}$$

and

$$Q'_3 = \left(F_b(k - 1; m, p)\right)^3 - A_1 + A_2 + A_3 - A_4, \tag{4.5}$$

where

$$A_1 = 2b(k; m, p)F_b(k - 1; m, p)\{(k - 1)F_b(k - 2; m, p)$$
$$- mpF_b(k - 3; m - 1, p)\},$$

$$A_2 = .5(b(k; m, p))^2\{(k - 1)(k - 2)F_b(k - 3; m, p)$$
$$- 2(k - 2)mpF_b(k - 4; m - 1, p) + m(m - 1)p^2F_b(k - 5; m - 2, p)\},$$

$$A_3 = \sum_{r=1}^{k-1} b(2k - r; m, p)(F_b(r - 1; m, p))^2,$$

$$A_4 = \sum_{r=2}^{k-1} b(2k - r; m, p)b(r; m, p)\{(r - 1)F_b(r - 2; m, p)$$
$$- mpF_b(r - 3; m - 1, p)\}.$$

There is also a series of approximations based on asymptotic results, the Erdös–Rényi-type law (see Chapter 13). These approximations can converge quite slowly.

The random variable V_0 denotes the length of the longest run of ones (*successes*), and $P(V_0 \geq m) = P'(m \mid m; N; p)$. The distribution of the length of the longest run of ones in a sequence of N Bernoulli trials is a classical problem in probability theory. A recursion relation going back to Abraham de Moivre (1738) is

$$P(V_0 \geq m; N + 1) = P(V_0 \geq m; N) + (1 - p)p^m(1 - P\{V_0 \geq m; N - m\}).$$
$$(4.6)$$

Various exact and approximate expressions are given for $P\{V_0 \geq m; N\}$ in Uspensky (1937, p. 79), Bradley (1968, p. 267), Bateman (1948, p. 112), and elsewhere. Bateman's exact formula is relatively simple and is

$$P\{V_0 \geq m; N\} = \sum_{j=1}^{[N/m]} (-1)^{j+1}\{p + ((N - jm + 1)q/j)\}\binom{N - jm}{i - 1}p^{jm}q^{j-1},$$
$$(4.7)$$

where $q = 1 - p$, and $[y]$ denotes the largest integer in y. Work on the distribution of the longest run and its variations continue through to today. Results are derived for both exact and limiting distributions. The book by Godbole and Papastavridis (1994) contains several papers focusing on the length of the longest success run for various models.

We could use the recursion relation (4.6) or the formula (4.7) to find the probability of getting a head run of length k in 200 tosses of a fair coin. For many cases of practical interest the number of trials N is large, and the length of the longest run of ones, m, is much smaller. For example, what is the probability of getting a run of at least 25 heads in $N = 200,000$ tosses of a fair coin? The exact formula (4.7) involves a sum of $[N/m] = 8000$ terms. For large N, various approximate and asymptotic formula and bounds have been developed.

Feller (1957, p. 310) gives a simple approximation

$$P'(m \mid m; N; p) \approx 1 - \exp\{-Nqp^m\}. \tag{4.8}$$

Approximation (4.3) gives

$$P\{V_0 \geq m; N\} = 1 - Q'(m \mid m; N; p) \approx 1 - Q_2'\{Q_3'/Q_2'\}^{((N/m)-2)}, \tag{4.9}$$

where we can apply (4.7) directly, for $(N/m) = 2, 3$ to find

$$
\begin{aligned}
Q_2' &= 1 - P'(m \mid m; 2m; p) = 1 - p^m(1 + mq), \\
Q_3' &= 1 - P'(m \mid m; 3m; p) = 1 - p^m(1 + 2mq) \\
&\quad + .5p^{2m}(2mq + m(m - 1)q^2).
\end{aligned} \tag{4.10}
$$

Comparisons with exact tables of runs (e.g., Grant (1947)), or with tight bounds such as the generating function bounds of Uspensky, the Chen–Stein bounds, or Glaz–Naus bounds (see Chapters 12 and 13) show that (4.9) is highly accurate over a wide range of the distribution. For example, $P'\{7 \mid 7; 50, .5\} = .1653$ from Grant's tables, .1653 from (4.9), as compared to .1774 from (4.8). By (4.9) the probability of getting a run of at least 25 heads in $N = 200,000$ tosses of a fair coin is .003.

Application 4.1 (The Distribution of the Length of the Longest Success Run). Schilling (1990) describes a classroom experiment by Revesz where half of the students each toss a coin 200 times and record the results; the other half are each asked to skip the tossing phase, and just write down what they believe is a random sequence of heads and tails. Revesz can usually pick out the random from the made up sequences. Schilling (1990) presents two illustrative sequences. One sequence is from tosses of a *fair* coin, the other sequence made up. The following are the first 50 tosses from each sequence:

```
Seq. 1:  THTHHTTTTHHTHTHHHHHHHHTTTHHTTHTTTHTT
         THTTHHTHHTHTHT
Seq. 2:  HHTHTTTHTTTTHHTHTTTHTTHHHHHTTHTHTHTT
         TTHHTTHHTTHHHT
```

One striking feature of the first sequence is the long run of eight heads. In the first sequence of 200 trials the longest run of heads (or tails) consists of eight consecutive heads. In the second sequence the longest run consists of five consecutive heads. Is the longest run of eight unusually long, or is the longest run of five unusually short?

Apply (4.9) to find the distribution of the length of the longest run of heads. To find the distribution of the length of the longest run of heads or tails, we can still apply (4.9) with the following known modification. If in the original sequence of

Table 4.1. Probability distribution of longest runs of heads or either type in 200 tosses of a fair coin.

k	P(longest run of heads $\geq k$)	P(longest run of either type $\geq k$)
5	.97	.9992
6	.80	.97
7	.54	.80
8	.32	.54
9	.17	.32
10	.09	.17

H's and T's, a letter is the same as the letter before it, then write an S under the letter, otherwise a D. Thus for the sequence:

$$H\ T\ H\ H\ T\ T\ T\ T\ H\ T\ H\ H\ T\ H\ H\ H\ H\ H\ T$$

$$D\ D\ S\ D\ S\ S\ S\ D\ D\ D\ S\ D\ D\ S\ S\ S\ S\ D$$

Note that a run of length 5 in the original sequence of N trials will appear as a run of four S's in the derived sequence of $N - 1$ trials. Thus, the probability of getting a run of either type of length k in the original sequence of 200 trials is equivalent to the probability of getting a run of heads of length $k - 1$ in 199 trials. Table 4.1 gives the probabilities for getting a longest run of length k for our example of 200 trials.

From Table 4.1, we see that there is only a 3% chance that the longest run of either type will be five or less. Thus, Sequence 2 has an unusually short longest run of either type. The longest run of eight of either type in Sequence 1 is not particularly unusual; we would expect to get a longest run at least this long more than half of the time. Revesz's experience was that most students making up an artificial sequence of random tosses will make the longest run too short.

Binswanger and Embrechts (1994) suggest some applications of the longest run to finance and gambling. Boldin (1993) develops a test of fit for regression models based on runs of positive (or negative) residuals.

Application 4.2 (Two Zone Control Charts for the Mean). In the classical control chart for the mean, the chart is centered at an ideal process value μ, and the standard deviation σ of the process is assumed known. The chart plots sample means each based on a small number, n, of observations. Three sigma limits are typically chosen for action lines, and if any sample mean falls outside $\mu - (3\sigma/n^{.5})$ to $\mu + (3\sigma/n^{.5})$ the process is viewed as being *out-of-control* and corrective action is taken.

Page (1955) studies more general control chart procedures with warning lines in addition to the usual action lines. These rules base action on either one extreme point (sample mean) or on a cluster of several moderately extreme points. Page considers rules of the form Rule 1: "Take action if any point falls outside the action lines, or if any k out of the last m points fall outside the warning lines."

One of the criteria by which different quality control plans are compared is the *Average Run Length* or ARL. This is the expected number of items inspected before taking action and is calculated for both in-control and various out-of-control situations. Page notes that the average run length of Rule 1 can be derived by an embedded Markov chain approach, but this approach becomes rapidly complex except for the simplest cases. He then derives the ARL for the special cases $k = 2$, and $k = m$, and tables a variety of plans.

Page's rules have been generalized in a variety of zone tests. Roberts (1958) develops a recursion formula and generating function for k consecutive *successes*, and k successes in $k + 1$ consecutive trials, and uses these to study the operating characteristics of the corresponding zone tests for control charts. These applications are typically set up from the prospective monitoring viewpoint of the present section. We discuss in this section how to use results on the scan statistics to find ARL's for the general case of Page's Rule 1.

Naus (1982) gives an accurate approximation for the expected waiting time till a k-in-m cluster in Bernoulli trials with probability p of *success* on an individual trial

$$E(T_{k.m}) \approx 2m + Q_2'/(1 - \{Q_3'/Q_2'\}^{1/m}), \qquad (4.11)$$

where Q_2' and Q_3' are written in terms of binomial probabilities in (4.4) and (4.5). More complicated formulas for the exact expectation and methods to find it are given in Huntington (1976a), Greenberg (1970a), and other approximations in Samuel-Cahn (1983). Equation (4.11) can be used to derive ARL in acceptance sampling for attribute plans and can be generalized to give ARL for quality control applications with two zone tests using Page's general Rule 1.

Let P_1 denote the probability that an individual sample mean (a point) falls in the action zone; that is, the point falls outside $\mu - (B_1\sigma/n^{.5})$ to $\mu + (B_1\sigma/n^{.5})$. Let P_2 denote the probability that an individual sample mean falls in the warning zone. That is, the point is inside $\mu - (B_1\sigma/n^{.5})$ to $\mu + (B_1\sigma/n^{.5})$, but outside $\mu - (B_2\sigma/n^{.5})$ to $\mu + (B_2\sigma/n^{.5})$. Here $B_2 < B_1$. It is usually assumed that each sample mean is based on n observations and that sample means are independent and approximately normally distributed. Different out-of-control situations are modeled by assuming that the process is centered at $\mu + C\sigma$; the larger C, the more the process is out of control. P_1 and P_2 are computed using normal tables (or formula) for specific values of B_1 and B_2, C and n.

Let $\mathcal{D}_{2\text{-zone}}$ denote the number of trials (waiting time) till either one point falls in the action zone, or that k-out-of-m consecutive points fall in the warning zone. The ARL of the 2-zone plan is n times the expected value of $\mathcal{D}_{2\text{-zone}}$:

$$\text{ARL} = nE(\mathcal{D}_{2\text{-zone}}) = n \sum_{T=0}^{\infty} P(\mathcal{D}_{2\text{-zone}} > T), \qquad (4.12)$$

$$P(\mathcal{D}_{2\text{-zone}} > T) = U_1 U_2, \qquad (4.13)$$

Table 4.2. ARL's for control chart for means based on five observations for different shifts in the centering to $\mu + \lambda\sigma$, for single and 2-zone plans.

C	$B_1 = 2.83$ 1-zone	$B_1 = 3.00, B_2 = 1.50$ $k = 3, m = 3$	$B_1 = 3.00, B_2 = 1.76$ $k = 3, m = 5$
0	1074	1074	1075
0.2	549	527	501
0.4	188	160	145
0.6	73	57	57
0.8	34	27	33
1.0	18	16	21

$$U_1 = P(\text{none of first } T \text{ points in action zone}) = (1 - P_1)^T, \qquad (4.14)$$

$$U_2 = P(\text{no } k\text{-in-}m \text{ consecutive points in warning zone given none}$$

$$\text{of } T \text{ points in action zone})$$

$$\approx Q_2'/\left(1 - \{Q_3'/Q_2'\}^{((T/m)-2)}, \qquad (4.15)$$

where for $T \geq 2m$, Q_2' and Q_3' are computed from (4.4) and (4.5), letting $p = P(\text{point falls in warning zone given it did not fall in action zone}) = P_2/(1 - P_1)$. For terms $T < 2m$, for many applications U_2 will be close to 1. (In cases where it is not, an exact formula for these cases can be used.)

Split (4.12) into two sums, and substitute (4.14) and (4.15) into (4.13) and the result into the split (4.12), and simplify to find

$$\text{ARL} \approx n \left\{ \sum_{T=0}^{2m-1} U_1 + \sum_{T=2m}^{\infty} U_1 U_2 \right\}$$

$$\approx \frac{n\{1 - (1 - P_1)^{2m}}{P_1} + \frac{Q_2'(1 - P_1)^{2m}\}}{1 - (1 - P_1)(Q_3'/Q_2')^{1/m}}, \qquad (4.16)$$

where Q_2' and Q_3' are computed from (4.4) and (4.5) letting $p = P_2/(1 - P_1)$.

Table 4.2 compares the ARL's of three plans all involving sample means based on $n = 5$ observations. The first plan is a traditional plan with out of control limits at 2.83 sigma, where the process is called out of control if any sample mean falls outside of the control limits $\mu - (2.83\sigma/5^{.5})$ to $\mu + (2.83\sigma/5^{.5})$.

The next two plans are 2-zone plans, with warning limits at $\mu \pm (B_2\sigma/5^{.5})$, and with action limits at $\mu \pm (3\sigma/5^{.5})$. The second plan comes from Table 1(a) in Page (1955) and calls the process out of control if any point is outside the action limits, or if any three consecutive points fall outside the warning limits, with $B_2 = 1.50$. The third plan calls the process out of control, if any point is outside the action limits, or if three points out of any five consecutive points fall outside the warning limits with $B_2 = 1.76$. The ARL's for the last plan are computed using (4.16). All three plans have about the same ARL when the process is in control.

In related work, Bauer and Hackl (1978) studied the power of the scan test based on moving sums of a fixed number of residuals in quality control. In an earlier paper they show that the moving sums (MOSUMS) procedure is superior to the cumulative sum (CUSUM) in the case of a sudden step function change in the mean.

Application 4.3 (Acceptance Sampling). In some acceptance sampling plans one looks at overlapping sets of items or batches of items, rather than just individual batches before passing sentence on individual batches. Anscombe, Godwin, and Plackett (1947) and Troxell (1972, 1980) consider such types of deferred sentencing acceptance sampling plans. Ahn and Kuo (1994) consider such types of deferred sentencing acceptance sampling plans. Ahn and Kuo (1994) consider the event that k successes out of m consecutive trials, occur for the first time at the jth trial, and note (p. 135):

> In view of the control chart and acceptance sampling system, we recall that most of signaling and switching rules in classical statistical quality control (SQC) procedures take the form of signal or switch as soon as k-out-of-m consecutive trials result in the occurrence of an event of interest.

Some products are costly to inspect, and other products may be destroyed in the testing process. For these types of items acceptance sampling plans are designed to use small samples. The problem with small samples for attributes (item defective or not defective) is that they do not discriminate well between good and bad quality. Consider an acceptance sampling plan that samples five items from a large lot, and only accepts the lot if none of the five items are defective. The purchaser may consider a lot that contains 10% defectives to be of unacceptable quality. However, a sample of five items drawn from such a lot has a 59% chance of having no defectives and the lot being accepted. From the view of the supplier, a lot might have only 1% defective (which might have been agreed by the buyer to be acceptable quality), and yet the large lot has a 5% chance of having at least one defective sampled item and being rejected. When a lot is rejected several actions can be taken. The individual lot can be sent back for inspection/rectification, but new lots will continue to be sampled. Alternatively, inspection can be suspended, and the supplier or manufacturer must take costly corrective action before any other shipments are made. The decision to suspend inspection needs to be based on more evidence than one defective item in a sample of five items.

Combining information from consecutive data can improve the effectiveness of the inspection system. Troxell (1980), building on suspension systems developed by Cone and Dodge (1963) in quality assurance, develops a class of *suspension rules* for attribute sampling. Troxell's plans suspend inspection when at any time there are k rejected lots within any m consecutive lots. Whenever any lot is rejected, the quality assurance specialist looks at the previous $m - 1$ lots and sees if $k - 1$ of them were also rejected. If so, inspection is suspended. Troxell tables operating characteristics of suspension systems of (k, m) plans for $k = 2, 3$ and

Table 4.3. Probability inspection is suspended in N trials for a (three to five) plan, for samples of five from each lot, and process proportion defective .01 and .1.

N Trials	Proportion defective .01	Proportion defective .10
10	.004	.65
15	.007	.82
50	.027	.998
100	.054	1.000

$m = k$ to $k + 8$, for samples of $n = 5, 10, 20, 50, 100, 200$, and fractions defective corresponding to Average Run Lengths (ARL).

Going back to our example, suppose that economics dictates that samples of size five are taken from each lot, and that individual lots are rejected if there are any defectives in the sample. Suppose further that it is agreed to suspend inspection whenever three out of five consecutive lots are rejected. If 1% of the processed items are defective, then $1 - (1 - .01)^5 = .049$ of lots will be rejected. If 10% of the processed items are defective, 41% of lots will be rejected. Table 4.3 uses (4.3) to find the probability that inspection will be suspended within N trials, given the probability an individual lot is rejected. We see that for 1% process defectives, about 5% of lots will be rejected, but inspection is unlikely to be suspended in 100 lots. However, for 10% process defective, about 41% of lots will be rejected, and it is highly likely that inspection will be suspended after 15 lots.

Application 4.4 (Hot Streaks in Sports). Sports commentators will often focus on winning or losing streaks of teams, or unusual hitting streaks of baseball players. Are the winning or hitting streaks evidence of an improvement in ability or are they just the results of chance bunching of successes in independent trials? For example, a batter might have been batting 250 (= 25%) during a season. At some point in the season the batter gets a hot streak of eight hits in 17 times at bat, a sensational 471 batting average. How should a manager or pitcher estimate the chance of the player getting a hit at the next time at bat? Has the chance of a hit by the player increased to .471 or is it still .25, or something in between? Casella and Berger (1994) use a Bayesian approach to estimate the probability p of the player getting a hit.

The scan distribution tells us to expect that a hitter with a 250 batting average will sometimes, in the course of 100 times at bat, get a streak of at least eight hits in 17 consecutive times at bat. Assuming success (hit) at the 100 different times at bat are independent, with probability .25, the chance is .749 that a player will get at least one such 8-hit-in-17-at-bat streak.

What would be an unusual streak for a batter with a 250 average in the course of 100 times at bat? Seven hits in seven at bats is unusual, but so is 8·in 9, and 9 in 10, and 9 in 11, and many other possibilities. There is a variety of testing procedures that measures unusualness, taking into account simultaneously many

Table 4.4. Critical streaks at the .01 level, for $p = .25$, $N = 100$.

Cluster of hits (k)	In window of (m) at bats	$P'(k\vert m; N, p)$
7	7	.004
8	9	.006
9	11	.006
10	13	.005
11	16	.009
12	18	.007
13	21	.009
	Total	.046

possibilities of interest in the practical situation. A simple approach is to consider a set of streaks that individually are highly significant, say more unusual than the .01 level, and that collectively are significant at better than the .05 level. For our example, with p(hit) = .250, and $N = 100$ trials, Table 4.4 lists the critical values for streaks in windows up to 21 that are individually significant at better than the .01 level.

For this case, $p = .25$ and $N = 100$, the table includes all the highly significant (.01) streaks for windows up to 21. Note that if 13 out of 21 is significant, then automatically 13 out of 20 will be significant, and so on. The chance that any one of these streaks will occur by chance, for a 250 batting player in 100 times at bat, is less than .046 (the sum of the probabilities). Of course, in theory one could look at windows longer than 21, but what is relevant is the range of window sizes that fans focus on. Karlin and Revesz and others have developed procedures that look at scan-type statistics for all possible window sizes that are useful in many applications. There is a cost in terms of power to look at all possible window sizes, which may be worth it if the range of window sizes of interest is large.

Application 4.5 (Studies of Learning). An educational psychologist is trying to determine the point at which learning takes place. A subject is given consecutive true–false questions. After each question the subject is given feedback and further training. The null hypothesis is that the subject has not learned anything (and is just guessing) and the probability of *success* (correct answer) on an individual question is .5. The researcher decides that the criterion to judge whether learning took place should be based on the number of correct answers in m consecutive questions. If the number correct is large enough, the training will stop. Bogartz (1965) notes that psychologists investigating learning and transfer of information sometimes base the criterion on disjoint sets of m questions, and sometimes on all overlapping sets of m consecutive questions. Bogartz derives, for the latter case, the probability of $m - 1$ successes within any m consecutive trials within N trials and also the probability of $m-2$, within m. This is the probability that $S'_m \geq m-1$ and $S'_m \geq m - 2$. Runnels, Thompson, and Runnels (1968) refer to these quotas as *near perfect runs*, and give additional tables for quotas of $m - 1$ in m. The formula in the present section allows the researcher to use more general criteria based on k-correct-answers-in-m consecutive trials.

Application 4.6 (Reliability Theory). Researchers evaluate the reliability of configurations of components, or design a system to have a certain reliability. Recently, researchers have been studying *consecutive-m-in-N failure systems*, and *k-within-consecutive-m-out-of-N systems*. These systems are viewed as a linearly ordered set of N independent components with possibly different individual probabilities of being defective. In the *consecutive-m-in-N failure system* the system fails if there is a run of m consecutive defective components in the system. In the *k-within-consecutive-m-out-of-N systems* the system fails if there is a quota of k defectives within any m consecutive components in the system. Papastavridis and Koutras (1993) derive asymptotic approximations and bounds for the reliability of consecutive k-within-m-out-of-N failure systems. Jain and Ghimire (1997) consider the number of random and correlated failures, and determine the optimum number of spare parts in the reliability of a system with N linearly ordered components that fails whenever there are k or more failed parts in any r consecutive components. Griffith (1994) suggests a Markov chain approach with taboo probabilities to find system reliability for k-within-m-out-of-N failure system. Recently, Hwang and Wright (1997) analyzed the level of computation of this approach, and found it efficient relative to some of the other exact approaches.

4.2.2   The Length of the Longest Quota

Note that (4.9) is of the basic approximation form of (4.3), and of similar form to (3.4):

$$Q'_L \approx Q'_2 \{Q'_3/Q'_2\}^{((N/m)-2)}. \tag{4.17}$$

Naus (1982) uses this same approach to approximate the distribution of the length of the longest quota. Substitute the values for Q'_2 and Q'_3 from (4.4) and (4.5) into (4.17) to approximate $Q'_L = 1 - P'\{k \mid m; N, p\}$. Approximation (4.17) appears highly accurate.

4.3   The Charge Problem

Scientists are currently studying protein (a chain of amino acids) sequences looking for associations between certain charge configurations and structural features and functional expressions of the protein. Some of the amino acids have positive charge, some negative charge, and some no charge. From this perspective, the protein can be viewed as a sequence of -1's, $+1$'s, and 0's. Charge configurations of particular interest include regions with a large positive or negative charge or net charge.

To test the unusualness of a cluster of many positive charges in a scanning window we can call a positive charge a one, and anything else a zero, and use the results of the previous sections. To test for the unusualness of a large positive net charge in a scanning window is more complicated, as the scores for any letter in the sequence can be a -1, 0, or 1, and we seek the distribution of the maximum moving sum of such scores.

Let $X_1, X_2, \ldots, X_N$ be a sequence of i.i.d. discrete random variables, where $P(X_i = -1) = p_{-1}$, $P(X_i = 0) = p_0$, $P(X_i = 1) = p_1$. For m an integer, and $t = 1, 2, \ldots, N - m + 1$, define the random variables

$$Y_t(m) = \sum_{i=t}^{t+m-1} X_j. \tag{4.18}$$

The $Y_t(m)$'s define a moving sum of m of the X's. The scan statistic, S'_m is defined as the maximum of the moving sums as the window of m trials scans the sequence. In this and the next sections we will be emphasizing the dependence of S'_m on N, by using the expanded notation

$$S'_m = S'_m(N) = \max_{1 \le t \le N-m+1} \{Y_t(m)\}.$$

We denote

$$G_{k,m}(N) = P(S'_m(N) < k). \tag{4.19}$$

Glaz and Naus (1991) give bounds and approximations for $G_{k,m}(N)$ for the general case of a sequence of i.i.d. integer values X's. These results are given in their general form in Chapter 13. Equation (4.20) gives a highly accurate approximation. To compute these bounds and approximations, one needs the simpler component probabilities $G_{k,m}(r)$ for $r = 2m - 1, 2m, 3m - 1$, and $3m$. Chapter 13 describes results for computing these (and some other) special case probabilities exactly for the charge problem.

Approximation (4.17) is of the same basic form as (3.4), as is

$$G_{k,m}(T) \approx G_{k,m}(2m)\{G_{k,m}(3m)/G_{k,m}(2m)\}^{((N/m)-2)}. \tag{4.20}$$

Glaz and Naus (1991) use this same approach to approximate the distribution of the largest net charge within a window of length m. They show simple cases where exact enumeration gives $G_{k,m}(2m)$ and $G_{k,m}(3m)$. Saperstein (1976) derives useful recursions for computing $G_{k,m}(T)$ for $T \le 2m$, and outlines a possible but computationally complex approach for $T > 2m$. Karwe (1993) derives new recursion formulas that are computationally more efficient than Saperstein's approach for $T \le 2m$, and computationally practical for $T = 3m - 1$ and $3m$. She develops programs, and extensive tables of $G_{k,m}(T)$ for $T = 2m - 1, 2m, 3m - 1$, and $3m$. The results are described in Chapter 13. Chapter 13 also discusses bounds, which when tight, can be used as approximations.

4.4   Binomial Distributed Events: Discrete Time, Conditional Case

Consider a sequence of N trials, where each trial results in either a *success* or *failure*. In the first part of this chapter we dealt with a model where the N trials are independent, and the total number of successes in N trials is treated as a random variable; we call this the *unconditional* or, in other applications, the *prospective* case.

In other applications the researcher conditions on a known given value for the total number of successes in the N trials. We call this the *conditional* or *retrospective* case. The maximum number of successes within any m contiguous trials within the N trials, denoted S'_m, is called the *scan statistic*. For the general case where $S'_m \geq k$, a *quota* of at least k successes within m consecutive trials has occurred. This section gives formula and applications for the distribution of S'_m given that there are exactly a successes in N trials. The distribution of S'_m is computed for the simple probability model where all $\binom{N}{a}$ sequences of a successes and $N-a$ failures are equally likely. For this case denote $P(S'_m \geq k)$ by $P(k \mid m; N, a)$.

Saperstein (1972) derives the exact distribution of $P(k \mid m; N, a)$ for the case $k > a/2$. Naus (1974) derives the exact distribution for all a and k for $m/N = 1/L$, L, an integer, and more generally for $m = cr$, $N = cL$, where c, r, and L are integers and $c > 1$. Details are given in Chapter 12. We mention here two simple methods to approximate $P(k \mid m; N, a)$.

For $k > a/2$, and $N/m = L$ an integer, Corollary 2 in Naus (1974) gives the exact result

$$P(k \mid m, N, a) = 2\sum_{s=k}^{a} H(s, a, m, N) + (Lk - a - 1)H(k, a, m, N), \quad (4.21)$$

where

$$H(s, a, m, N) = \binom{m}{s}\binom{N-m}{a-s} \bigg/ \binom{N}{a}$$

is the hypergeometric probability. Naus (1974) points out that for small values ($<$ .1) of $P(k \mid m; N, a)$, (4.21) provides a good approximation even when $k \leq a/2$.

The limit of $P(k \mid m; N, a)$, as m and N tend to infinity, is $P(k; a, \rho)$, where $\rho = m/N$. Formula and approximations for $P(k; a, \rho)$ are given in Chapter 2. The probability for the continuous scan can be used to approximate the discrete when m, N are large relative to k and a.

Application 4.7 (A Generalized Birthday Problem). Stewart (1998) points out how people are struck and fascinated by coincidences. He refers to an article by Matthews and Stones (1998) on a surprising but common coincidence, people sharing the same birthday (month and day). The classical birthday problem asks the following question: How likely is it to find (at least) two people who share a birthday in a group of 23 people? Most people feel that it is not very likely; in fact the chance is greater than 50%. Mosteller (1965) gives an explanation as to why people tend to underestimate the probability of a match.

The mathematical proof is simple. Assuming N days of the year are equally likely, and given a people, the probability of no match is $(N!/(N-a)!)/N^a$. The denominator is the unrestricted number of ways to assign birthdays to the a people, and the numerator the number of ways to assign days so each person has different birthdays. For $a = 23$, $N = 365$, the probability of at least one match is about .51. Since people's intuition is so strongly contrary, an empirical example is handy. Matthews and Stones studied 10 soccer games played on the same day in 1997. Each soccer match involved 11 players on each team plus one referee, a total of 23 people. In six out of the 10 soccer games there were birthday matches.

One generalization of the birthday problem is to find the probability of no two birthdays within any d consecutive days. In this case, the N day period can be viewed as a line, or as a circle. In terms of the application to nearness of birthdays, the circle is more natural because December 31 and January 1 are adjacent days. Naus (1968) gives the probability of no two out of a people having birthdays within m days within a circular N day period as $\mathcal{R}_c$, and within a linear N day period as $\mathcal{R}$ where

$$\mathcal{R}_c = (N - am + a - 1)!/(N - am)!\, N^{a-1}, \qquad N \ge am, \qquad (4.22)$$

and

$$\mathcal{R} - (N - (a-1)(m-1))!/(N - (a-1)(m-1) - a)!\, N^a, \quad (4.23)$$
$$N \ge (a-1)(m-1).$$

These results can be used to illustrate the birthday coincidence problem in small samples.

Application 4.8 (Generalized Birthday Problem). Given a family consisting of a mother, father, and two children, there are four birthdays and one wedding anniversary. Assuming independence of dates, is it unusual for two of the five dates to fall within the same 7 day period? From (4.22), with $N = 365$, $a = 5$, $m = 7$, the probability is .31, and we see that the event is not unusual.

Application 4.9 (Clusters of Wins in Chess). A chess grandmaster played 20 tournaments over 1 year, and won nine. Seven of the won tournaments occurred within 10 consecutive tournaments. Assuming that the nine wins occurred independently of each other and completely at random over the 20 tournaments, how likely is it for there to have been 10 consecutive tournaments containing at least seven wins? Here $a = 9$, $N = 20$, $k = 7$, and $m = 10$, and (4.21) gives the exact result easily computed with a calculator

$$P(7 \mid 10;\, 20,\, 9) = 2\sum_{s=7}^{9} H(s, 9, 10, 20) + (14 - 9 - 1)H(7, 9, 10, 20) = .20.$$

The cluster of seven wins within 10 consecutive tournaments, given nine wins over 20 tournaments is not unusual. If we had approximated the conditional problem, by the unconditional problem where there are $N = 20$ trials, and on each trial the probability of success is $p = 9/20 = .45$, the chance of a cluster of seven wins within 10 consecutive tournaments is .32.

4.5   Related Statistics

4.6   Longest Run of any Letter in a Sequence of r Letters

Suman (1994) looks at a generalization to the case where on each of N independent trials, any of r equally likely possible letters can occur, and looks at the distribution of the longest run of any letter. On page 128, Suman relates this problem to that of the longest success run in $N - 1$ Bernoulli trials. The trick in the relationship is to observe that in the sequence of r-letter alphabets, each letter (from the second onward) is the same (success) or different (failure) as the letter that precedes it. The probability of success, $p = 1/r$. Thus, in the five letter alphabet, the sequence

| A | B | B | E | C | B | C | E | E | E | E | A | D | D | corresponds to |
| | f | s | f | f | f | f | f | s | s | s | f | f | s. | |

The longest run in the five letter alphabet is of length 4(EEEE), corresponding to the longest success run of size 3(sss). As an application of this relation, Suman (1994, p. 129) notes that the limiting (for N large) result for the variable, $\zeta_r =$ size of the longest run of any letter from an equally likely r letter alphabet, in a sequence of N independent trials, is

$$E(\zeta_r) \approx +.5 + \log_e\{(N - 1)(r - 1)/r)\} + \gamma)/\log_e r \qquad (4.24)$$

and

$$\mathrm{Var}(\zeta_r) \approx \{(\pi^2)/2(\log_e r)^2\} + (1/12), \qquad (4.25)$$

where $\gamma = .577\ldots$ (Euler's constant).

From the above correspondence, the expected size of the longest success run in N Bernoulli trials, with probability of success $p = 1/r$ is

$$E(V_0) \approx -.5 + \log_e\{N(r - 1)/r)\} + \gamma)/\log_e r, \qquad (4.26)$$

and $\mathrm{Var}(V_0) \approx \mathrm{Var}(\zeta_r)$. See also Schilling (1990) and Gordon, Schilling, and Waterman (1986) for interesting discussion, background, and insight into these formula.

4.7   Moments of Scan Statistics

4.7.1   The Expectation and Variance of S'_m, the Size of the Largest Cluster

To find $E(S'_m)$, apply (4.3) for $P(S'_m \geq k)$:

$$E(S'_m) = \sum_{k=1}^{\infty} P(S'_m \geq k). \tag{4.27}$$

The expression $P(S'_m \geq k)$ will be close to one for $k < K_1$ and be close to zero for $k > K_2$, where (K_1, K_2) is a relatively narrow range. The range can easily be found by trying values somewhat bigger than pm. (Chapter 13 discusses the range under Erdös–Rényi laws). We only need to apply (4.3) for values in this range. For example, for $N = 10,000$, $p = .1$, and $m = 59$, (4.3) gives the following values for $P(S'_m \geq k)$:

k	12	13	14	15	16	17	18	19	20
$P(S'_{59} \geq k)$	1.00	.980	.799	.449	.183	.060	.017	.0046	.0011

From (4.24), $E(S'_m) = 12 + (.980 + .799 + \cdots + .0011) = 17.7$.
To find $\mathrm{Var}(S'_m)$, one can use values from (4.3) to compute

$$P(S'_m = k) = P(S'_m \geq k) - P(S'_m \geq k + 1), \tag{4.28}$$

find $E\{(S'_m)^2\}$ by averaging $(S'_m)^2$ over the probability (4.28), and substituting in

$$\mathrm{Var}(S'_m) = E\{(S'_m)^2\} - \{E(S'_m)\}^2. \tag{4.29}$$

A simpler approach is to compute

$$\mathrm{Var}(S'_m) = 2 \sum_{k=1}^{\infty} k P(S'_m \geq k) - E(S'_m)(1 + E(S'_m)). \tag{4.30}$$

4.7.2   The Expectation and Variance of W'_k, the Size of the Smallest Interval

To find $E(W'_k)$, we can substitute values from (4.3) into

$$E(W'_k) = \sum_{m=1}^{\infty} P(W'_k \geq m), \tag{4.31}$$

$$\mathrm{Var}(W'_k) = 2 \sum_{m=1}^{\infty} m P(W'_k \geq m) - E(W'_k)(1 + E(W'_k)). \tag{4.32}$$

For example, for $p = .3, k = 5, N = 100$:

m	5	6	7	8	9	10	11	12
$P(W_k' \geq m)$	1	.8474	.5799	.3324	.1692	.0806	.0372	.0171

m	13	14	15	16	17	18	19
$P(W_k' \geq m)$	.0080	.0038	.0019	.0009	.0005	.0003	.0001

From (4.31) and (4.32):

$$E(W_k') = 5 + .8474 + .5799 + \cdots + .0001 = 7.0784,$$
$$\mathrm{Var}(W_k') = 2(15 + 6(.8474) + 7(.5799) + \cdots + 19(.0001))$$
$$- (7.0784)(8.0784) = 2.74.$$

4.7.3 The Expected Waiting Time until a Cluster

Huntington (1976a) derives the exact expected waiting time till a k-in-m quota. The result is expressed in terms of the ratios of determinants of matrices. Denote the expected waiting time till a k-in-m quota, by $T_{k,m}$.

Naus (1982) illustrates how to use the approximate values for Q_2' and Q_3', together with (4.3) to approximate the expected waiting time. The approach is to write $E(T_{k,m})$ as an infinite sum (over N) of $P(S_m' \geq k)$, substitute in the approximation for $P(S_m' \geq k)$ based on Q_2' and Q_3', and simplify the resulting geometric sum

$$E(T_{k,m}) = \sum_{N=0}^{\infty} (1 - P(S_m' < k)) \approx 2m + Q_2'(1 - \{Q_3'/Q_2'\}^{1/m}). \qquad (4.33)$$

Approximation (4.33) appears quite accurate. For example, $P(S_6' \geq 5)$ is 25,250 for $p = .1$, and 1025.50 for $p = .2$, both by the exact and approximate formulas.

Samuel-Cahn (1983) gives approximations and bounds for the expectation and variance of the waiting time until a cluster, and bounds for the expectation, for general point processes with i.i.d. interarrival times between the points. Details are given for the Poisson, Bernoulli, and compound Poisson processes (see Chapters 11 and 13).

5
Higher-Dimensional Scans

5.1 Introduction

The previous chapters describe one-dimensional scan statistics for clusters of events over time, or over a sequence of trials. The present chapter describes and applies scan statistics for two and higher dimensions.

Researchers in many fields scan for unusual clusters in two or more dimensions. An epidemiologist is drawn to a spatial cluster of cancer cases. A geologist scans a region to find clusters of mineral deposits. An astrophysicist scans the heavens for sources of concentration of gamma ray bursts. A traffic specialist looks at clusters of accidents on a highway that are close in time and space. Two-dimensional clusters are investigated in medical imaging, mine detection, reliability of systems.

A wide variety of scan statistics has been developed for two and higher dimensions. In one dimension one uses an interval as the scanning window for scanning a continuous-time interval or discrete sequence of trials. In two dimensions results have been derived for square, rectangular, circular, triangular, and other shaped scanning windows. The two-dimensional regions scanned include rectangles, the surface of a sphere, and more generally, irregularly shaped geographical areas. Scan distributions have been derived for uniform, Poisson, and other distributed points in continuous space, and binomial, hypergeometric, and other distributions on two-dimensional grids.

Some of the approaches and techniques for handling one-dimensional scan statistics are applied to handling two-dimensional and higher cases. In some applications a two-dimensional scan statistic is applied, and its distribution is approximated. In other applications, a two-dimensional problem is handled by applying a one-dimensional scan statistic. We first illustrate this latter approach with a geologic aerial reconnaissance problem. We then proceed to describe the development of two-dimensional scan statistics.

Application 5.1 (Scanning for Uranium Deposits). Conover, Bement, and Iman (1979) apply a one-dimensional scan statistic to a two-dimensional region. They were motivated by an aerial search for uranium deposits under the National Uranium Resource Evaluation Program. They divide a two-dimensional mapping of bismuth-214 anomalies into disjoint parallel strips, and scan all the strips with a scanning window.

In one variation an airplane flies over a rectangular region starting in the northwest corner, and crosses the region (horizontally) flying west to east. The plane then turns south for a distance, and then makes a horizontal pass from east to west, and so on till the whole region has been surveyed. The plane will detect points of high interest. The results will be plotted on a map, with parallel horizontal lines representing the series of passes of the plane, and points on each of the lines representing spots of high interest detected by the plane on its passes. Divide the map into a series of disjoint strips each of width w; each strip can contain several lines. The number of points on each line is assumed Poisson distributed, as is the number in each strip. Now scan each strip with a square window of width w. Since the width of the scanning window is the same as the width of the strip, the distribution of the scan statistic is given by the one-dimensional case. Whenever the number of points in the scanning window exceeds a critical value, the region on the map covered by the window is shaded in. The critical value is computed based on the distribution of the one-dimensional scan statistic. Conover, Bement, and Iman note that using the scan statistic this way, the clusters they identified were related to both known uranium deposits and formations in the region.

In another surveillance application, a plane makes parallel horizontal passes. The plane has a detector/register on board that can measure signals within a distance $w/2$ on either side of the plane, and will cumulate the signals for the latest t minutes. The plane's flight path is viewed as one long continuous strip. A moving rectangular window of width w and length t scans the strip. Whenever the detector registers a cumulative signal above some threshold k, the area covered by the window is noted to be of high interest, and a field team is sent down for detailed investigation.

We next describe some two-dimensional generalizations of the conditional one-dimensional scan statistic. In one dimension, N points are randomly distributed over the unit interval (or unit circle). The scan statistic S_w denotes the largest number of points to be found in any subinterval of $[0, 1)$ of length w. Another scan statistic, W_k, is the size of the smallest subinterval of $[0, 1)$ that contains k points. The interval W_{r+1} is the minimum rth-order gap, and represents the *smallest rth-nearest–neighbor distance* (i.e., the smallest distance between any point and its rth nearest neighbor). The distributions of the statistics S_w and W_k

are related, $P(S_w \geq k) = P(W_k \leq w)$. We denote the common probability, $P(k; N, w)$.

In two dimensions, the N points are randomly distributed over a two-dimensional region of some given shape. The unit square is a natural generalization of the unit interval; the surface of a sphere, or of a torus is a natural generalization of the unit circle. The scanning window, an interval in one dimension, can be a rectangular, circular, elliptical, or other shape. The scan statistic S_w can be generalized to be the largest number of points in any window of diameter w; the scan statistic W_k generalizes to the diameter of the smallest scanning window that contains k points. The distributions of the statistics S_w and W_k are still related, $P(S_v \geq k) = P(W_k \leq w)$. However, in more than one dimension, W_{k+1} is not equivalent to the smallest kth-nearest–neighbor distance among the N points. This is illustrated in Application 5.3.

In scanning a two-dimensional region, one can look for the largest cluster within a scanning window of a given shape. Eggleton and Kermack (1944) and Mack (1950) consider the problem of scanning the unit square with a subrectangle with sides of length u and height v, that are parallel to the sides of the square. Section 5.2 discusses the conditional version of the problem where there is a fixed number of N points distributed over the unit square. In the unconditional version of the problem the number of points in the unit square is a Poisson distributed random variable. The results for the unit square give the results for an $a \times b$ scanning window within an $S \times T$ rectangular region, by choosing the units of measurement for the x- and y-axes to make $S = 1$ unit on the x-axis, and $T = 1$ unit on the y-axis, and setting $u = a/S$ and $v = b/T$.

5.2 The Conditional Problem

Given N points distributed at random over the unit square, let $S_{u,v}$ denote the maximum number of points in any subrectangle with sides of length u and height v parallel to sides of the unit square. Let $P(k; N, u, v)$ denote $P(S_{u,v} \geq k)$, the probability that at least one $u \times v$ scanning subrectangle with sides parallel to sides of the square contains at least k points. Naus (1965b) derives bounds for $P(k; N, u, v)$, that converge for u and v small, and for this case gives the approximation

$$P(k; N, u, v) \cong k^2 \binom{N}{k} (uv)^{k-1}. \tag{5.1}$$

The lower bound is fairly simple

$$\max\{P(k; N, u)P(k; k, v); P(k; N, v)P(k; k, u)\} \leq P(k; N, u, v). \tag{5.2}$$

For the case $k = N$, the lower bound is equal to a simple (but in general poor) upper bound, $P(k; N, u)P(k; N, v)$, and we have the exact result

$$P(N; N, u, v) = P(N; N; u)P(N; N, v). \tag{5.3}$$

Neff (1978) gives an exact formula for $P(N-1; N; u, v)$ (see Chapter 16). For the case where both $u \leq .5$ and $v \leq .5$, the formula can be written as a simple function of one-dimensional scan probabilities

$$
\begin{aligned}
P(N-1; N, u, v) = {} & P(N; N, u)P(N-1; N, v) \\
& + \{P(N-1; N, u) - B_{12}\}P(N-1; N-1; v) \\
& + \{B_{12} - P(N; N, u)\}\{2P(N-1; N-1, v) - P(N; N, v) \\
& - (2(Nv^{N-1} - (N+1)v^N)/N(N-1))\},
\end{aligned} \tag{5.4}
$$

where

$$
B_{12} = 2Nu^{N-1}(1-u),
$$
$$
P(N; N, u) = Nu^{N-1} - (N-1)u^N,
$$
$$
P(N-1; N-1, v) = (N-1)v^{N-2} - (N-2)v^{N-1},
$$
$$
P(N-1; N, u) = 2u^N + N(N-1)u^{N-2}(1-u)^2, \qquad u \leq .5.
$$

Example 5.1. For $N = 5$, $u = .2$, $v = .3$, (5.4) gives $P(4; 5, .2, .3) = .0101787$, which the reader can check also equals $P(4; 5, .3, .2)$.

Loader (1990a, 1991) gives the following approximation based on large deviation theory

$$
P(k; N, u, v) \cong (\{N^2 w(1-u)(1-v)E^3/(1-w)^3(1+E)\} + C)b(k; N, w), \tag{5.5}
$$

where

$$
b(k; N, w) = \binom{N}{k} w^k (1-w)^{N-k},
$$
$$
w = uv,
$$
$$
E = (k/Nw) - 1,
$$
$$
C = \{Nv(1-u)E/(1-w)\} + \{Nu(1-v)E^2/(1+E)(1-w)^2\}
$$
$$
+ \{(1+E)(1-w)/E\}.
$$

The C term combines Loader (1990a) correction terms (25), (26), and (27).

Approximation (5.5) can be further refined, but appears to give good accuracy for $P(k; N, u, v)$ small. For example, for $N = 20$, $k = 12$, and $u = v = .5$, Loader's approximation (5.5) gives .064, as compared to his simulation of .066. For $N = 50$, $k = 24$, $u = v = .5$, the approximation and simulations are each .043; and for $N = 100$, $k = 42$, $u = v = .5$, the approximation is .026, the simulation is .025. For the case $N = 5$, $k = 4$, $u = .2$, $v = .3$, (5.4) gives the exact result .01018; Loader's approximation (5.5) gives .01024.

Application 5.2 (Cluster of Cancer Cases). The public is very concerned about above-average rates of cancers in their local areas. Public health officials looking for possible causes for the excess rates take great efforts to follow up these clusters. It is understood that a random distribution of cancer cases over space does not imply an even dispersion; rather one expects that there will be some clustering due to both chance and the uneven spread of the population. In one investigation of excess brain cancer cases in New Mexico, Kulldorff, Atlas, Feurer, and Miller (1998) applied a scan statistic and found the cluster not significant. They noted that the "scan statistic accounts for the preselection bias and multiple testing inherent in a cluster alarm."

Hjalmars, Kulldorff, Gustafsson, and Nagarwalla (1996) looked at clusters of childhood (ages up to 15 years) acute leukemia cases in Sweden diagnosed in the 20 year period ending in 1993. Their approach uses overlapping scan windows of a variety of sizes. We use a simplified piece of their data to illustrate the use of a two-dimensional scan statistic test. In Sweden during the period, there were 1534 cases of acute childhood leukemia among a population of 1,703,235 children. Hjalmars et al. found a cluster of three cases of acute leukemia among a population of 133 children in Okome (in the southwest of Sweden). This was about 25 times the average incidence rate for Sweden. Was this cluster significant? Since the population is not spread evenly, we will apply a variation of Weinstock's approach and stretch the map to give a uniform distribution.

View the map of Sweden as stretched so that there is a grid of 1,703,235 squares with one person in the center of the square. For simplicity, view the map as a 1305 by 1305 square (1305 being the square-root of 1,703,235). View the population of Okome as falling roughly within an 11.5 by 11.5 subsquare (11.5 being the square-root of 133). Given 1534 leukemia cases in the whole square, how likely is it to get a cluster of three cases within a subsquare with sides $u = v = 11.5/1305$? This is $P(3; 1534, .0088, .0088)$. Loader's approximation (5.5) for $P(k; 1534, .0088, .0088)$ is greater than one for $k = 3, 4$; $P(5; 1534, .0088, .0088)$ is about .052, and $P(6; 1534, .0088, .0088)$ is .0015. Thus, the observed cluster of three cases within a population of 133 children is not significant; this is consistent with Hjalmars et al. finding of a p-value for this case to be .697.

In another study, Kulldorff, Feurer, Miller, and Freedman (1997) used a spatial scan statistic to find a highly significant geographical clustering of breast cancer in the New York City/Philadelphia Metro area. In this area there was a 7.4% higher mortality rate compared to the rest of the northeast. These clusters remained significant even after they adjusted for race and urbanicity. Looking further within the New York City/Philadelphia Metro area, they found four highly significant subclusters.

5.2.1 Effect of the Shape of the Scanning Rectangle

In scanning a region for cancer clusters, does the shape of a scanning window (of given area) make a difference on the probability of a large cluster? Using the exact result for $P(N; N, u, v)$, we find that $P(5; 5, .1, .9) = .00042$, while $P(5; 5, .3, .3) = .00095$. One can show that in scanning the unit square, for uv

fixed, $P(N; N, u, v)$ is maximized for $u = v$. Using the exact formula (5.4), we find $P(4; 5, .15, .4) = .00962$; $P(4; 5, .2, .3) = .01018$ and $P(4; 5, .2449489, .2449489) = .01029$. The square scanning window leads to a slightly higher probability of cluster than the rectangular windows.

Anderson and Titterington (1997) give a rich discussion of the application of scan statistics in two dimensions to investigate the spatial clustering of disease. They apply their approach to data involving laryngeal cancer patients. The paper describes the use of both square and circular scanning windows, as well as studies the effects of different orientations of the scanning square. They point out that some shapes, such as ellipses or rectangles, can be oriented to yield greater power, for example, by taking into account the direction of wind in spreading pollutants. They note that no matter which shape window is used there is a need for efficient algorithms to reduce the computational complexities of simulations of scanning in two dimensions. They give algorithms for carrying out the scanning procedure; these algorithms are useful, both for simulations to study the operating characteristics of the test and for the scanning for clusters in an observed set of data. A variety of simulation algorithms has been developed to estimate scan probabilities in two dimensions. Kulldorff (1999), Anderson and Titterington (1997), and Naiman and Priebe (1998) give sampling approaches to developing efficient Monte Carlo algorithms for one and two dimensions (see Chapter 16).

Anderson and Titterington (1997) describe a Monte Carlo approach to estimate scan statistic probabilities for different shaped windows. They note that simulations can be computationally intensive when N is large. For example, to estimate a true probability of .05, within .01 of the true value (with 95% confidence) one would need about 1900 replications of the Monte Carlo procedure. Each replication would generate the x- and y-coordinates of N points, where the coordinates are independent uniform $[0, 1)$ random variables. Then one must check all possible positions of the scanning window. One might try to move the window in small incremental steps, but this is a ratchet scan, which is not the same as a regular scan. Anderson and Titterington note that "the computational challenge is to design an efficient algorithm for the scan statistic," and they describe useful algorithms for a square, and for a circular scanning window.

The algorithm is simpler for the case of a square scanning window with a fixed orientation (sides parallel to the top and side of the page on which the map is drawn). Given that the observed maximum scan within a square is k, the simulation seeks to estimate the p-value $P(k; N, u, v)$. Order the points by the X-coordinates, with $X_1 < X_2 < \cdots < X_N$. For each $i = 1, \ldots, N - k + 1$, check whether $(X_{k+i-1} - X_i \leq u)$, and if so, whether the corresponding y's fall within a distance v. This essentially uses each of the N points as a reference point. For the case of a circular scanning window of radius r, the algorithm looks at pairs of points within a distance $2r$, finds the two circles of radius r on which the two points fall on the circumference, and counts the number of points in each of the circles. The next application deals with a circular scanning window.

Application 5.3 (A Star Cluster). In Chapter 1 we discussed Sir Ronald A. Fisher's (1959) example of a scan statistic test in two dimensions. This example is instructive in that it illustrates aspects and approaches in computing and approximating scan statistic probabilities in higher dimensions.

The example went back to 1767 when the Reverend Michell scanning the heavens, noted the visual closeness of six of the stars in the *Pleiades*. The *Pleiades*, also called the *Seven Sisters* (according to one legend, daughters of the mythological Atlas), consists of six stars easily seen with the naked eye, and a fainter star. The six stars are Atlas, Maia, Alcyone, Merope, Electra, and Taygeta. Michell notes

> we may take the six brightest of the *Pleiades*, and supposing the whole number of those stars, which are equal in splendor to the faintest of these, to be about 1500, we shall find the odds to be near 500,000 to 1, that no six stars, out of that number, scattered at random in the whole heavens, would be within so small a distance from each other as the *Pleiades* are.

Assuming that the 1500 stars are distributed at random over the celestial sphere, Fisher notes that Michell tried to calculate the probability that the smallest distance between any star and its fifth nearest neighbor was within 49 minutes arc (an angle of 49/60 of a degree). This is equivalent to the event of a cluster of six stars all within a small circle (of radius 49 minutes arc), centered on one of the stars. Fisher found Michell's calculations "obscure." Fisher then went on to derive an upper bound to the probability. Fisher first calculates the fraction of the celestial sphere within a scanning circle of ϕ minutes arc, as approximately $p = (\phi/6875.5)^2$.[1]

Fisher observes that "the number of minutes from Maia [one of the stars] to its fifth nearest neighbor, Atlas" is 49 minutes. This implies that the circle centered at Maia, with radius $\phi = 49$ minutes, contains the other five stars. Fisher approximates the probability that at least five stars out of the 1499 stars (other than Maia) randomly distributed over the celestial sphere would fall in the circle of radius 49 minutes centered at Maia. He uses a Poisson approximation (to the binomial) distribution of X, the number of stars out of the 1499 that fall within the circle centered at Maia,

$$E(X) = 1499, \qquad p = 1499(49/6875.5)^2 = .076135 = \lambda,$$
$$P(X \geq 5) = \sum_{x \geq 5} p(x; \lambda) = 2.001 \times 10^{-8}.$$

Fisher concludes:

---

[1] One minute $= (1/60)$ degree $= 2\pi/(60 \times 360)$ radians $= 1/3437.75$ of a radian. The surface of the celestial sphere with radius r is $4\pi r^2$. A small subcircle with radial arc ϕ minutes, on the surface of the celestial sphere, has approximate surface area $\pi(\phi \text{ minutes})^2 = \pi(\phi r/3437.75)^2$. Dividing this, by the surface of the celestial sphere with radius r, gives $(\phi/6875.5)^2$.

Since 1500 stars have each this probability of being the centre of such a close cluster of six, although these probabilities are not strictly independent, the probability that among them any one fulfils the condition cannot be far from 30 in a million, or one in 33,000. Michell arrived at a chance of only one in 500,000, but the higher probability indicated by the calculations indicated above is amply low enough to exclude at a high level of significance any theory involving a random distribution.

Fisher's calculation gives a Bonferroni upper bound to the probability. Let J_i denote the event that a circle centered at star i contains at least five other points. $P(J_i) = 2.0 \times 10^{-8}$. The probability that the maximum number of stars in the scanning circular window (of radius 49 minutes) is at least six, is equivalent to $P(\bigcup J_i)$. The upper Bonferroni bound gives $P(\bigcup J_i) \leq \sum P(J_i) = 1500 P(J_i) = 3 \times 10^{-5}$.

Fisher's statistic is the size of the smallest circle, among circles centered on a star, that contains five other stars. Note that there may be an even smaller circle not centered on a star that contains all six stars. Maia is not at the center of the six stars, and the six stars can be contained in a circle with radius 31 minutes, see Figure 5.1. Given 1500 stars, we approximate that the probability that there are at least six stars within a circle of 31 minutes radius by $P(6; 1500, u, v)$, where $u = v = (31/6875.5)$. We use approximation (5.5) using a scanning square of the same area as a circle with radius 31 minutes; $P(6; 1500, .00451, .00451) = 1/500,000$.

Michell's estimate was on target by coincidence, as his calculation was for a different statistic than either the size of the smallest circle centered on a star that contains six stars (Fisher's statistic), or the size of the smallest circle that contains six stars (the standard scan statistic). Michell's cluster statistic was based on the joint distribution of five nearest-neighbor distances to a star. He noted the distance between Maia, and each of Atlas ($\phi_5 = 49$ minutes), Alcyone ($\phi_4 = 27$ minutes), Merope ($\phi_3 = 24.5$ minutes), Electra ($\phi_2 = 19.5$ minutes), and Taygeta ($\phi_1 = 11$ minutes). He then tried to derive the probability that there exists a fixed star, j, among 1500 randomly distributed stars, such that there exists at least one star within distance 11 minutes, one star within distance 19.5 minutes, one star within 24.5 minutes, one star within 27 minutes, and one star within 49 minutes of the fixed star j. Mitchell's estimate was $1/496000$.[2] Michell notes,

---

[2]Michell's calculation was as follows: He first noted the distance between Maia, and each of Atlas ($\phi_5 = 49$ minutes), Alcyone ($\phi_4 = 27$ minutes), Merope ($\phi_3 = 24.5$ minutes), Electra ($\phi_2 = 19.5$) minutes, and Taygeta ($\phi_1 = 11$ minutes). He then computed

$$q_i = \{1 - (\phi_i/6875.5)^2\}^{1500}, \qquad p_i = 1 - q_i, \qquad p^* = p_1 p_2 p_3 p_4 p_5,$$

and the probability "that no five stars would be within the distance above specified from a sixth..." to be $1 - (1 - p^*)^{1500} = 1/496,000$. q_i approximates the probability of the event $E_{i(Maia)}$, that none of the 1499 stars (other than Maia) would be within distance ϕ_i from a fixed star, Maia. p_i approximates the probability that at least one of the 1499 stars (other than Maia) would be within ϕ_i from Maia. Michell uses, p^*, the product of the p_i's, to approximate the probability that there exists at least one

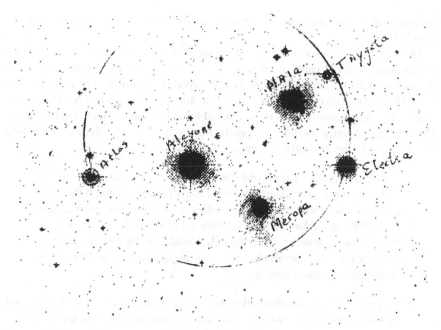

Figure 5.1. Royal Conservatory Edinburgh/Anglo-Australian Observatory photograph from UK Schmidt plates by David Malin.

> But it must be observed that this number is smaller than it ought to be upon two accounts; for, in the first place, this method of computation gives only the probability, that no five stars would be within the distance above specified from a sixth, *if they occupied the largest space, the possibly could do, under that limitation.* . . .

The goal of Michell's calculation using a scan-type statistic was to indicate that the stars were not distributed at random. Astronomers focusing on how stars are distributed use a variety of statistical models and tests to find that stars are not distributed at random, but rather cluster into clusters of clusters. Darling and Waterman (1986) describe a discrete version of a two-dimensional scan statistic on the lattice to test for super-clustering of galaxies. We describe this in Application 5.7. Astronomers also use scan statistics to search the heavens for clustered particles, signals, or radiation sources. Tu (1997) derives results for scan statistics

---

the probability that at least one of the 1499 stars (other than Maia) would be within ϕ_i from Maia. Michell uses, p^*, the product of the p_i's, to approximate the probability that there exists at least one star within 11 minutes, one star within 19.5 minutes, one star within 24.5 minutes, one star within 27 minutes, and one star within 49 minutes of the fixed star Maia. $(1 - p^*)^{1500}$ approximates the probability that there is no fixed star, j, such that there exists at least one star within 11 minutes, one star within 19.5 minutes, one star within 24.5 minutes, one star within 27 minutes, and one star within 49 minutes of the fixed star j. The events $E_{i(j)}$ are not independent, and the approximations rough.

muons against the background of cosmic radiation." We discuss this in Application 5.4.

Orford (2000) reviews approaches for analyzing cosmic-ray data in one and two dimensions, with extensive discussion of the scan statistic. He discusses methods to analyze unusual bursts of high-energy arrival direction data from space. He notes the importance of these analyses for satellite gamma rays and X-rays and for very high-energy cosmic rays not deflected by the magnetic field in our Galaxy. He compares several methods for analyzing large bursts, or clusters, including fixed grid and scan methods. He notes:

> Simple methods rely on a grid placed on the events and counts in the grid cells taken as independent Poisson-distributed events. If the cells are fixed absolutely, there is no problem in ascribing suitable Poisson probability to the largest number detected in any cell. If there is freedom to incrementally move the cell containing the largest count, a larger number is generally found . . . simple application of Poissonian probabilities is inappropriate.

Orford goes on to discuss alternative methods of spatial analysis, with a detailed discussion of the use of the two-dimensional scan statistic. He concludes that

> it is a preferred general statistic for those cases where events are located randomly on a plane, within fixed bounds, and where there is no a priori expectation such as a known source with known instrumental spread function.

Consider scanning the r-dimensional unit cube with a scanning rectangular block with sides of length $u_1, \ldots, u_r$, oriented parallel to sides of unit cube. Let $w = \prod u_i$, denote the volume of the scanning rectangle. Let $P(k; N, u_1, u_2, \ldots, u_r)$ denote the probability that at least one scanning rectangular block with sides $(u_1, u_2, \ldots, u_r)$ parallel to those of the unit cube contains at least k points. Tu (1997) in his Corollary 2.3, gives the approximation for $r = 1, 2, 3$:

$$P(k; N, u_1, u_2, \ldots, u_r) \cong \left(1 - \{Nw/k(1-w)\}\right)^{2r-1}(k^r/w)b(k; N, w),$$
(5.6)

where $w = \prod u_i$, and $b(k; N, w)$ is the binomial probability in (5.5). For the case $r = 2$, (5.6) does not reduce exactly to (5.5) either with or without the correction C in (5.5). For example, for $u_1 = u_2 = .25$, $k = 7$, $N = 20$, it follows that $w = .0625$, $b(7; 20, .0625) = 1.24796E-4$, and $P(7; 20, .25, .25)$ is, by Loader's (5.5), .042 (and with $C = 0$ in (5.5), is .037)). Tu's approximation (5.6) gives .052. Anderson and Titterington (1997, Table 2) give a Monte Carlo simulated value of .032; (the Monte Carlo was based on 1000 simulations, so the bound on the error of the estimate is .011).

For $u_1 = u_2 = 1/32$, $n = 5$, $N = 150$, it follows that $w = 9.765625E-4$, and $b(5; 150, w) = 4.56039E-7$. Loader's (5.5) approximates $P(5; 150, .03125,$

.03125) as .010 (with or without correction term C), which is very similar to Tu's (5.6) value of .011. Anderson and Titterington give a Monte Carlo based on 1000 trials of .011 (with bound on error of estimate of .007).

Application 5.4 (Scanning for Source of Muons). When high-energy cosmic radiation particles strike nuclei, various other particles are formed. One such particle, the muon, was detected in 1937. The muon is negatively charged like the electron, but has 200 times its mass, and unlike the electron, the muon is unstable and decays into electrons and neutrinos. Researchers have been seeking to pinpoint locations in space from which high concentrations of muons come. The Soudan 2 is a sensitive shielded underground detector of cosmic muons. A detector focuses a *window* on the sky and observes the total number of muons in a fixed time. The window is then shifted by a small (relative to the size of the window) amount in longitude or latitude, and the number of muons is measured in this scanning window.

Unusually large values in the scanning window are of particular interest. The distribution of the maximum number in the scanning window is used to determine what is unusually large. Tu models the window as a rectangle. In Tu's application, the window size is 29 by 56 units as compared to the whole sky as being 1160 by 4480 units.

One unit is the shifting amount in positions of overlapping rectangles, so that Tu is workiing with a two-dimensional ratchet scan problem. As he notes, the shifting amount is sufficiently small relative to the window size, that there is not much difference between a ratchet scan and a continuous scan for this application. Tu gives an approximation for both the ratchet and continuous scan problems. In this application we deal with the continuous scan approximation.

Consider the case where the average density per square unit is .002 muons. Then in the 1160 by 4480 units of sky there are 10,394 muons. Tu then calculates that a scan statistic of 17 or more within a 29 by 56 window would be significant at better than the .05 level. (In a 29 by 56 window, one would expect $(29)(56)(.002) = 3.248$ muons.)

To apply approximations (5.5) and (5.6) take $u_1 = u = 29/1160 = .025$, $u_2 = v = 56/4480 = .0125$, $N = 10,394$, and $n = 17$. We use a Poisson approximation for the binomial $b(17; 10394, .0003125) = 54427E-8$, and this gives $P(17; 10394, .025, .0125)$ to be .026 by Loader's approximations (with or without correction), and .027 by Tu's approximation.

If the average density per square unit is .02 muons, $N = 103,936$, we would expect 32.48 in a fixed window. $n \geq 68$ for the maximum scan to be unusual; $P(68; 103936, .025, .0125) \cong .040$ by Loader's, and .041 by Tu's approximations.

Application 5.5 (Estimating Population Size in Time or Space). Researchers use a variety of quadrat and other sampling techniques to estimate the size of wildlife population (see Chapter 10 of Scheaffer, Mendenhall, and Ott, 1996). Consider the case where an unknown number N of animals (or fish or mines) are distributed over an area of A units. In the quadrat methods, the region of area A

units is divided into a grid of quadrats each of area 1 unit. A random sample of n quadrats is picked from the A quadrats. In one method the number of animals in each sampled quadrat is counted. N is estimated by multiplying the sample mean per quadrat by the total number of quadrats in the area. An estimate of the bound on the error of this estimate is computed by taking $(1.96An^{-.5})$ times the sample standard deviation per quadrat. In another method, appropriate where the points are Poisson distributed, only the sample mean per quadrat is computed. In the Poisson process the population standard deviation of the number of points per quadrat is equal to the square-root of the population mean. The estimate of N is A times the sample mean, and the estimated bound on the error is $1.96A$ (sample mean/n)$^{.5}$. In a third method, the *stocked quadrat method*, a random sample of n quadrats is picked, and the number of sampled quadrats that have no animals (that are not stocked) is recorded. The fraction of sample quadrats that are not stocked is used to estimate $e^{-\mu}$, where μ is the population mean number of animals per quadrat. The methods using the observed counts in cells can sample fewer quadrats than the stocked quadrat method to achieve the same bound on the error. The stocked quadrat method is more cost-effective in applications where it is much easier to determine whether a quadrat is stocked than to count the number of animals in the quadrat.

In some applications it may be easier to locate a subregion that has a high concentration of points, and just count the number of points in that subregion. We present an estimation procedure based on $S_{u,v}$, the maximum number of points (animals) in a rectangular scanning window with sides of width u and height v parallel to the sides of the square. As in the two quadrat methods that assume a Poisson distribution for points over the region, the method of estimation based on $S_{u,v}$ is appropriate, given that the N points are distributed completely at random over the region. We illustrate the approach to compute the maximum likelihood estimate (MLE) of N based on the distribution of $S_{u,v}$ for a simple example.

Mines are distributed at random over a one square mile field. A helicopter-suspended detector scans the field with a moving subsquare of size .1 by .1 miles. The subsquare with the highest reading on the detector is located, and a ground search finds and counts the number of mines in that subsquare. Given that six mines are found in the subsquare ($S_{.1,.1} = 6$), what is a reasonable estimate of the number of mines in the whole field? One approach is to estimate N by the MLE. The MLE is the value of N that maximizes the likelihood that $S_{.1,.1} = 6$. We seek the value of N that maximizes

$$P(S_{.1,.1} = 6 \mid N) = P(S_{.1,.1} \geq 6 \mid N) - P(S_{.1,.1} \geq 7 \mid N).$$

Using Loader's approximation for $P(k; N, .1, .1)$ for $k = 6, 7$ and different values of N, we find the (approximate) likelihood is maximized for $N = 104$. We could similarly approximate the MLE for N given other observed values of $S_{.1,.1}$. We can evaluate the MLE for different values of N. For example, for a .1 $\times$ .1 scanning square, and $N = 100$, the following is the approximate distribution of the MLE estimator.

Table 5.1. Approximating* the likelihood $P(S_{.1..1} = 6|N)$ for $N = 102(1)104$.

N	$P(6; N, .1..1)$	$P(7; N, .1..1)$	$P(S_{.1..1} = 6|N)$
102	.93	.19	.74
103	.97	.20	.77
104	1.00	.21	.79

*The values of $P(k; N, .1..1)$ are approximate. See comments at the end of Aplication 5.5.

Table 5.2. The approximate maximum likelihood estimate of N based on $S_{.1..1} = k$.

k	2	3	4	5	6	7	8	9	10
MLE	9	24	46	73	104	139	178	219	263

Averaging the MLE in Table 5.3 over the distribution of $S_{.1..1} = k$, given $N = 100$, shows that the average value of the MLE for this case is 106.3. The MLE in this case is biased upward. The distribution of the MLE given in Table 5.3 similarly allows us to compute the variance (499) and the mean square error (539) of the MLE based on $S_{.1..1}$ when $N = 100$. The bound on the error of the estimate is $1.96(539)^{.5} = 45.5$. By comparison, if we had used the stocked quadrat approach we would have to take a sample of 32 out of the 100 quadrats to achieve the same bound on the error of estimate. For the quadrat method that uses A times the sample mean count of n quadrats we have to count the number of observations in 19 randomly chosen quadrats to achieve the same bound on error (given a Poisson model). Depending on the nature of the detector in the application, an overall scan to detect the high-scoring region, followed by a careful ground survey of that one region, may be more cost effective than a careful ground survey of 32 or even 19 randomly chosen regions.

A similar approach can be used in the one-dimensional case to estimate the number of trucks (or potholes) on a highway, or the number of events occurring in time. For example, given an unknown umber, N, of points distributed over a time period (taken as the unit of time) we observe the maximum scan in a window of one-tenth the time period, $S_{.1} = 9$. The approximate likelihood of this observation for different values of N is given in Table 5.4. The approximations and exact bounds for $P(k; N, .1)$ are computed from the web site http//c3.biomath.msmm.edu/scan.html. The likelihood $P(S_{.1} = 9 | N) = P(9; N, .1) - P(10; N, .1)$; the lower bounds for the likelihood are computed by taking the lower bound for $P(9; N, .1)$ and subtracting the upper bound for $P(10; N, .1)$; and the upper bound by taking the upper bound for $P(9; N, .1)$ and subtracting the lower bound for $P(10; N, .1)$. The bounds on

Table 5.3. Distribution of the maximum likelihood estimate based on $S_{.1,.1} = k$ when $N = 100$.

k	5	6	7	8	9	10
MLE given $S_{.1,.1} = k$	73	104	139	178	219	263
$P(S_{.1,.1} = k\|N = 100)^*$	.1546	.6770	1411	.0236	.0033	.0004

*Approximate probabilities.

Table 5.4. Approximating the likelihood $P(S_{.1} = 9\|N)$ for $N = 37(1)49$.

N	$P(9; N, .1)$	$P(10; N, .1)$	$P(S_{.1} = 9\|N)$ {Bounds}
37	.34	.13	.21
38	.39	.16	.23
39	.44	.18	.26
40	.49	.22	.27
41	.55	.25	.30
42	.60	.29	.31
43	.6539	.3329	.3210 {.3154 to .3221}
44	.7046	.3770	.3276 {.3195 to .3293}
45	.7523	.4233	.3290 {.3178 to .3318}
46	.7964	.4712	.3252 {.3099 to .3294}
47	.8361	.5202	.3159 {.2955 to .3224}
48	.8710	.5695	.3015 {.2749 to .3111}
49	.90	.62	.28

Based on the approximation we take the MLE to be 45. (Based on the bounds it could be between 43 and 47.) We can similarly find the approximate MLE given $S_{.1} = k$, for another k.

$P(k; N, .1)$ are fairly tight. For example, $.6966 \leq P(9; 44, .1) \leq .7056$ and $.3763 \leq P(10; 44, .1) \leq .3771$.

These one- and two-dimensional estimation applications of the scan statistic require reasonably accurate approximation for moderate-to-large values of $P(k; N, w)$ and $P(k; N, u, v)$. Most of the work on approximations have concentrated on approximating small values of these probabilities and this is useful for most of the hypothesis testing applications of this chapter. For the one-dimensional case more accurate approximations and exact results exist even for moderate-to-large values of $P(k; N, w)$. For the estimation application there is a need for accurate approximations and bounds for large values of the two-dimensional scan probabilities. Alternatively, one can use Monte Carlo techniques (see Naiman and Priebe, 1998).

Table 5.5. The approximate maximum likelihood estimate of N based on $S_{\cdot 1} = k$.

k	1	2	3	4	5	6	7	8	9
MLE	1	5	9	14	20	25.5	32	38.5	45

5.3   The Unconditional Problem

Let the number of points in the unit square be a Poisson distributed random variate with mean λ. Scan the unit square with a subrectangle with sides of length u and height v, that are parallel to the sides of the square. Let $P^*(k; \lambda, u, v)$ denote the probability that at least one $u \times v$ scanning subrectangle contains at least k points. Alm (1999) gives several approximations for $P^*(k; \lambda, u, v)$. His rough approximation is

$$P^*(k; \lambda, u, v) \cong 1 - \exp\left\{-k\lambda(1 - u)(1 - v)p(k - 1; \lambda uv)\right\}, \qquad (5.7)$$

where

$$p(k - 1; \lambda uv) = \exp\{-\lambda uv\}(\lambda uv)^{k-1}/(k - 1)!. \qquad (5.8)$$

Aldous (1989) gives the similar approximation

$$P^*(k; \lambda, u, v) \cong 1 - \exp\left\{-(k - 1)^2\lambda(1 - u)(1 - v)p(k - 1; \lambda uv)/k\right\}. \qquad (5.9)$$

Alm (1999) gives the better approximation

$$P^*(k; \lambda, u, v) \qquad (5.10)$$
$$\cong 1 - F_p(k - 1; \lambda uv) \exp\left\{-\zeta - (1 - (\lambda uv/k))\lambda v(1 - u)p(k - 1; \lambda uv)\right\},$$

where

$$F_p(k - 1; \lambda uv) = \sum_{i=0}^{k-1} p(i; \lambda uv) \qquad (5.11)$$

and

$$\zeta = (1 - (\lambda uv/k))\lambda u(1 - v)\{P^*(k - 1; \lambda, v, u) - P^*(k; \lambda v, u)\}, \qquad (5.12)$$

where $P^*(k; \lambda v, u)$ is the one-dimensional scan statistic. Alm has an approximation for $P^*(k; \lambda v, u)$, but any accurate approximation, such as (3.4), can be substituted into (5.12). Similarly, one can approximate

$$P^*(k; \lambda, u, v) \cong 1 - \{1 - P^*(k - 1; \lambda v, u)\} \exp(-\zeta), \qquad (5.13)$$

where ζ is defined in (5.12).

Example 5.2. $u = v = 1/30$, $\lambda uv = 5$, $k = 19$. $\lambda = 4500$, and we seek $P^*(19;$ 4500, 1/30, 1/30). Approximation (3.4) gives the quantities $P^*(18; 150, 1/30) =$ .00151927; $P^*(19; 150, 1/30) = .000430589$. Approximation (5.13) gives

$$\zeta = (1 - (5/19))150(29/30)\{P^*(18; \lambda v, u) - P^*(19; \lambda v, u)\} = .11632,$$

$P^*(19; 4500, 1/30, 1/30) \cong 1 - \{1 - P^*(18; 150, 1/30)\} \exp(-\zeta) = .11$. This agrees with the result for (5.10) given in Table 5.3 of Alm (1999), and with Alm's simulation (10,000 trials) of .11 for this case.

The above approximations handles the case of screening a rectangular region by a rectangular window. For the case of scanning an $S \times T$ rectangular region by a circular window of radius r, let $r\pi^{.5}/S = u$, $r\pi^{.5}/T = v$, and choose the X- and Y-scales so that $S = 1$ and $T = 1$. Let $P_c^*(k; \lambda, u, v)$ denote the probability that the maximum number of points in the scanning window is at least k, where λuv denotes the expected number of points in a circle of radius r. Aldous (1989) has given the approximation

$$P_c^*(k; \lambda, u, v) \cong 1 - \exp\{-k\lambda(1 - 2u)(1 - 2v)p(k - 1; \lambda uv)\}, \qquad (5.14)$$

A comparison of approximations (5.7), (5.9), and (5.14) suggests that for u, v small, the circular window case can be approximated by a square window of the same area. We used this approach for the conditional problem in Application 5.3. Alm has done simulations that show for u, v small, $P_c^*(k; \lambda, u, v) \cong P^*(k; \lambda, u, v)$.

For higher than two dimensions, Alm (1999) gives approximations, and Auer, Hornik, and Revesz (1991) give strong limit theorems for the maximum number of points in a scanning cube of fixed volume.

5.4 Clustering on the Lattice

An agricultural expert looks for clusters of diseased plants in a field where the plants are evenly spaced. A market researcher looks for clusters of houses in a development that have cable TV. In certain applications the events can naturally occur only at a discrete set of points in space. In other applications the underlying events can occur anywhere in space, but the method of observation limits the observed events to occurring on a grid or lattice of points. Application 5.7 is of this form. Given a lattice of points in space where events can occur, the researcher may seek to scan for unusual clusters of events. For simplicity, we focus on a rectangular $R \times T$ lattice of points, and consider scanning the lattice by a rectangular $m_1 \times m_2$ sublattice, where the sides of the sublattice are parallel to those of the lattice. We deal with the model where events are independent and equally likely to occur at any point of the lattice.

Let X_{ij}, $i = 1, \ldots, R$, $j = 1, \ldots, T$, denote a rectangular lattice of independent and identically distributed (i.i.d.) Bernoulli random variables, where

$P(X_{ij} = 1) = p = 1 - P(X_{ij} = 0)$. View the lattice with position $(1, 1)$ in the lower left corner. Let

$$Y_{r,s}(m_1, m_2) = \sum_{i=r}^{r+m_1-1} \sum_{j=s}^{s+m_2-1} X_{ij}. \qquad (5.15)$$

$Y_{r,s}(m_1, m_2)$ is the number of events (ones) in an $m_1 \times m_2$ subrectangle whose lower left corner is at (r, s) in the lattice. Define the *two-dimensional discrete scan statistic* to be

$$S'_{m_1,m_2} = \max\{Y_{r,s}(m_1, m_2); \text{ for } 1 \le r \le R - m_1 + 1; 1 \le s \le T - m_2 + 1\}. \qquad (5.16)$$

S'_{m_1,m_2} denotes the maximum number of events in the scanning subrectangle when we scan the $R \times T$ lattice with an $m_1 \times m_2$ rectangle of points (with sides oriented to sides of lattice).

Sheng and Naus (1994) give approximations for $P(S'_{m_1,m_2} \ge m_1 m_2)$. The event $(S'_{m_1,m_2} \ge m_1 m_2)$ is equivalent to there being a $m_1 \times m_2$ subrectangle all of ones. Nemetz and Kusolitsch (1982) give limit laws for the size of the largest rectangle all of ones; generalizing results of Revesz for the largest square. Darling and Waterman (1985) give algorithms to find the largest rectangle all of ones in the lattice, and generalize the limit laws to higher dimensions, and to allow for some zeros in the subrectangle. Chen and Glaz (1996) give approximation for $P(S'_{m_1,m_2} \ge k)$. These results are detailed in Chapter 16. For simplicity, we give the approximation for the special case of square lattice, $R = T$, and square scanning subrectangle, $m_1 = m_2 = m$.

Chen and Glaz (1996, 1999) give the following simple approximation for $P(S'_{m,m} \ge k)$. Let B_s denote the event $\{Y_{1,s}(m, m) < k\}$. Then,

$$P(S'_{m,m} \ge k) \cong 1 - q(2m - 1)\{q(2m)/q(2m - 1)\}^{(T-2m+1)(T-m+1)}, \qquad (5.17)$$

where

$$q(2m - 1) = P(B_1 \cap B_2 \cap \cdots \cap B_m),$$
$$q(2m) = P(B_1 \cap B_2 \cap \cdots \cap B_{m+1}). \qquad (5.18)$$

The terms $q(2m-1)$ and $q(2m)$ can be evaluated using an algorithm of Karwe and Naus (1997) applied to the maximum moving sum of binomial[3] random variables. See Chapter 13 for details.

Chen and Glaz (1999) find the product-type approximation (5.17) superior to competing Poisson and compound Poisson approximations. Glaz (1996) and Chen and Glaz (1999) compare approximation (5.17) with simulated values based on 10,000 trials. Table 5.6 gives some examples.

---

[3]Given that the X_{ij} are i.i.d. Bernoulli, $Y_{1,s}(m, m)$ has a binomial distribution with parameters m^2 and p. $q(2m - 1)$ is the probability that the maximum of m identically (but not independently) distributed binomial random variables is less than k.

Table 5.6. Simulations and approximate values for $P(S'_{m,m} \geq k)$.

				$P(S'_{m,m} \geq k)$	
T	m	p	k	Simulation	(5.17)
25	5	.05	7	.04	.04
25	5	.10	10	.02	.02
25	10	.05	14	.03	.02
50	5	.02	6	.01	.01
100	5	.02	6	.04	.05
100	10	.05	17	.03	.04
100	10	.10	25	.04	.06
100	10	.10	26	.01	.02

*Given that the X_{ij} are i.i.d. Bernoulli, $Y_{1.s}(m, m)$ has a binomial distribution with parameters m^2 and p. $(2m - 1)$ is the probability that the maximum of m identically (but not independently) distributed binomial random variables is less than k.

Application 5.6 (Minefield Detection). A two-dimensional rectangular region on land (or sea) is being checked for minefields. The region is viewed as being divided into grid of small squares (quadrats). An aircraft flies over the region and processes information from a sensor. When the sensor gives a reading above a specified threshold for a quadrat, the score for the quadrat is recorded as either high or not. An unusual number of contiguous quadrats that score high suggest a possible minefield. Glaz (1996) investigates the use of the discrete scan statistic in two dimensions to measure what is unusual clustering.

Example 5.3. A large region is divided into 10,000 quadrats and, on average, about 2% of quadrats score high. In scanning the map with a 5×5 square of quadrats, we observe a square 25 quadrat area that contains six high quadrats. Is this unusual evidence of nonrandom clustering? Use approximation (5.17) with $T = 100$ (the square-root of 10,000), $m = 5$, $p = .02$, $k = 6$, to find $P(S'_{5,5} \geq 6)$ is approximately .05. This might be sufficiently unusual that we would want to tag the area as a potential minefield subject to more careful investigation.

For the case where T and m are large, we could try to approximate the probability for the discrete scan statistic by that for the continuous. To illustrate the approach for the simple Example 5.3, approximate $P(S'_{m,m} \geq k)$ by $P^*(k, pT^2; m/T, m/T)$, substitute $k = 6$, $m = 5$, $T = 100$, and $pT^2 = 200$ into (5.13). First use (3.4) to find $P^*(5; 10, .05) = .01362$, $P^*(6; 10, .05) = .00139$. From (5.12) and (5.13):

$$\zeta = (1 - (.5/6))10(.95)\{P^*(5; 10, .05) - P^*(6, 10, .05)\} = .1065,$$
$$P^*(6, 200; .05, .05) \cong 1 - \{1 - P^*(5; 10, .05)\} \exp(-\zeta) = .11.$$

This compares to the discrete approximation of .05. For Example 5.3, m is small and the continuous approximation to the discrete case is too rough.

Application 5.7 (Testing for Super-Clusters of Galaxies). Darling and Waterman (1986) apply a two-dimensional discrete scan test for super-clustering of galaxies. The following is a simplified illustration of their application.

A photograph shows 500 galaxies of a certain brightness. Divide the photographic plate by an evenly spaced $T \times T$ grid consisting of T^2 cells. Let $X_{ij} = 1$, iff there is at least one galaxy in cell (i, j). Given that the galaxies are distributed completely at random over the photograph, $P(X_{ij} = 1) = p = 1 - (1 - (1/T)^2))^{500}$. (Here the X_{ij} are not independent, but for an approximation assume they are.) An unusually large square consisting of many ones is evidence of clustering of the clusters of galaxies, where $P(S'_{m,m} \geq k)$ measures unusualness.

For example, if $T = 100$ then $p = .05$. Choosing $m = 10$, we observe 17 galaxies within a 10×10 scanning square. $S'_{10,10} = 17$. From Table 5.6, (5.17), $P(S'_{10,10} \geq 17)$ is approximately .04.

Application 5.8 (Reliabiliity of Two-Dimensional Systems). Barbour, Chryssaphinou, and Roos (1996) derive results for a *two-dimensional consecutive k-out-of-n system*. Given a system composed of a square lattice of components, the system fails if there is a subsquare of defective components within the larger square. Salvia and Lasher (1990) give an application to a group of connector pins in an electronic device. There is built-in redundancy so that the device will work unless there is a defective square of four components.

6

Scan Statistics in DNA and Protein Sequence Analysis

6.1 Introduction

Scientists in fields ranging from evolution to medicine compare protein or DNA sequences from several biological sources. DNA is a long molecule, deoxyribonucleic acid, that contains genetic codes that control biological processes. The DNA molecule most often consists of two strands of nucleotides each consisting of a deoxyribose residue, a phosphate group, and a nucleotide base. The four nucleotide bases (or bases for short) are denoted A, C, G, T corresponding to adenine, cytosine, guanine, and thymine. The deoxyribose residues linked by phosphate bonds are like the backbone of a single strand of a long necklace with the bases being attached beads. The two strands are linked by hydrogen bonds between pairs of bases, where an A on one strand links with T on the other strand, and a C on one strand links with a G on the other strand. Knowing the sequence of bases in one strand automatically gives the sequence in the complementary strand.

In studying patterns of sequence on one strand, one can look at the sequence of bases (the four-letter alphabet) or of other related alphabets. Triplets of bases are called *codons*, and the 64 ($= 4^3$) possible codons map into 20 amino acids and stop and start codons. (Several codons correspond to the same amino acid.) Proteins are made up of strings of amino acids. Many of the applications in this chapter deal with patterns in DNA or protein sequences, viewed as a linear (one-dimensional) sequence on one of the strands. The strands are oriented by the deoxyribose residues with the convention that one strand goes from the 5' end to the 3' end, the complementary strand goes from 3' to 5'. Sometimes researchers look at the secondary (two-dimensional) structure of the protein as a sequence of three states H, E, L (representing helix, beta-sheets, and loops). The full biological functioning of proteins is determined by the three-dimensional structure of the folded strand.

We will be concentrating on applications of the scan statistic to one-dimensional sequences of letters, and looking at words (patterns of consecutive letters). The letters could be from a four-letter alphabet (the nucleotides A, C, G, T), or a 20-letter alphabet (the 20 amino acids). The alphabet could consist of 64 letters (the 4^3 possible codons). It could be a variety of two-letter alphabets such as purine (A, G) versus pyrimidines (T, C). The alphabet could consist of three letters representing charges; certain amino acids have positive charges, others negative charges, and others neutral.

Some scientists study individual sequences looking for clusters of patterns important to understanding biological functions. Other scientists look for similarities between different sequences to suggest commonality of functions, or genetic material that is preserved. Still other scientists use matches between segments of DNA to help reconstruct longer portions of a genome. See the book by Waterman (1989), and the articles by Karlin and Macken (1991), Karlin and Brendel (1992) for useful additional background. Scan statistics play an important role in these applications. This chapter discusses and illustrates these roles.

6.2   Scanning for Clusters of Patterns in Individual DNA or Protein Sequences

Scientists studying protein sequences look for clustering of certain types of patterns, net charges, or events in the sequence. These patterns have or are hypothesized as having biologically important effects. Examples are clusters of genes, DAM sites, leucine zippers, regions of high positive net charge, clusters of palindrome patterns. The next three applications illustrate the use of the scan statistic in measuring the unusualness of such clusters of patterns in individual sequences.

Application 6.1 (Clusters of DAM Sites in *E. Coli* DNA). A molecular biologist is investigating a long DNA sequence looking for unusual patterns. The DNA can be viewed from many perspective representations and dimensional structures. In the present example (Karlin and Brendel, *Science*, 1992) the scientists are studying a string of 4.7 million letters (the DNA of *E. coli*), and are viewing the DNA as a linear sequence of a four-letter alphabet A, C, G, T. The scientists are looking for occurrences of a particular pattern, GATC, in the sequence. This pattern is important in regulatory processes related to repair and replication of DNA. The points in the sequence where this pattern occurs are called DAM sites. The scientists estimate that there are in the *E. coli* genome sequence, on average, about 1.1 DAM sites per 250 letters. In studying the DNA they note that in a particular sequence of 245 consecutive letters, there are eight DAM sites. The scientists seek to determine whether such clustering of the eight DAM sites within 245 letters anywhere within a sequence of 4.7 million letters is unusual or not. Unusual is measured relative to assuming that the number of DAM sites per 250 letters is approximately Poisson with mean 1.1, the time period $T = 4.7$ million, and the scanning window $w = 245$. The scientists use an approximation to the scan probability equivalent to the Newell–Ikeda approximation (3.1) discussed in Chapter 3 to estimate the unusualness of this cluster. Here $k = 8$, $w = 245$, $T = 4,700,000$, and $\lambda = (1.1/250) = .0044$. The Newell–Ikeda approximation gives

$$P^*(k = 8; \lambda T, w/T) \approx 1 - \exp\{-.0044^k(245^{k-1})4,700,000/(k-1)!\} = .999.$$

For this case, the accurate approximation (3.4) gives $P^*(k = 8; \lambda T, w/T) \approx .66$. The researchers correctly conclude that the cluster of eight DAM sites within 245 consecutive letters somewhere in the 4.7 million letter genome of E. coli is not particularly unusual.

Had the researchers observed $k = 9$ DAM sites the Newell–Ikeda approximation gives $P^*(9) \approx .0987$, the more accurate approximation gives .124. For $k = 10$, the corresponding values are .011 and .015. In this application, the Newell–Ikeda approximation leads to basically similar conclusions as use of the more accurate approximations.

Application 6.2 (Clusters in the Epstein–Barr Virus). This example comes from a molecular biology application by Karlin and Brendel (1992). In that example, the DNA sequence of a strain of the Epstein–Barr virus was being studied. The sequence consisted of about 172,000 positions where an event could take place, and there were 342 events that took place. Six of the events occurred within a stretch of 255 positions. That is, six of the events occurred within $255/172,000 = 1/674.51$ of the sequence. We approximate the discrete, conditional on $N = 342$ points situation here, by a continuous Poisson model.

The Newell–Ikeda approximation takes $k = 6$, $\lambda = 342(255)/172,000 = .50703$, $w = 1$, $T = 674.51$, and gives an approximation value of .0911. Approximations (3.3), (3.4), and (3.7) all give the value .051. In this example, depending on the level of significance chosen by the researcher, the Newell–Ikeda approximation may not lead to the same concluson as do the more accurate approximations.

Application 6.3 (Palindrome Clusters in the Search for the Origin of Replication in Human Cytomegalovirus). Leung, Schachtel, and Yu (1994) apply the scan statistic to search the DNA sequence of a virus for patterns related to its replication. The description that follows is summarized from their paper. They focus on the human cytomegalovirus (HCMV). This virus, a member of the herpes virus family, poses a major risk in therapies or conditions that suppress the immune system. Many people have dormant herpes viruses in their systems, and only become ill when the virus enters a replication cycle. The replication process is activated when certain initiating proteins attach to certain signal subsequences of the virus'

DNA. The regions that contain these subsequences are called the origin of replication (ORI) of the virus.

Previous studies on other herpes viruses have observed certain types of symmetric and repeat patterns associated with the origin of replication. In herpes simplex there is one long palindrome; the Epstein–Barr virus has clusters of short palindromes and close repeats.

In general usage, a palindrome means a word or phrase that reads forward and backward the same (a classic example might have been the first introduction: MADAM IM ADAM). In DNA sequence analysis a palindrome is defined somewhat differently. For simplicity, we have described DNA as a sequence of letters (bases) from the alphabet A, C, G, T. There are actually two strands (sequences) consisting of complementary base pairs, with A in one sequence linked with T in the other sequence, and similarly C and G. A palindrome pattern (PLP) is a sequence of bases followed by the complementary sequence in reverse order. For example, CCACGTGG is a palindromic pattern of eight bases. This pattern in the two complementary strands is

CCACGTGG

GGTGCACC

Note that in terms of complementary base pairs, the palindromic pattern looks the same in either direction, and their signal to the DNA-binding protein can be recognized on either strand. A dyad is a generalization of a palindromic pattern that allows some intervening bases (the loop) between the two symmetric parts of the palindrome, CCACtatGTGG. If the number of intervening bases is not too large (< 150 base pair) the dyad is called a close dyad.

Leung, Schachtel, and Yu (1994) illustrate their approach for palindromic patterns (PLP's). They first screened the entire HCMV sequence of 229,354 base pairs (bp) looking for PLP's of at least 10 letters length (call these PLP*'s). They chose the length 10 so that roughly .001 of all starting positions would, by chance, start with a PLP of length 10. (They show that for an equally likely alphabet, independent and identically distributed (i.i.d.) case, the probability of a PLP is at its maximum, and for this case the probability of a PLP of length 10 is just $.25^5$).

They then screened the whole sequence with a window of 1000 bases looking for clusters of PLP*'s. (They used a version of the ratchet scan statistic, in that they slid forward in steps of 500 bp.) They found a maximum cluster of 10 PLP*'s in a particular region. They also used other window lengths, as well as other repeat patterns, and found unusual clusters in all of them for this same region. Biological experimental assays were focused on this region, and an important origin of replication of the virus was found.

The importance of the findings led the authors to consider automating their underlying approach. To this end they ask "How can we tell if a peak really represents a nonrandom cluster, or could an observed peak be just due to chance?" They choose to "use the scan statistic to establish a set of quantitative criteria in the evaluation of clusters." Their Example 3.1 is as follows: There are $N = 296$

PLP*'s in the HCMV sequence of $T = 229,354$ bases. The maximum cluster within a window of $w = 1000$ bases is $S_w = 10$ PLP*'s. Use approximation (2.3) or approximation (3.4) to find $P(S_w \geq 10) \approx .0017$. The observed palindrome cluster is highly significant.

For clusters of individual types of patterns (say palindromes) one can use one of the variations of the standard scan statistics. For the more general problem of evaluating the unusualness of simultaneous clusters of several types of patterns one needs to solve more general scan-type problems. Given k types of events occurring over a continuous time period $[0, T)$ (or a sequence of T trials), we seek the probability that there exists a window of length w somewhere in $[0, T)$ that contains, simultaneously for all $i = 1, 2, \ldots, k$, at least r_i of type i events. For the discrete trial problem, Huntington (1976) described a Markov chain embedding approach to finding these probabilities. Recent results, by Hwang and Wright (1997), Koutras and Alexandrou (1995), Stefanov and Pakes (1997), and others, extend the range of computability of the Markov chain embedding approach. Naiman and Priebe (1998) use importance sampling to improve on simple Monte Carlo simulations. An alternative scan statistic that deals with the number of multiple-type clusters can be developed from generalizations of the approaches on the double scan statistic in Naus and Wartenburg (1997) (see Chapter 18). A different type of multiple clustering is discussion in Section 6.4.

Application 6.4 (Clusters of High Negative Net Charge in the Epstein–Barr Virus). Of the 20 amino acids, three have positive charges (arginine, histidine, and lysine), two have negative charges (aspartic and glutamic acid), and the rest are neutral. Proteins are linked chains of amino acids, and researchers are currently studying the relation between their charge configurations and functions. Researchers scan protein sequences looking for unusually large net charges.

Karlin, Blaisdell, Mocarski, and Brendel (1989) looked for unusual (at the 1% level of significance) regions of negative or positive net charges in the polypeptides of the Epstein–Barr virus. They note that this virus causes infectious mononucleosis and is associated with certain cancers. In one of the polypeptides (a portion of the protein molecule), glycoprotein, gp350, the sequence length is 907 residues of which 6.6% are positively charged, and 6.7% negatively charged. Scanning the 907 residues with a window of 33 residues, the authors deemed unusual a region of high negative net charge that contained nine negative charges and one positive charge. From the methods of Chapter 4, the p-value for the net charge is .046.

6.3 Matching in DNA Sequences

With the explosive growth of molecular biology, large data banks of sequenced DNA are being accumulated at an exponential rate. Scientists in many fields compare sequences of DNA from several biological sources. The scientists look for similarity between different sequences to suggest commonality of functions, or genetic material that is preserved. Unusually large matches between viral DNA and host DNA provides clues to understanding and treating diseases.

Researchers with newly sequenced segments search the data banks looking for similarities. Computer algorithms have been developed to scan two long DNA sequences, searching for subsequences or fragments that match perfectly or almost perfectly. In the process of comparing two long sequences, one would expect to find, purely by chance, some matching subsequences. To search efficiently, the researcher seeks to determine, for various chance models, what is an unusually large match.

In some applications, a newly sequenced contiguous fragment (contig) of DNA is compared with other identified sequences in GenBank or other pools, searching for matching subsequences. The matching can either be perfect or with a certain number of mismatches or insertion/deletions (indels). Homologies in proteins express clues to common biological functioning. If the goal is to compare a new segment of DNA with previously identified sequences in DNA data banks, some molecular biologists suggest that such comparisons might be made on the newly identified fragments, even without sequencing the fragments together into a larger contig. In several of these applications one would be looking at matches between parts of relatively short fragments, or between short fragments and somewhat longer sequences in the data bank.

Many of the existing asymptotic formula to estimate the unusualness of matches are based on large sample approximations; various authors note that the convergence of these formula can be slow. For the cases of multiple (nonoverlapping) matches by probes, the probability of an individual match might be high, and for this case many of the asymptotic formula lose accuracy. For applications dealing with shorter fragments, or with longer fragments but matches on several probes, accurate approximations to the probability of matches provide useful information.

One problem area is where two sequences are aligned by an overall criteria, and then the scientists highlight matching subsequences with common location in the two sequences. The scientists seek to determine what is an unusually long match in this *aligned case*. A second problem area is where the two sequences are compared under all possible alignments, and searched for matching fragments. The scientists seek to determine which are the unusually long *matches* in this *nonaligned case*. Various research seeks to estimate accurately the probability of perfect or almost perfect matches for specific alignments and for all possible alignments, for general scoring schemes and various underlying chance models.

To compare the letters in fragments for a particular alignment, the scientist can use a 0–1 scoring (corresponding to: doesn't match, matches). Alternatively, the scientist can use a scoring system using biologically meaningful measures of similarity between different letters. Leontovich (1992) notes that the 0–1 scoring is often used to measure how well polynucleotide sequences match, while more general scoring, an important example being the Dayoff matrix, is often used for the similarity measures of how closely amino acid residues match.

In some applications, two sequences are aligned by global criteria, and the researcher looks for perfectly or almost perfectly matching fragments (subsequences) with a common location in the two aligned sequences. Piterbarg (1992) notes that an established search method for similar fragments is Staden's method. This method can be viewed as starting with a given alignment of the two sequences, and comparing each pair of aligned letters to get a sequence of similarity scores. The method then computes a moving sum of these scores in a window of fixed length m as the window scans the sequence of similarity scores.

For the 0–1 similarity scoring, the maximum sum in any window of length m, for two aligned sequences each of length N, is the scan statistic S'_m. A perfect match is a run, and an almost perfect match is a quota.

Piterbarg (1992) deals with a particular independent (null) model and derives various approximate results for the distribution of the maximum similarity score under Staden's method both for the aligned and nonaligned cases. Under this usual null model, it is assumed that the sequence of similarity scores for the aligned sequences are mutually independent. Arratia, Gordon, and Waterman (1990) note that even though the letters within a DNA sequence are not independent, the proportion of time that large matches were observed in a study of unrelated DNA sequences letters is close to that estimated from the independence model. For the independence model, and 0–1 scoring, the sequence of similarity scores is assumed to follow a Bernoulli process.

For the case of 0–1 similarity scoring, there is a variety of results. In the aligned version of the problem one looks for unusually long almost perfectly matching words. This is the unconditional discrete scan statistic; its distribution for the independence null model is detailed in Chapters 4 and 13. To evaluate the power of the test, for a specific alternative, more complicated bounds and approximations are developed in Wallenstein, Naus, and Glaz (1994); see Chapter 14.

For the case of integer scoring, for the aligned version of the problem, various asymptotic results have been derived in Karlin and Altschul (1990) and Karlin and Dembo (1992). The general form of the Naus (1982) approximation and tight bounds of Glaz and Naus (1991) apply. However, the component quantities needed to evaluate the approximation and bounds required more efficient recursion methods. These are described in general in Karwe and Naus (1997), and developed there in detail for the case of a 0–1–2 scoring system. Additional recursions are given in Naus and Sheng (1996). This latter scoring system has additional applications of interest to molecular biologists (the charge problem and three-sequence alignment). See Applications 6.4 and 6.7.

For the nonaligned version of the problem, with 0–1 scoring, various asymptotic results have been developed in Arratia and Waterman (1985, 1989), Goldstein and Waterman (1992), and others, for statistical significance of perfect of almost perfect matches. The powerful Chen–Stein approach provides measures on the errors of some of the approximations; see Arratia, Goldstein, and Gordon (1990) for a description of the approach. To get more accurate approximations for shorter sequences, Mott, Kirkwood, and Curnow (1990) developed approximations for the case of perfect matches, and Sheng and Naus (1994) gave approximations and bounds for perfect or almost perfect matches. These more accurate approximations require more computationally complex components.

For the nonaligned problem, with 0–1 scoring, Application 6.9 illustrates a useful approximation to the probability of a perfectly matching word of length k between two independent i.i.d. sequences. Section 6.4 generalizes this to words in common, to more than two sequences.

A more general form of the problem deals with similarity scoring systems where the scores can take values other than 0 or 1; the scores depend on the biological closeness of the match between two letters. The tight bounds in Glaz and Naus (1991) apply to integer scoring schemes for the i.i.d. variable case. Karwe and Naus (1997) develop procedures to compute the components for this case.

Application 6.5 (Almost Perfect Matching in Two Aligned Amino Acid Sequences). Waterman (1986) develops an algorithm for aligning multiple sequences. His Table 1 gives an alignment by his algorithm of 34 rRNA sequences. For the purpose of illustration, we list parts of two aligned sequences:

Wheat. mt	A A A C C G G G C A C T A C T T T G A G A C G T G A
Th. aquat	A A T C C C C C G T G C C C T T A G C G G C G T G G
Score	1 1 0 1 1 0 0 0 0 0 0 0 0 1 1 1 0 1 0 1 0 1 1 1 1 0

Under the aligned letters, we place a 1 if the letters match, a 0 if they do not. We note that the longest word with at most one mismatch is of length six letters (underlined). How unusual is it to get such a long almost perfectly matching word (at most 1 mismatch)? The answer depends on the appropriate randomness model.

Model 6.1. If the sequences of letters can be viewed as i.i.d. sequences of letters from an equally likely four-letter alphabet, then the sequence of zeros and ones are outcomes of 26 Bernoulli trials, with the probability of a one on any trial being .25. In this case, the answer is given by the unconditional discrete scan probability, $P'(5 \mid 6; N = 26, p = .25) = .055$ by approximation (4.3).

Model 6.2. Same as Model 6.1, except the four letters are not equally likely. Using the observed frequencies as estimates of the probabilities of A, C, G, T in each of the sequences, we have the estimates: For the first sequence (Wheat): $P_{A1} = 5/26$, $P_{C1} = 6/26$, $P_{G1} = 7/26$, $P_{T1} = 5/26$; and for the second sequence: $P_{A2} = 3/26$, $P_{C2} = 10/26$, $P_{G2} = 8/26$, $P_{T2} = 5/26$. The probability of a matching letter (score of one) on any trial is $p = (P_{A1}P_{A2} + P_{C1}P_{C2} + P_{G1}P_{G2} + P_{T1}P_{T2}) = .244$. The unconditional discrete scan probability is $P'(5 \mid 6; N = 26, p = .244) = .050$.

Model 6.3. Given that there are 13 one's in 26 trials, assume that all positions of the one's are equally likely. Given this, how likely is it that there is an almost perfectly matching word of six letters (at most one mismatch)? This is the discrete conditional scan statistic probability $P(k \mid m; N, \mathbf{a}) = P(5 \mid 6; 26, 13)$ given in Section 4.3 of Chapter 4. From approximation (4.21), the probability is .71; it is not at all unusual to get such a word. (Note that using the unconditional model with a $p = 13/26 = .50$, gives a similar p-value of .63.)

If the alignment was based on a method that caused a higher probability of matching, one might want to use Model 6.3, for the scan.

Application 6.6 (Perfect Matching in Multiple Aligned Sequences). Karlin and Ghandour (1985) compare sections of immunoglobulin amino acid sequences for three species: human, mouse, and rabbit. Consider the following aligned sequences where the letters represent amino acids:

Mouse	A	D	A	A	P	T	V	S
Rabbit	D	P	V	A	P	T	V	L
Human	T	V	A	A	P	S	V	F
Score	0	0	0	1	1	0	1	0

Under each column of letters, enter a one if all three letters in a column match. Otherwise enter a zero. For this case, the largest aligned common word consists of two letters (AP). Assume for simplicity of illustration the independence of the three sequences and the letters within them. Without any additional complexity, the letters can have different probabilities for different species. Denote probabilities of the various amino acids within the sequence to be M_i, R_i, and H_i for the ith letter in the alphabet for, respectively, mouse, rabbit, and human. Then the probability of all three letters in a given column matching is $p = \sum M_i R_i H_i$. The probability of a perfectly matching aligned word of length at least k letters is the probability of a run of at least k one's in the sequence of scores. Given the independence assumptions the scores are distributed as Bernoulli trials, with probability of *success* (a one) equal to p.

Application 6.7 (Almost Perfect Matching in Three Aligned Sequences). For the case of three (or more sequences), even if we are only focusing on match versus mismatch, there are still various alternative ways to score mismatches within a column in the alignment. For the example in the previous application, how should we count the mismatches in the third column AVA? Mouse and human match, but rabbit differs. One approach is to count the number of matches in the column. ADT has zero matches, and AVA has one match, AAA can be counted as two or three matches, depending on the scoring system chosen ($score_2$ or $score_3$). A related scoring would count the number of mismatching letters $score_0$:

Mouse	A	D	A	A	P	T	V	S
Rabbit	D	P	V	A	P	T	V	L
Human	T	V	A	A	P	S	V	F
$Score_2$	0	0	1	2	2	1	2	0
$Score_3$	0	0	1	3	3	1	3	0
$Score_0$	3	3	1	0	0	1	0	3

The last scoring system illustrates how there is a four-letter aligned fragment that agrees on all but one letter.

Application 6.8 (Nonaligned Imperfect Matching to Two Contigs of *E. Coli*). Cardon, Burge, Schachtel, Blaisdell, and Karlin (1993) apply scan approaches for several comparative analyses of two long sections (contigs) of DNA from *E. Coli*. One sequence is denoted (in abbreviation) as UW85, the other as MORI. The former is about 91,000 bases (91 kb), the latter about 111 kb. They used the *r*-scan to test for unusualness of clusters of special markers, direct or inverted repeats, and dyads. They also used a ratchet-type scan histogram where they looked at counts in windows of 500 bases shifted in steps of 250 bases.

One of the highlighted statistically significant findings involved an unusual match between the two contigs. This was a word of 29 letters (bases) that matched almost perfectly, with only three mismatches. (The word was not in the same position in the two sequences. It started in UW85 at position 4813, and in MORI at position 86,467.) We illustrate the method of approximating the probability of such a match anywhere in the two long sequences, assuming two independent sequences of i.i.d. letters of lengths $T > M$.

There are $(T - w + 1)$ possible words of length w in sequence 1, and $(M - w + 1)$ possible words of length w in sequence 2. There are thus $(T - w + 1) * (M - w + 1)$ opportunities for match-ups in words between the two sequences. The probability of any one match-up for independent sequences of i.i.d. letters is $b(k; w; p)$. Here p is the probability of two aligned letters matching. Application 6.5 illustrates how p can be computed for unequal and different letter probabilities in the two sequences. For illustration, we take $p = .25$. For a small probability of a nonaligned match, and for large sequences, the number of possible positions where words can match is extremely large; the probability of any particular match is extremely small. For this case, Poisson approximation is excellent.

The probability of at least one k-in-w match between the two sequences is approximately

$$1 - \exp\{-\vartheta\}, \tag{6.1}$$

where ϑ is the expected number of matches

$$\vartheta = (T - w + 1)(M - w + 1)b(k; w; p).$$

This approximation is in general highly accurate. For our example, $T = 111,000$; $M = 91,000$; $w = 29$; $k = 26$, and for illustrative purposes $p = .25$. From the binomial, $b(26; 29; .25) = (3.42289) \times 10^{-13}$. $\vartheta = (90,972)(110,972)3.42289 \times 10^{-13} = .0034$. P(at least one match) $\cong 1 - \exp\{-\vartheta\} = .00345$.

Application 6.9 (Nonaligned Matching in Encoding Genes of Amitochondrial Protozoa). Katiyar, Visvesvara and Edlind (1995) compare sections of the *r*RNA-encoding genes for certain primitive protozoa. The authors noted that for certain internal transcribed spacers, the alignment was not clear. Naus and Sheng (1996) applied nonaligned matching to two of these sequences, the internal transcribed spacer ITS2 from two protozoa parasites that came from different phyla and hosts. The first was *Archamoeba entamoeba invadens* (EIN) from a snake host; the other was *Parabasalia tritrichomonas foetus* (TFO) from cattle host. The following are the nucleotide sequences:

EIN (51 letters: 34 A, 4 C, 8 G, 5 T)
AAAAGAAGACAAGAAA<u>AAT*AACAAAT*</u>GTATACGAAAACAGG
AAGAAAAATA

TFO (62 letters: 30 A, 8 C, 5 G, 19 T)
TTAATTT<u>AATACCAAAT</u>TCTCTTTTTAAGCAAAAGAGCGA<u>AA*AACAAAT*</u>
ATGTATTAACAAA

The largest perfect match between the two sequences is of length seven bases, underlined *and* in italics. (There is another seven-letter perfect match not displayed.) The longest almost perfectly matching sequences with just one mismatch is of length 10 bases, underlined in the two sequences. (There are two in TFO that almost match the one in EIN.) Neither the perfect nor almost perfect match are unusual. From approximation (6.1), the p-values are .82 and .66, respectively.

6.4 Matching in Multiple Random Letter Sequences

Given an alphabet consisting of B different letters, there are B^m possible different m-letter words. Consider R sequences each consisting of N letters chosen from the B-letter alphabet. If all the R sequences share a common m-letter word, we say that there is a *perfect m-word match* between the R sequences. The common word could appear in different positions in the R sequences; (this is called the *nonaligned case*). Sometimes we are looking for a common m-letter word in the same position in all R sequences; this is called the *aligned case*. Researchers are also interested in almost-perfect m-word matches. There may be a common m-letter word that appears with up to s letters changed in any match word. This is referred to as the *almost-perfect matching word allowing s mismatches*. There are several other variations in how the number of mismatches can be counted.

The classical scan statistic is directly related to perfect or almost-perfect m-word matches in the aligned case. View the R sequences of N letters as R rows aligned one above the other. Below the last row, add an $(R+1)$st row consisting of the sequence $X_1, X_2, \ldots, X_N$ where $X_i = 1$ if the R letters above it are identical, and $X_i = 0$ otherwise. Now scan the sequence of X's with a window of m consecutive letters. If the window contains m ones this is equivalent to their being an aligned perfectly matching m-word. If the window contains k ones this is equivalent to their being an aligned almost perfectly matching m-word with at most $m - k$ mismatches. For the case where the R sequences are mutually independent sequences of independent (but not necessarily identically distributed) letters, the results for the discrete scan statistic S'_m give the probability of aligned matching words allowing for mismatches. Exact results, highly accurate approximations, and tight bounds exist for this aligned case, see Chapters 4 and 13.

The generalization that we discuss in this section involves the length of the longest word in common to all R (nonaligned) sequences. Here we are scanning the R sequences looking for a word in common to all. In Application 6.9 we deal with the nonaligned case for two sequences; we describe there how to approximate accurately the probability of a matching common word. Researchers also seek to determine the unusualness of a common word in several sequences. We illustrate the approximation for a simple case. Given R independent sequences each of T i.i.d. letters from a four-letter equally likely alphabet, what is the probability that there exists a w-letter word in common to all R sequences?

The reasoning of the approximation for two sequences can be generalized, by arguing that there are $(T - w + 1)^R$ possible sets of positions where the common w-letter word can appear, and for each set of positions, the probability of a perfect match is $(.25)^{w(R-1)}$. The expected number of matches is $\vartheta = (T - w + 1)^R (.25)^{w(R-1)}$. The probability of at least one w-letter word in common to all sequences is approximately $1 - \exp(-\vartheta)$. Naus and Sheng (1997) show that this approximation, as well as some related asymptotic formula for the probability, deteriorates as R gets larger than two. We now discuss their results including their alternative accurate approximation.

For simplicity we illustrate the reasoning for the case of R independent sequences each of length T i.i.d. letters from an equally likely four-letter alphabet. Let $R(w, T)$ denote the probability that a common word of length w appears in all R sequences. Generalizing the reasoning for the case of two nonaligned sequences, we might argue that given R sequences, each of T letters, there are $(T - w + 1)$ possible positions for a w-letter word in each sequence. There are $(T - w + 1)^R$ possible combinations of positions where the common word of length w could appear in all R sequences. Consider one combination of positions: the first w letters in all R sequences. The probability that the first letter in all R sequences match is $\theta = (1/4)^{R-1}$.

The probability that the first w letters of all R sequences are the same w-letter word is θ^w. In practice, the number of possible combinations of positions is huge, and the probability of a common word is very small. The expected number of matches is $(T - w + 1)^R \theta^w$. Applying the Poisson approximation, the probability of at least one occurrence of a w-letter word in common to all R sequences is approximately

$$R(w, T) = 1 - \exp\{-(T - w + 1)^R \theta^W\}. \tag{6.2}$$

The Poisson approximation does not take into account dependence between different combinations of positions. For example, if the first $w + 1$ letters of all R sequences match, then there are two related sets of common w-letter words (the first w letters, and letters 2 to $w + 1$). To eliminate this type of overlap, Karlin and Ost (1988) applied declumping to the Poisson approximation, and give the asymptotic result

$$R(w, T) \cong 1 - \exp\{-(1 - \theta)T^R\theta^W\}. \tag{6.3}$$

As a limiting result (as T gets large) this is correct, though a better approximation is defined by replacing T by $(T - w + 1)$:

$$R(w, T) \cong 1 - \exp\{-(1 - \theta)(T - w + 1)^R\theta^W\}. \tag{6.4}$$

For $R = 2$, approximations (6.4) and (6.2) both give excellent accuracy. However, as R gets larger, these approximations fail for many practical applications. The reason the approximation deteriorates for larger R is that it does not take into account a different type of dependence between combinations of positions. For example, consider the case where $R = 10$, $w = 5$, and T is large. One combination of positions is where the first five letters of all 10 sequences are the same word. A different combination is where the first five letters of the first nine sequences, and the last five letters of the tenth sequence are the same word. These two combinations are highly related, but the above approximation does not account for this. Naus and Sheng (1997) give an alternative approximation that adjusts for this type of association.

View the first w letters of sequence 1 as a random word. Let δ denote the probability that this word appears somewhere in sequence 2. Then δ^{R-1} is the probability that the first w letters of sequence 1 appear somewhere in all the $R - 1$ sequences. Given T^* different words in sequence 1, the expected number of these words that will result in R-sequence matches is $T^*\delta^{R-1}$. The probability of at least one such R-sequence (w-letter word) match is from a Poisson approximation

$$R(w, T) \cong 1 - \exp\{-T^*\delta^{R-1}\}. \tag{6.5}$$

We can further estimate δ by a Poisson approximation. There are $(T - w + 1)$ starting positions for the matching word somewhere in sequence 2. The probability that in a given position j in sequence 2, there (starts) a word that matches the first w letters of sequence 1 is $\theta = (1/4)^{R-1}$. The probability that at least one of these $(T - w + 1)$ positions in sequence 2 starts the word (that matches the first w letters of sequence 1) is approximately

$$\delta \cong 1 - \exp\{-(T - w + 1)\theta\}. \tag{6.6}$$

We note that T^*, the number of distinct words in sequence 1, is usually less than $(T - w + 1)$. Let $V = 4^w$, denote the number of possible w-letter words from a four-letter alphabet. Given $(T - w + 1)$ words are picked at random (with replacement) from the V possible words, let $E(T^*)$ denote the expected number of distinct words. This is just the expected number of V cells that are occupied when $(T - w + 1)$ balls are distributed at random

$$E(T^*) = V\left(1 - \{(V - 1)/V\}^{T-w+1}\right). \tag{6.7}$$

Table 6.1. Probability of a w-letter word in common to R independent sequences each consisting of T independent letters from an equally likely four letter alphabet.

w	R	T	(6.3)	(6.4)	(6.5) N& S	Simulation
4	6	55	.025	.018	.010	.010
4	6	74	.139	.110	.050	.050
4	8	87	.045	.034	.010	.010
4	8	111	.274	.227	.049	.051
4	10	118	.105	.082	.010	.010
4	10	145	.581	.506	.049	.050

Substitute $E(T^*)$ for T^* and (6.6) and (6.7) into (6.5) to approximate $R(w, T)$.

Table 6.1 compares the approximations with simulations for the case of a matching w-letter word in common to R sequences.

6.5   Sequencing Fragments to Reconstruct a Genome

In studying polypeptide or polynucleotide sequences, molecular biologists sometimes search for fragments of the two sequences that when aligned match on most of the positions. The scientists frequently seek to distinguish unusual matching from chance matching under a specified chance model.

In the *shotgun approach* of genome sequencing, multiple copies of a long sequence of DNA are fragmented into many shorter strips. The parts are decoded, and then matched up via overlapping parts to reassemble the longer sequence. A variety of protocols and algorithms have been developed to reconstruct the long DNA sequence from multiple randomly selected strips. For recent research, see Siegel, Roach, and Van Den Engh (1998).

The positions of these strips in the sequence are initially unknown, but enough overlapping copies are taken and decoded to multiply cover the sequence (in some protocols, seven or more times). One approach is to reconstruct the sequence by linking together segments into a contig through long matching words.

Several laboratories have developed chips containing probes that include all k-mers of letters. Use of multiple chips can allow for expanding the value of k. If the same k-mer probe matches two different fragments, the match between the fragments is used to help sequence the fragments. The measure of unusualness of matches (either individual probes or in combination) in fragments is of use in the effective choice of probe sizes, k.

We have been exploring the use of scan statistics to compare protocols with different probe sizes, as well as to study the effects of errors in coding. Given a segment with an end probe word of k letters, and given M other sequences each with T letters, how likely is it to find the probe by chance in at least one of the other sequences? This is an application of a generalization of the scan statistic and can be derived from the probability that a probe can be found by chance in a specific sequence. Naus and Sheng (1996) give exact results for perfect or almost perfect matching in short segment sequences.

6.6 Using Double Scans for More Effective Searches for Homologies

This generalization of the simple scan statistic deals with two types of matchings between sequences. We have described the DNA sequence as a linear sequence of letters. This is a simplification of the three-dimensional structure of DNA. Proteins can sometimes have very similar structures but dissimilar sequences. Brenner, Chothia, and Hubbard (1998) note the example of hemoglobin and myoglobin, and observe that "comparing structures is a more powerful (if less convenient) way to recognize distant evolutionary relationships than comparing sequences."

Scientists are interested in studying the three-dimensional structural similarity between DNA sequences. Wallqvist, Fununishi, Murphy, Fadel, and Levy (1999) look at an approach that compares two protein sequences, first in an amino acid alphabet (of 20 letters), and then in a secondary structure (linearly strung out) of a three-letter alphabet H, E, L (representing helix, beta-sheets, and loops). This approach suggests several generalizations of scan statistics both for aligned and nonaligned problems. These statistics would take into account unusual clusters of multiple types of matching.

6.7 Correlated Descendant Sequences Scan Statistics

Chen (1996) describes a variety of correlated sequence models that lead to generalized scan statistic distributions. We describe one such simple model. An ancestor has a DNA sequence that contains markers distributed over the sequence according to a Poisson process. The ancestor has several *children*. Each marker of the ancestor's sequence is passed on to a child with probability p, independently of other markers, and of other children.

One scan statistic looks at the largest number of markers within any window of length w, among any of the children. Chen derives approximate null distributions of this generalized scan statistic for this and other models.

A different set of problems involves *identical by descent* (IBD) models in genetic linkage analysis. Linkage analysis is an important approach used to find the gene, or more typically the genes, related to a trait or causing a disease. Tu (1997) describes several models corresponding to different relationships between individuals (e.g., siblings, half-siblings, mixture of siblings, and first cousins). The following is based on his work.

A gene is a subsequence of DNA that has certain functions, and can appear in alternative forms called alleles. Individuals who inherit the same allele from their common ancestor are said to be IBD. A person has pairs of alleles (one on each of the two strands of DNA) that define the person's genotype.

An individual's two strands come from a process that starts with one strand coming from the father and one from the mother. When these two strands pair up (in meiosis) there may be a shift of genetic material with them through a process that can be viewed as the two strands crossing and then splitting (a crossover process). In this process, two alleles that were originally on one strand (the one inherited from the mother), may be split with one on one strand of the child, and the other on the other strand of the child; in this case we say there is recombination. In one model (Haldane's) the occurrence of crossovers along the strand follows a Poisson process. Given that two genes are inherited independently, there is a fifty–fifty chance of recombination. When the genes tend to be inherited together (less than 50% chance of recombination), we say they are linked.

Given a pair of descendants (say, half-sibs who have the same mother but different father), let $X_t = 1$ if the pair share an allele IBD at location t on the sequence, and 0 otherwise. (The genetic distance is scaled to take into account the expected number of crossovers between points.) Given no linkage, the Haldane crossover model, X_t, follows a stationary Markov chain with $P(X_t = 1) = .5$. Tu details the various nonstationary Markov chain model for various types of linkage. Given N independent pairs of descendants, he computes $X_t(i)$ for the ith pair, and lets $Y_t = \sum X_t(i)$, and describes a scan-type score statistic $\max_t Y_t$.

Scan statistics have been used in a variety of approaches for linkage analysis. Hoh and Ott (2000) apply scan statistic approaches to screen a genome for susceptibility to a complex trait. They use both fixed and variable size windows. They note that in linkage analysis for autism a scan statistic of fixed length 60 centimorgans (a measure of genetic distance) performed well. They also look at scan methods that use a range of window sizes and take as their scan statistic the smallest P-value among these. They measure the overall significance of this multiple-comparison scan statistic by a Monte Carlo permutation test. (Computer programs are available from Hoh and Ott, Laboratory of Statistical Genetics, Rockefeller University, 1230 York Avenue, New York, NY 10021.) They note

> The scan statistic developed here provide additional support for linkage above and beyond what is conveyed by the maximum lod [logarithm of odds] score. They are powerful when a susceptibility locus exerts an effect over multiple marker loci, which is generally the case for genetic linkage in today's genome screen.

Part II

Scan Distribution Theory and its Developments

7

Approaches Used for
Derivations and Approximations

7.1 Introduction

This chapter provides background on different approaches, results, and techniques that are used in several of the chapters. Some of the topics: order statistics and direct integration; random walks and the reflection principle; ballot problems; the Karlin–McGregor theorem; Poisson and compound Poisson approximation; Bonferroni bounds; the Q_2/Q_3 Markov-type approximation.

7.2 Order Statistics and a Direct Integration Approach

Parzen (1960), Elteren and Gerritis (1961), Frosini (1981), Huffer and Lin (1997b), and other researchers have applied the direct integration/order statistic approach for specific cases of the scan statistic distribution. We illustrate the order statistic direct integration approach to deriving the distribution of scan statistics for independent and identically distributed (i.i.d.) uniform random variates. The same approach can be applied for other distributions, and may prove useful for special cases of N, k, w. For general N, k, w the integration approach poses a certain complexity even for the simple uniform case.

The complexity in the uniform case does not arise from the integrands, which can always be expanded into simply polynomial forms. The complexity arises from the bounds of integration, which cause us to split the multiple integral into many parts.

Let $X_1, X_2, \ldots, X_N$, be i.i.d. random variables, with common density

$$f(x) = \begin{cases} 1, & 0 \le x \le 1, \\ 0, & \text{elsewhere.} \end{cases}$$

Let $X_{(1)} \le X_{(2)} \le \cdots \le X_{(N)}$, denote the ordered values of the X's. Let

$$W_k = \min_{1 \le i \le N-k+1} \{X_{(i+k-1)} - X_{(i)}\},$$

$$Q(k; N, w) = 1 - P(k; N; w) = P(W_k > w)$$

$$= P\left(\min_{1 \le i \le N-k+1} \{X_{(i+k-1)} - X_{(i)}\} > w\right)$$

$$= P\left\{\bigcap_{i=1}^{N-k+1} (X_{(i+k-1)} - X_{(i)} > w)\right\}.$$

Using the distribution for order statistics from a uniform distribution, $Q(k; N, w)$ can be written as the iterated integral of $N!$ with respect to $X_{(1)}, X_{(2)}, \ldots, X_{(N)}$ over the region: $0 \le X_{(1)} \le X_{(2)} \le \cdots \le X_{(N)} \le 1$ and $\{X_{(i+k-1)} - X_{(i)} > w\}$ for all $i = 1, 2, \ldots, N - k + 1$.

Example 7.1. To compute $1 - P(2; 4, w)$, we integrate 4! over the values, $0 \le X_{(1)} \le X_{(2)} \le X_{(3)} \le X_{(4)} \le 1$ and $X_{(2)} - X_{(1)} > w$, $X_{(3)} - X_{(2)} > w$, $X_{(4)} - X_{(3)} > w$. Since $\min\{X_{(2)}, X_{(2)} - w\} = X_{(2)} - w$, the bounds of integration satisfy $0 \le X_{(1)} < X_{(2)} - w < X_{(3)} - 2w < X_{(4)} - 3w \le 1 - 3w$:

$$1 - P(2; 4, w) = \int_{3w}^{1} \int_{2w}^{x_4 - w} \int_{w}^{x_3 - w} \int_{0}^{x_2 - w} (4!)\, dx_1\, dx_2\, dx_3\, dx_4,$$

let $y_1 = x_1, y_2 = x_2 - w, y_3 = x_3 - 2w, y_4 = x_4 - 3w$:

$$= \int_{0}^{1-3w} \int_{0}^{y_4} \int_{0}^{y_3} \int_{0}^{y_2} (4!)\, dy_1\, dy_2\, dy_3\, dy_4 = (1 - 3w)^4.$$

Example 7.2. To compute $1 - P(3; 4, w)$, we integrate 4! over the values, $0 \le X_{(1)} \le X_{(2)} \le X_{(3)} \le X_{(4)} \le 1$ and $X_{(3)} - X_{(1)} > w$, $X_{(4)} - X_{(2)} > w$. Here the bounds of integration are somewhat more complex: $0 \le X_{(1)} < \min\{X_{(2)}, X_{(3)} - w\}$; $0 \le X_{(2)} < \min\{X_{(3)}, X_{(4)} - w\}$; $w \le X_{(3)} \le X_{(4)}$; $w \le X_{(4)} \le 1$. Make the change of variable $y_3 = x_3 - w, y_4 = x_4 - w$, to find

$$1 - P(3; 4, w) = \int_{0}^{1-w} \int_{0}^{y_4} \cdots \int_{0}^{\min(y_3 + w; y_4)} \int_{0}^{\min(x_2; y_3)} (4!)\, dx_1\, dx_2\, dy_3\, dy_4.$$

We can remove the min$\{$; $\}$ from the upper limits of integration of x_1 and x_2 by splitting up the regions of integration of x_2 and y_3, respectively. There will be four integrals when we are through, with ranges of integration:

Integral	x_1	x_2	y_3	y_4
1	$[0, x_2)$	$[0, y_3)$	$[0, y_4)$	$[0, 1 - w)$
2	$[0, y_3)$	$[y_3, y_3 + w)$	$[0, y_4 - w)$	$[w, 1 - w)$
3	$[0, y_3)$	$[y_3, y_4)$	$[0, y_4)$	$[0, \min\{w, 1 - w\})$
4	$[0, y_3)$	$[y_3, y_4)$	$[y_4 - w, y_4)$	$[w, 1 - w)$

The second and fourth integrals are zero, when $w \geq 1 - w$ (i.e., $w \geq .5$). Evaluating the integrals for the two cases, $w \geq 1 - w$ and $w \leq 1 - w$ gives

$$P(3; 4, w) = 12w^2 + 24w^3 + 14w^4, \qquad\qquad w \leq 1/2,$$

$$= -1 + 8w - 12w^2 + 8w^3 - 2w^4, \qquad w \geq 1/2.$$

For this example, we see that $P(3; 4, w)$ is piecewise polynomial in w, with one polynomial for $w \leq 1/2$, and a different polynomial for $w \geq 1/2$, Elteren and Gerritis (1961) use the direct integration approach to find $P(3; N, w)$ for $N = 6$, 7, 8.

7.3   Combinatorial Approach: Random Walks, the Reflection Principle, Ballot Problems

This repeated splitting of the integrals in the direct integration/order statistic approach hints at the combinatorial nature of the problem. To see how combinatorics applies, consider the example $P(6; 9, .5)$. Split the unit interval into the two subintervals $[0, .5)$ and $[.5, 1)$. Let n_1 denote the number of points in $[0, .5)$, and let $n_2 = 9 - n_1$ denote the number of points in $[.5, 1)$. If either n_1 or $n_2 \geq 6$, then there is automatically a cluster of at least six points within an interval of length .5. $P\{(n_1 \geq 6) \cup (n_2 \geq 6)\} = 2G_b(6; 9, .5)$. However, there is another way to get a cluster of at least six points within an interval of length .5. Figure 7.1 illustrates a case where $n_1 < 6$ and $n_2 < 6$, and yet there is a cluster of at least six points within an interval of length .5.

We denote the four points in $[0, .5)$, d's, and the five points in $[.5, 1)$, u's. Figure 7.1 illustrates a situation where three d's and three u's combine to form a cluster of six points within an interval of length .5. This is because these three u's are closer to the beginning of their interval, than the three d's are to the beginning of their interval. If we order the d's and u's in terms of nearness to the beginning of their interval, the sequence corresponding to Figure 7.1 is: $duuuddduu$. Since conditional on $n_1 = 4$, $n_2 = 5$, the points are uniformly distributed over their respective subintervals, all $\binom{9}{3}$ orders of the four d's and five u's are equally likely. Our problem reduces to the combinatorial problem of how many of these orders correspond to an overlapping interval containing six or more points. The theory of random walks gives the answer.

For our example of $n_1 = 4$, $n_2 = 5$, consider an interval $[t, t + .5)$ that as t takes values in the range $[0, .5)$ *scans* the interval $[0, 1)$. Let $Y_t(.5)$ denote the number of points in $[t, t + .5)$. $Y_t(.5)$ can be viewed as following a random path. The path starts at height 4 at time zero, and ends at height 5. At each step the

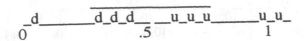

Figure 7.1.

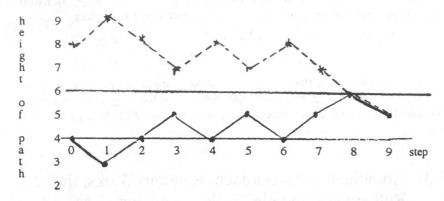

Figure 7.2. The reflection principle: A path in $\mathcal{D}$ and its mirror image (reflected at height = 6).

The path starts at height 4 at time zero, and ends at height 5. At each step the particle can either move up by one or down by one. There are a total of four down moves and five up moves. (As the interval $[t, t + .5)$ scans $[0, 1)$, four points drop out and five points come in.) The order of the four downs and five ups is random in the sense that all $\binom{9}{4} = 126$ orders are equally likely. The orders correspond to paths. How many of these orders (paths) hit the height level 6 (corresponding to the scanning interval containing six points)?

The reflection principle (see Feller, 1958) finds the answer via a one-to-one correspondence between the set of paths $\mathcal{D}$ and a set of reflected paths $\mathcal{R}$. For our example, $\mathcal{D}$ is the set of paths that start at $(0, 4)$ and end at $(9, 5)$ and somewhere reach a height 6. $\mathcal{R}$ is the set of paths that start at $(0, 8)$ and ends at $(9, 5)$. Figure 7.2 illustrates the reflection principle for this case; shown is one of the paths in $\mathcal{D}$ (solid line) and the corresponding reflected path (dashed line) in $\mathcal{R}$. To find the number of paths in $\mathcal{R}$ (and thus the number in $\mathcal{D}$), note that in $\mathcal{R}$ the total number of moves = up + downs = 9, while the change in height = up − down = 8 − 5 = 3. Add the two equations and solve for the number of ups and downs in $\mathcal{R}$, to find that ups = 3, downs = 6, and the total number of paths in $\mathcal{R}$ is (ups + downs)!/ups! downs! = $\binom{9}{3}$ = 84. (See Chapter 8 for a general formula.)

The random walk problem is related to the classical problem. In this problem, two candidates, C_1 and C_2 compete in an election. Given that C_1 gets u votes, and C_2 gets d votes, and the votes come in sequentially, what is the probability that throughout the election C_1 is always ahead of C_2? Think of the two candidates as two intervals, and the votes as points in the interval. Both problems deal with the relative order of votes (points) and the problems are connected. The above example for $P(6; 9, .5)$ deals with the case of splitting $[0, 1)$ into two intervals, and scanning with a window of length $w = 1/2$.

A generalization of the Ballot problem to L candidates provides the key to find probabilities for scanning with windows of length $1/L$. Barton and Mallows (1965) in a corollary to a theorem of Karlin and McGregor (1959) provide the needed ballot problem result.

7.3.1 The Karlin–McGregor Theorem

This result and variations are used to solve a variety of scan problems. We give the theorem here, together with Barton and Mallows' corollary.

Karlin–McGregor (1959) Theorem. *Let L labeled particles follow L independent processes with identical transition probabilities $P_{u,v}(t)$. The processes must satisfy the strong Markov property, be one-dimensional (linear ordered state space), and have paths that do not make jumps over states (transitions are only to adjacent states). The ith particle starts (at time 0) at position u_i, $i = 1, 2, \ldots, L$. Without loss of generality assume that the particles are ordered by $u_1 > u_2 > \cdots > u_L$. Then the probability that at time t, particle i is in state v_i, $i = 1, 2, \ldots, L$, and $v_1 > v_2 > \cdots > v_L$, without any two of the particles coinciding anywhere in $[0, t)$ is the determinant of the $L \times L$ matrix whose entries are $P_{u_i, v_j}(t)$. Denote this determinant $\det|P_{u_i, v_j}(t)|$.*

Barton and Mallows (1965, p. 243) describe the following generalization of a classical L-candidate ballot problem. Given L candidates in an election, assume n people each cast their vote for only one candidate. Let $J_i(m)$ denote the number of votes received by the ith candidate after a total of m votes has been counted. Let the candidates each start off with 0 votes, and let candidate i end up with $J_i(n) = a_i$ votes, $i = 1, \ldots, L$, where $\sum a_i = n$. Assume that the candidates are ordered by $a_1 > a_2 > \cdots > a_L$. The ballots are drawn one vote at a time, and randomly in the sense that all $(\sum a_i)!/a_1!a_2! \ldots a_L!$ orders in which ballots might occur are equally likely. A classical L-candidate ballot problem seeks the probability that the ending order of the candidates was also the order throughout the balloting, $P(J_1(m) > J_2(m) > \cdots > J_L(m), m = 1, 2, \ldots, n)$.

Barton and Mallows consider the generalization of this L-candidate problem to allow the candidates to start off with differing leads. Now assume that candidate i starts off with α_i votes, and ends up with $a_i + \alpha_i$ votes, $i = 1, 2, \ldots, L$. Assume further that $a_1 > a_2 > \cdots > a_L$, and also that the candidates who start out ahead also end up ahead, so that $a_1 + \alpha_1 > a_2 + \alpha_2 > \cdots > a_L + \alpha_L$. Let $X_i(m) + \alpha_i$ denote the accumulated number of votes for candidate i after m votes have been counted. Barton and Mallows (1965, equation 19) prove that

$$P\left(X_1(m) + \alpha_1 > X_2(m) + \alpha_2 > \cdots > X_L(m) + \alpha_L; m = 1, 2, \ldots, n \mid \{a_i, \alpha_i\}\right)$$
$$= \det \mid a_i! / (a_i + \alpha_i - \alpha_j)!. \tag{7.1}$$

7.4 Bonferroni-Type Inequalities

The following classical Bonferroni inequalities for the probability of a union of n events have been derived in Bonferroni (1936). Let $A_1, \ldots, A_n$ be a sequence of events and let $A = \bigcup_{i=1}^{n} A_i$. Then for $2 \le k \le n$:

$$\sum_{j=1}^{k} (-1)^{j-1} s_j \le P(A) \le \sum_{j=1}^{k-1} (-1)^{j-1} s_j, \tag{7.2}$$

where k is an even integer and for $1 \le j \le n$:

$$s_j = \sum_{1 \le i_1 < \cdots < i_j \le n} P\left(\bigcap_{m=1}^{j} A_{i_m}\right). \tag{7.3}$$

The orders of these inequalities is given by the upper index of the sums in (7.3). The first-order Bonferroni upper bound is referred to in the statistical literature as Boole's inequality and has been derived earlier in Boole (1854). These classical lower (upper) Bonferroni inequalities have a shortcoming of not necessarily increasing (decreasing) with the increase of the order of the inequality (Schwager, 1984). Moreover, these inequalities can be wide for a low order and the computational complexity increases rapidly with the increase of the order of the inequalities. Therefore attempts have been made to derive simpler inequalities that are more accurate than the classical Bonferroni inequalities. We refer to these inequalities as Bonferroni-type inequalities.

In this book we make use of the following class of upper Bonferroni-type inequalities proposed in Hunter (1976). The basic idea of this approach is to represent the event $A = \bigcup_{i=1}^{n} A_i$ as a union of disjoint events:

$$A = A_1 \cup \left\{\bigcup_{i=2}^{n}\left[A_i \cap \left(\bigcap_{j=1}^{i-1} A_j^c\right)\right]\right\}.$$

Therefore,

$$P(A) = P(A_1) + \sum_{i=2}^{n} P\left[A_i \cap \left(\bigcap_{j=1}^{i-1} A_j^c\right)\right].$$

For $2 \le k \le n - 1$:

$$P(A) \le P(A_1) + \sum_{i=2}^{k} P\left[A_i \cap \left(\bigcap_{j=1}^{i-1} A_j^c\right)\right] + \sum_{i=k+1}^{n} P\left[A_i \cap \left(\bigcap_{j=i-k+1}^{i-1} A_j^c\right)\right].$$

This inequality can be rewritten for $k = 2$ as

$$P(A) \leq s_1 - \sum_{i=2}^{n} P(A_i \cap A_{i-1}) \qquad (7.4)$$

and for $k \geq 3$ as

$$P(A) \leq s_1 - \sum_{i=2}^{n} P(A_i \cap A_{i-1}) - \sum_{j=2}^{k-1} \sum_{i=1}^{n-j} P\left\{A_i \cap \left[\left(\bigcap_{j=i+1}^{i+j-1} A_j^c\right) \cap A_{i+j}\right]\right\}. \qquad (7.5)$$

Note that these upper inequalities are of order k and they decrease as the order of the inequalities is increasing.

The inequality (7.4) is a member of a class of second-order inequalities derived in Hunter (1976). The following concepts from graph theory have to be introduced. A *graph* $G(V, E)$, or briefly G, is a combinatorial structure comprised of a set of vertices V and a set of edges E. Each edge is associated with two vertices referred to as the endpoints of the edge. The graph G is called *undirected* if both endpoints of an edge have same relationship for each of the edges. A *path* is a sequence of edges such that two consecutive edges in it share a common endpoint. A *tree* is an undirected graph such that there is a unique path between every pair of its vertices. Let $v_1, \ldots, v_n$ be the vertices of a tree T, representing the events $A_1, \ldots, A_n$, respectively. The vertices v_i and v_j are joined by an edge e_{ij} if and only if $A_i \cap A_j \neq \phi$. The following inequality has been derived in Hunter (1976):

$$P(A) \leq s_1 - \sum_{\{(i.j):e_{ij} \in T\}} P(A_i \cap A_j). \qquad (7.6)$$

The optimal inequality in the class of inequalities (7.6) can be obtained via an algorithm in Kruskal (1956). Incquality (7.4) is the most stuingent within the class of inequalities (7.6) if the events $A_1, \ldots, A_n$ are exchangeable or if they are ordered in such a way that for $1 \leq i_1 < i_2 < n$, $P(A_{i_1} \cap A_{i_2})$ is maximized for $i_1 - i_2 = 1$ (Worsley, 1982, Examples 3.1 and 3.2).

Inequality (7.5) is a member of the following class of inequalities investigated in Hoover (1990):

$$P(A) \leq P\left(\bigcup_{i=1}^{k} A_i\right) + \sum_{j=k+1}^{n} P\left\{A_j \cap \left(\bigcap_{m \in T_j} A_m^c\right)\right\}, \qquad (7.7)$$

where for $j \geq k+1$, T_j is a subset of $\{1, \ldots, j-1\}$ of size $k-1$. For $k \geq 3$ there is no efficient algorithm to obtain the optimal inequality in the class of inequalities (7.7). In the case where the events $A_1, \ldots, A_n$ are naturally ordered in such a way that $P(\bigcap_{j=1}^{k-1} A_{i_j})$ is maximized for $i_j - i_{j-1} = 1, 2 \leq j \leq k - 1$, and $3 \leq k \leq n - 1$, the natural ordering with $T_j = \{j - 1, \ldots, j - k + 1\}$ is recommended. In this case, inequalities in (7.7) reduce to inequalities (7.5). If the events $A_1, \ldots, A_n$ are exchangeable, inequalities in (7.7) reduce to inequalities (7.5) and have the following simplified form

$$P(A) \leq nP(A_1) - (n-1)P(A_1 \cap A_2)$$
$$- \sum_{j=2}^{k-1}(n-j)P\left\{A_1 \cap \left[\left(\bigcap_{i=2}^{j} A_i^c\right) \cap A_{j+1}\right]\right\}. \tag{7.8}$$

It is tedious but quite routine to verify that the Bonferroni-type inequalities (7.5) and (7.8) for $P\left(\bigcap_{i=1}^{n} A_i^c\right) = 1 - P\left(\bigcup_{i=1}^{n} A_i\right)$ are given by

$$P\left(\bigcap_{i=1}^{n} A_i^c\right) \geq \sum_{i=1}^{n-k+1} \alpha_{i,i+k-1} - \sum_{i=1}^{n-k} \alpha_{i+1,i+k-1} \tag{7.9}$$

and

$$P\left(\bigcap_{i=1}^{n} A_i^c\right) \geq (n+k-1)\alpha_{1,k} - (n-k)\alpha_{2,k}, \tag{7.10}$$

respectively, where

$$\alpha_{m,n} = P\left(\bigcap_{i=m}^{n} A_i^c\right).$$

In some examples it is easier to evaluate the terms $\alpha_{m,n}$, in which case inequalities (7.9) and (7.10) will be used. The following inequality is given in Galambos and Simonelli (1996, Inequality I8, p. 27) for $b = \min\{2 + [3s_3/s_2], n-1\}$:

$$P(A) \leq s_1 - \frac{2(2b-1)}{(b-1)(b-2)}s_2 + \frac{6}{b(b+1)}s_3. \tag{7.11}$$

A second-order lower Bonferroni-type inequality for $P\left(\bigcup_{i=1}^{n} A_i\right)$ had been derived in Dawson and Sankoff (1967). Let s_1 and s_2 be given in (7.3) above. Then

$$P(A) \geq \frac{2s_1}{a} - \frac{2s_2}{a(a-1)}, \tag{7.12}$$

where a is the integer part of $2 + 2s_2/s_1$. Kwerel (1975), using a linear programming approach, has proved that inequality (7.12) is optimal in the class of all linear inequalities of the form

$$P(A) \geq b_1 s_1 + b_2 s_2.$$

In particular, it outperforms the Bonferroni inequality $P(A) \geq s_1 - s_2$, whenever $a > 2$.

Lower Bonferroni-type inequalities for $P\left(\bigcup_{i=1}^{n} A_i\right)$ of order $k \geq 3$, for arbitrary events $A_1, \ldots, A_n$, are discussed in Galambos and Simonelli (1996). We present now a third-order inequality given in Galambos and Simonelli (1996, Inquality IV.1(ii), p. 118):

$$P(A) \geq \max_{1 \leq i \leq n-2} \left\{ \frac{i+2n-1}{n(i+1)} s_1 - \frac{2(i+n-2)}{ni(i+1)} s_2 + \frac{b}{ni(i+1)} s_3 \right\}. \quad (7.13)$$

Fourth- or higher-order inequalities are discussed there and are not presented here, because of their complexity and impracticality from the computational point of view. For the case of exchangeable events, these inequalities simplify considerably, since for $1 \leq j \leq n$:

$$s_j = \binom{n}{j} P\left(\bigcap_{i=1}^{j} A_i \right).$$

In this case even the classical Bonferroni inequalities given in (7.2) are easy to evaluate, if one can evaluate $P(\bigcap_{i=1}^{j} A_i)$.

7.5 The Q_2/Q_3 Approximation for Scan Statistics

The following approach provides remarkably good approximations for a variety of problems involving scan statistics. For continuous time, consider a point process on $[0, T)$ and scan $[0, T)$ with a moving subinterval $[t, t+w)$, $0 \leq t \leq T-w$. For discrete time consider a sequence of T i.i.d. random variates and scan the discrete sequence with a moving sequence of w consecutive trials. Call the moving subinterval, or moving sequence, a *sliding window*. In both cases we are interested in extremal values within the sliding window. Let Q_V denote the probability of the event E_V^* that nowhere in $[0, V)$ is the extremal value as large as (small as) a specified value. Naus (1982) gives the following approximation:

$$Q_T \approx Q_{2w} (Q_{3w}/Q_{2w})^{(T/w)-2}. \quad (7.14)$$

The reasoning behind the approximation can be illustrated for the case $T = Lw$, for L an integer. Divide the time interval (or sequence) into L disjoint intervals each of length w. Consider pairs of adjacent intervals, where the ith pair in the continuous time case are the two halves of $[(i-1)w, (i+1)w)$, and in the discrete sequence case fall in trials $\{(i-1)w+1, \ldots, (i+1)w)\}$. Let E_i denote the event that nowhere within the ith pair is the extremal value as large as (small as) the specified value. The event E_T^* is equivalent to the intersection of the $(L-1)$ E_i's:

$$Q_T = P(E_1)P(E_2 \mid E_1)P(E_3 \mid E_2 \cap E_1) \ldots P\left(E_{L-1} \mid \bigcap_{i=1}^{L-2} E_i \right). \quad (7.15)$$

In certain cases where the dependence due to overlapping intervals has limited impact on distant intervals, one can approximate $P(E_3 \mid E_2 \cap E_1)$ by $P(E_3 \mid E_2)$, approximate $P(E_4 \mid E_3 \cap E_2 \cap E_1)$ by $P(E_4 \mid E_3)$, and so on. In many problems there is exchangeability that implies that

$$P(E_4 \mid E_3) = P(E_3 \mid E_2) = P(E_2 \mid E_1) = P(E_1 \cap E_2)/P(E_1) = Q_{3w}/Q_{2w}. \tag{7.16}$$

Substituting (7.16) into (7.15) gives (7.14).

One can sharpen the approximation further by allowing a greater range of dependence, and use approximations of the form

$$P(E_{i+3} \mid E_{i+2} \cap E_{i+1} \cap E_i) = P(E_{i+3} \mid E_{i+2} \cap E_{i+1})$$
$$P(E_{i+3} \cap E_{i+2} \cap E_{i+1})/P(E_{i+2} \cap E_{i+1}) = Q_{4w}/Q_{3w}, \tag{7.17}$$
$$Q_T \approx P(E_1 \cap E_2)P(E_3 \mid E_2 \cap E_1)P(E_4 \mid E_3 \cap E_2)\dots$$
$$= Q_{3w}(Q_{4w}/Q_{3w})^{(T/w)-3}. \tag{7.18}$$

Similarly, one could develop still sharper (but more difficult to evalute) approximations such as

$$Q_T \approx Q_{4w}(Q_{5w}/Q_{4w})^{(T/w)-4}.$$

For the case of points on a circle (either continuous time, or a circular sequence), the above approach is easily modified. Here, the event E_T^* is equivalent to the intersection of the L E_i's. To modify to the circle, the first-order approximation of the form of (7.14), note that the Lth pair of adjacent windows involves the first and last intervals. The key change is to recognize the adjacency of the $(L - 1)$st and first pairs to the Lth pair of windows, and to approximate

$$P(E_L \mid E_1 \cap E_2 \cap E_3 \cap \dots \cap E_{L-1}) \approx P(E_L \mid E_1 \cap E_{L-1}) = Q_{4w}/Q_{3w}. \tag{7.19}$$

Tables of Q_{4w}, Q_{3w}, and Q_{2w} are given in Neff and Naus (1980).

7.6   Poisson and Compound Poisson Approximations

Let $A_1, \dots, A_n$ be a sequence of arbitrary events. For $1 \le j \le n$, define the indicator random variables

$$I_j = \begin{cases} 1 & \text{if the event } A_j \text{ occurs,} \\ 0 & \text{otherwise.} \end{cases} \tag{7.20}$$

We are interested in approximating the distribution of

$$W = \sum_{j=1}^{n} I_j, \tag{7.21}$$

the number of occurrences of the events $A_1, \dots, A_n$. If the events $A_1, \dots, A_n$ are independent and equally probable then the random variable W has a binomial distribution with parameters n and p, where $P(A_1) = p$. It is well known that for any integer $k \geq 0$, when $n \to \infty$ and $p \to 0$ such that $np \to \lambda$, where $\lambda > 0$ is a constant,

$$\lim_{\substack{n \to \infty \\ p \to 0}} P(W = k) = e^{-\lambda} \frac{(np)^k}{k!} \tag{7.22}$$

(Casella and Berger, 1990, Sect. 2.3). The distance between the binomial and the limiting Poisson distribution in (7.22) has been investigated by many authors (Barbour, Holst, and Janson, 1992, Chap. 1) and one of the interesting results has been obtained by Kerstan (1964): For $0 < p \leq .25$:

$$\max_{j \geq 0} |P(W \leq j) - F_\lambda(j)| \leq 1.05p, \tag{7.23}$$

where $\lambda = np$ and

$$F_\lambda(j) = \sum_{k=0}^{j} e^{-\lambda} \frac{(np)^k}{k!} . \tag{7.24}$$

Results of this nature shed light on the accuracy of the Poisson approximations for the distribution of W.

For the case when the events $A_1, \dots, A_n$ are not independent and not necessarily equally probable, Freedman (1974) and Serfling (1975) have shown that

$$\max_{j \geq 0} |P(w \leq j) - F_\lambda(j)| \leq \sum_{i=1}^{n} \{[E(P_i)]^2 + E|P_i - E(P_i)|\}, \tag{7.25}$$

where

$$P_i = P[I_i = 1 \mid I_1, \dots, I_{i-1}],$$

$$\lambda = \sum_{i=1}^{n} E(P_i),$$

and W and $F_\lambda(j)$ are given in (7.21) and (7.24), respectively. Note that for the independent and equally probable events, the estimate of the error of the Poisson approximations in (7.25) reduces to np^2, which for $\lambda > 1.05$ is larger than the estimate of error given in (7.23).

Stein (1972) introduced an ingenious and powerful method for approximating distributions of sums of dependent random variables. This method has been extended to Poisson approximations for the distribution of W in Chen (1975). A nice survey of these results is presented in Arratia, Goldstein, and Gordon (1990) and in Barbour, Holst, and Janson (1992, Chap. 1). The following version of the Poisson approximation for the number of occurrences of dependent events has been presented in Arratia, Goldstein, and Gordon (1989, 1990, Sect. 3). For $1 \leq i \leq n$, let $i \in B_i \subset \{1, \dots, n\}$ and denote by $p_i = P(I_i = 1)$

and $p_{ij} = P(I_i = 1, I_j = 1)$, where I_i are defined in (7.20). B_i is a set of indices for the indicator random variables that are dependent with I_i. Let $\lambda = E(W) = \sum_{i=1}^{n} p_i$ and define

$$b_1 = \sum_{i=1}^{n} \sum_{j \in B_i} p_i p_j,$$

$$b_2 = \sum_{i=1}^{n} \sum_{i \neq j \in B_i} p_{ij},$$

and

$$b_3 = \sum_{i=1}^{n} E\left|E[I_i - p_i \mid I_j; j \in B_i^c]\right|.$$

From Arratia, Goldstein, and Gordon (1989) it follows that

$$\max_{j \geq 0} |P(W \leq j) - F_\lambda(j)| \leq (b_1 + b_2)\lambda^{-1}(1 - e^{-\lambda}) + b_3 \min\{1, 1.4\lambda^{-.5}\}$$

$$(7.26)$$

and

$$|P(W = 0) - e^{-\lambda}| \leq (b_1 + b_2 + b_3)\lambda^{-1}(1 - e^{-\lambda}). \qquad (7.27)$$

In many applications I_i is independent of $\{I_j; j \in B_i^c\}$, in which case $b_3 = 0$ and $b_2 - b_1 = \text{Var}(W) - \lambda$. Therefore, when $b_3 = 0$ and b_1 is small, the estimate of the error of the Poisson approximation for the distribution of W is comparable to the difference of variances for these two distributions. Barbour, Holst, and Janson (1992) present many interesting results related to inequalities for the distribution of W and the rate of convergence of the distribution of W to the Poisson distribution with mean $\lambda = E(W)$. For scan statistics discussed in this book Poisson-type approximations are of importance, rather than the inequalities. Therefore we do not discuss Poisson-type inequalities here.

Usually we will be interested in Poisson approximations for $P(W \geq 1)$. It follows from (7.27) that

$$P(W \geq 1) \approx 1 - e^{-\lambda}, \qquad (7.28)$$

where $\lambda = E(W)$. For the scan statistics discussed in this book approximation (7.28) can be inaccurate. The reason for this is that the events $A_1, \ldots, A_n$ associated with the scan statistics tend to clump. Suppose that we are able to evaluate $P\left(\bigcap_{i=1}^{j} A_i\right)$ for $1 \leq j \leq m$. The following method of *local declumping* of order m has its roots in Arratia, Goldstein, and Gordon (1990) and Glaz, Naus, Roos, and Wallenstein (1994). For $1 \leq j \leq n$ and $2 \leq m < n/2$, let

$$I_j^* = \begin{cases} 1 & \text{if the event } A_j \cap \left[\bigcap_{i=j+1}^{\min\{j+m-1,n\}} A_i^c\right] \text{ occurs,} \\ 0 & \text{otherwise.} \end{cases} \qquad (7.29)$$

The indicators $I_1^*, \ldots, I_n^*$ discount events that occur within a distance less than m from another event that has occurred and that has been accounted for. Then

$$\sum_{j=1}^{n} I_j = 0 \quad \Leftrightarrow \quad \sum_{j=1}^{n} I_j^* = 0.$$

Let

$$W^* = \sum_{j=1}^{n} I_j^*$$

and set $\lambda^* = E(W^*) = \sum_{j=1}^{n} P(I_j^* = 1)$. The Poisson approximation for $P(W^* \geq 1)$ is used to approximate $P(W \geq 1)$:

$$P(W \geq 1) \approx 1 - e^{-\lambda^*} \tag{7.30}$$

and is referred to as an improved Poisson-type approximation. For scan statistics discussed in this book, approximation (7.30) is more accurate than the usual Poisson approximation given in (7.28) (Glaz, Naus, Roos, and Wallenstein (1994) and Chen and Glaz (1997)).

Compound Poisson approximations is another class of approximations that takes into account the clumping of the events $A_1, \ldots, A_n$. The distribution of W is approximated by a compound Poisson distribution with parameters $\{\lambda_j\}_{j=1}^{\infty}$, $\sum_{j=1}^{\infty} \lambda_j = E(W) < \infty$, defined on a lattice of nonnegative integers and has the form $\sum_{j=1}^{\infty} j N_j$, where for $j \geq 1$, N_j are independent Poisson random variables with mean λ_j, respectively. The following equivalent and widely known representation for this compound Poisson distribution is presented in Feller (1968). Let $\{X_i\}_{i=1}^{\infty}$ be a sequence of i.i.d. nonnegative integer valued random variables. Let M be a Poisson random variable with mean equal to λt and assume that it is independent of $\{X_i\}_{i=1}^{\infty}$. Then the random sum

$$\sum_{i=1}^{M} X_i$$

is said to have a compound Poisson distribution (Feller, 1968, p. 288). If we denote by $\lambda_j = \lambda P(X_i = j)$, using the method of generating functions, we can show that

$$\sum_{i=1}^{M} X_i = \sum_{j=1}^{\infty} j N_j,$$

where N_j are independent Poisson random variables with mean λ_j, respectively.

In practice, only a finite number of the λ_j's are used in the approximation (Barbour, Chen, and Loh (1992) and Roos (1993a,b, 1994)). The determination of the λ_j's used in the approximations for the distribution of scan statistics will be discussed for each case separately. The general form of the compound Poisson approximation for $P(W \geq 1)$ is given by

$$P(W \geq 1) \approx 1 - \exp\left(-\sum_{i=1}^{m} \lambda_i^*\right),$$

where λ_i^* is defined in terms of the finite set of λ_j's.

8

Scanning N Uniform Distributed Points: Exact Results

8.1 Introduction

Let $X_1, X_2, \ldots, X_N$, be independent and identically distributed (i.i.d.) random variables, with common density $f(x) = 1, 0 \leq x \leq 1, f(x) = 0$, elsewhere. Let $Y_t(w)$ denote the number of X's in the interval $\{t, t + w)$. The statistic $S_w = \max_{0 \leq t \leq 1-w} \{Y_t(w)\}$. Let $X_{(1)} \leq X_{(2)} \leq \cdots \leq X_{(N)}$ denote the ordered values of the X's.

The statistic W_k equals $\min_{0 < w < 1} \{w : S_w \geq k\} = \min_{1 \leq i \leq N-k+1} \{X_{(i+k-1)} - X_{(i)}\}$. For $k = 2$, the quantity $X_{(i+k-1)} - X_{(i)} = X_{(i+1)} - X_{(i)}$, the distance, called *gap* or *spacing*, between the ith and $(i+1)$st point. W_2 is the smallest gap between any two of the N points. The quantities $X_{(i+k-1)} - X_{(i)}$ are called *higher-order gaps* or *quasi-ranges*. For $k = N, i = 1$, the quantity $X_{(i+k-1)} - X_{(i)} = X_{(N)} - X_{(1)}$, which is the sample range of the N points. For $k = N - 1, i = 1, 2$ there are two *quasi-ranges*, $X_{(N)} - X_{(2)}$ and $X_{(N-1)} - X_{(1)}$. W_{N-1} is the minimum of these two quasi-ranges.

The distributions of the statistics S_w and W_k are related, $P(S_w \geq k) = P(W_k \leq w)$. We denote the common probability, $P(k: N, w)$, and let $Q(k; N, w) = 1 - P(k; N, w)$. This chapter reviews approaches to derive exact expressions for $P(k; N, w)$.

8.2   The Direct Integration Approach

Exact formulas and proofs for two special cases, $P(2; N, w)$ and $P(N; N, w)$, appear in various probability texts, and have been long known. Silberstein (1945, p. 322) notes that $P(k; N, w)$ is a polynomial in w of order N. Mack (1948, p. 783) notes that $P(k; N, w)$ is piecewise polynomial, that is, the polynomial expressions change for different ranges of w. An exact formula for $P(N; N, w)$, the cumulative distribution function (c.d.f.) of W_N, the sample range of the N points, is derived in Burnside (1928, p. 22):

$$P(N; N, w) = Nw^{N-1} - (N - 1)w^N, \qquad 0 \le w \le 1. \qquad (8.1)$$

An exact formula for $P(2; N, w)$, the cumulative distribution function of W_2, the smallest distance between any of the N points, is derived in Parzen (1960, p. 304), by a direct integration approach.

$$
\begin{aligned}
P(2; N, w) &= 1 - (1 - [N - 1]w)^N, & 0 \le w \le 1/(N - 1), \\
&= 1, & 1/(N - 1) \le w \le 1. \qquad (8.2)
\end{aligned}
$$

Frosini (1981) illustrates the direct integration approach for $P(3; 4, w)$, notes the difficulty of applying this method in general, and carries out extensive Monte Carlo simulations of $P(k; N, w)$. Chapter 7 illustrates the direct integration approach for $P(2; 4, w)$ and $P(3; 4, w)$. Elteren and Gerritis (1961) used the direct integration approach to derive exact formulas for three special cases, $(k, N) = (3; 6), (3; 7),$ and $(3; 8)$. The direct integration approach becomes complicated even for simple cases such as these

$$
\begin{aligned}
1 - P(3; 6, w) &= 5(1 - 2w)^6 - 4(1 - 3w)^5, & 0 \le w \le 1/3, \\
&= 5(1 - 2w)^6, & 1/3 \le w \le 1/2, \\
&= 0, & 1/2 \le w, \\
& & (8.3)
\end{aligned}
$$

$$
\begin{aligned}
1 - P(3; 7, w) &= (1 - 4w)^7 + 7w(1 - 2w)(4 - 7w)(1 - 3w)^4, & 0 \le w \le 1/4, \\
&= 7w(1 - 2w)(4 - 7w)(1 - 3w)^4, & 1/4 \le w \le 1/3, \\
&= 0, & 1/3 \le w \le 1, \\
& & (8.4)
\end{aligned}
$$

$$
\begin{aligned}
1 - P(3; 8, w) &= 14(1 - 3w)^8 - (1 - 4w)^6(13 - 24w), & 0 \le w \le 1/4, \\
&= 14(1 - 3w)^8, & 1/4 \le w \le 1/3, \\
&= 0, & 1/3 \le w \le 1. \\
& & (8.5)
\end{aligned}
$$

Naus (1963) derived, by an integration approach that conditioned on the sample range, the exact formula for the case $k = N - 1$. However, this approach did not eliminate the complexity for the other k:

$$
\begin{aligned}
P(N-1; N, w) &= N(N-1)w^{N-2} - 2N(N-1)w^{N-1} \\
&\quad + (N^2 - N + 2)w^N, \qquad 0 \le w \le 1/2, \\
&= N(N-1)w^{N-2} - 2N(N-1)w^{N-1} + (N^2 - N + 2)w^N \\
&\quad - (2w-1)^N, \qquad\qquad 1/2 \le w \le 1.
\end{aligned} \tag{8.6}
$$

8.3 The Combinatorial Approach

For any specific k and N, the direct integration approach can in theory be carried out. However, even for simple examples the direct integration route appears overly complicated by the repeated splitting of the integral over many regions. Naus (1963, 1965a) developed an alternative combinatorial approach to derive simple formula for $P(k; N, w)$ for $k > (N+1)/2$. For $k > (N+1)/2$, $P(k; N, w)$ is piecewise polynomial, with different polynomials for $w \le 1/2$ and $w \ge 1/2$. The polynomials are written in terms of binomials and cumulative binomials. Let

$$
b(k; N, w) = \binom{N}{k} w^k (1-w)^{N-k}, \tag{8.7}
$$

$$
F_b(k; N, w) = \sum_{i=0}^{k} b(i; N, w),
$$

$$
G_b(k; N, w) = 1 - F_b(k-1; N, w),
$$

$$
\begin{aligned}
P(k; N, w) &= C(k; N, w), & w \le 1/2, \quad k > N/2, \tag{8.8} \\
&= C(k; N, w) - R(k; N, w), & w \ge 1/2, \quad k > (N+1)/2, \tag{8.9}
\end{aligned}
$$

where

$$
\begin{aligned}
C(k; N, w) &= (N-k+1)b(k-1; N, w) - (N-k)b(k; N, w) \\
&\quad + G_b(k; N, w) + G_b(k+1; N, w),
\end{aligned}
$$

$$
R(k; N, w) = U(k; N, w)b(k; N, w) + \sum_{y=k}^{N} b(y; N, w) F_b(N-k; y, (1-w)/w),
$$

$$
\begin{aligned}
U(k; N, w) &= \{k(1-w)/w\} F_b(N-k; k-1, (1-w)/w) \\
&\quad - (N-k+1) F_b(N-k+1; k, (1-w)/w).
\end{aligned}
$$

The reasoning underlying the combinatorial approach to (8.8) is as follows. From the direct integration approach it can be shown that $P(k; N, w)$ is a polynomial in w for $0 \le w \le 1/C$, for C sufficiently large. Neff (1978) gives a formal proof. Given enough values of the polynomial for different w, we could fit the polynomial exactly. In particular, if we can find the polynomial expression for

$P(k; N, w)$ for $w = 1/L$, for all integer $L > C$, then this same polynomial will apply for $P(k; N, w)$ for all $0 \leq w \leq 1/C$.

We first illustrate the combinatorial approach for the example $P(N; N, w), 0 \leq w \leq 1$. The reader can apply the approach to derive the formula for $P(3; 4, w)$, $0 \leq w \leq .5$.

Example 8.1 (Combinatorial Approach to Derive $P(N; N, w)$). To find $P(N; N, 1/L)$, L an integer, divide the unit interval into L disjoint intervals $\{[i - 1)/L, i/L\}$, $i = 1, 2, \ldots, L$. Let $\mathcal{A}_i$ denote the event that there are at least k points in the ith interval, where for this example $k = N$. Let B_i denote the event that no $\mathcal{A}_i$ occurs, and that there exists an interval of length $1/L$, over-lapping the ith and $(i + 1)$st intervals, that contains at least k (here $= N$) points. Let $\mathcal{A} = \bigcup \mathcal{A}_i$ and $B = \bigcup B_i$. $\mathcal{A}$ and B are mutually exclusive events, and $P(N; N, 1/L) = P(\mathcal{A} \cup B) = P(\mathcal{A}) + P(B)$. For this example (and, in general, for $k > (N + 1)/2$), the $\mathcal{A}_i$ are mutually exclusive events

$$P(\mathcal{A}) = LP(\mathcal{A}_i) = LG_b(N; N, 1/L) = L(1/L)^N = (1/L)^{(N-1)}.$$

For $k = N$, the B_i's are mutually exclusive events, and

$$P(B) = (L - 1)P(B_1).$$

To find $P(B_1)$, condition on the number of points, n_1 and n_2 that fall, respec-tively, in the first and second intervals $[0, 1/L)$ and $[1/L, 2/L)$. When $k = N$, for B_1 to occur, $n_1 + n_2 = N$, and $1 \leq n_1, n_2 \leq N - 1$. In addition, in order for some interval overlapping the first two intervals to contain N points, the n_1 points in the first interval must all come later in their interval than the n_2 points in the sec-ond interval do (relative to the beginning of their interval). Conditional on n_1 and n_2, all $\binom{N}{n_1}$ relative orders of the points are equally likely, and only one of these relative orders satisfy the condition needed for B_1. Chapter 7 discusses this ap-proach in more detail. Averaging the conditional probability over the multinomial distribution of n_1 and n_2 gives

$$P(B_1) = \sum_{n_1=1}^{N-1} (1/L)^N = (N - 1)(1/L)^N.$$

Combining results for $P(\mathcal{A})$ and $P(B)$ gives

$$P(N; N, 1/L) = (1/L)^{(N-1)} + (L - 1)(N - 1)(1/L)^N$$
$$= N(1/L)^{(N-1)} - (N - 1)(1/L)^N. \tag{8.10}$$

Given that $P(N; N, w)$ is a polynomial in w, $0 \leq w \leq 1$, it follows from substi-tuting w for $1/L$ in the right-hand side of (8.10), that

$$P(N; N, w) = Nw^{(N-1)} - (N - 1)w^N.$$

This completes the combinatorial proof of (8.1). The same approach yields (8.8) once we have generalized the approach to count relative order of points and take into account the intersection of the B_i events.

8.4　The Derivation of $P(k; N, w)$ for $k > (N + 1)/2$, $w \leq 1/2$

For $k > (N + 1)/2$, $w \leq 1/2$, $P(k; N, w)$ is a polynomial in w. We first find $P(k; N, 1/L)$ for $k > (N + 1)/2$, $L \geq 2$, L an integer. Divide the unit interval into L disjoint intervals, $[i - 1)/L, i/L), i = 1, 2, \ldots, L$. Let $\mathcal{A}_i$ denote the event that there are at least k points in the ith interval. Let B_i denote the event that no $\mathcal{A}_i$ occurs and that there exists an interval of length $1/L$, overlapping the ith and $(i + 1)$st intervals, that contains at least k points. Let $\mathcal{A} = \bigcup \mathcal{A}_i$ and $B = \bigcup B_i$. $\mathcal{A}$ and B are mutually exclusive events, and

$$P(k; N, 1/L) = P(\mathcal{A} \cup B) = P(\mathcal{A}) + P(B). \tag{8.11}$$

For $k > (N + 1)/2$, the $\mathcal{A}_i$ are mutually exclusive events

$$P(\mathcal{A}) = L P(\mathcal{A}_i) = L G_b(k; N, 1/L). \tag{8.12}$$

For $(N + 1)/2 < k < N$, the B_i's are not mutually exclusive events; B_i and B_{i+1} can simultaneously happen. For example, if the first and third intervals each contain one point, and the second interval contains $N - 2$ points, then it is possible for B_1 and B_2 to both happen. Whether they both happen depends on the relative nearness of the points to the beginning of their interval. Figure 8.1 illustrates a situation where $B_1 \cap B_2$ occurs. However, for $k > (N + 1)/2$, $B_i \cap B_j$ cannot occur for $|i - j| > 1$:

$$P(B) = (L - 1)P(B_1) - (L - 2)P(B_1 \cap B_2). \tag{8.13}$$

We first find $P(B_1)$ and then find $P(B_1 \cap B_2)$.

8.4.1　Finding $P(B_1)$

To find $P(B_1)$, condition on the number of points, n_1 and n_2, that fall, respctively, in the first and second intervals, $[0, 1/L)$ and $[1/L, 2/L)$. The remaining $N -$

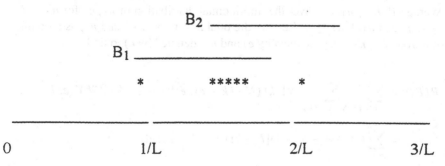

Figure 8.1. $N = 6$, $k = 5$, and $B_1 \cap B_2$ occurs. Points denoted by $\star$.

$n_1 - n_2$ points fall in $[2/L, 1)$. Let $w = 1/L$. Given that the N points have a uniform distribution on $[0, 1)$, (n_1, n_2) have the multinomial distribution

$$P(n_1, n_2) = (N!/n_1! \, n_2! \, (N - n_1 - n_2)!) w^{n_1} w^{n_2} (1 - 2w)^{N - n_1 - n_2}.$$

The term $\binom{n_1 + n_2}{n_1}$ in the binomial expression is usually explained as follows: We only care for the number of points falling in the first two intervals (cells), and not their order of falling; therefore, we add probabilities for all orders corresponding to cell counts n_1, n_2. The quantity $\binom{n_1 + n_2}{n_1}$ counts the number of these orders. In the present approach, the points are viewed as being ordered, not by their time of falling in the interval, but by their relative nearness to the beginning of the interval. If the n_2 points in the second interval are closer to the beginning of their interval than the n_1 points are to the beginning of their interval, then the n_2 points come into the scanning interval before the n_1 points drop out. This makes for a large cluster in the scanning interval.

Slide an interval of length w over the interval $[0, 2w)$. The number of points in this scanning interval define a path that starts at n_1 (when the scanning interval's left-most point is zero) and ends at n_2 (when the scanning interval's left-most point is w). As the scanning interval slides from left to right, the points in $[0, w)$ drop out, and the points in $(w, 2w)$ come in. The corresponding path has n_1 moves down and has n_2 moves up. Conditional on n_1 and n_2, all $\binom{n_1 + n_2}{n_1}$ orders of the ups and downs (paths) are equally likely. To find $P(B_1)$ we seek the number of paths that correspond to the scanning interval containing k or more points. This is the number of paths that touch or pass through k. We first translate the path to the origin (starting at a height 0, and ending at a height $n_2 - n_1$). We then apply the reflection principle (see Chapter 7 for details) to find that there are $\binom{n_1 + n_2}{k}$ paths that touch k. For $k > N/2$, if $n_1 < k$, $n_2 < k$, and $n_1 + n_2 \geq k$, then none of the L disjoint intervals, $[iL, (i + 1)L)$, can contain k or more points

$$P(B_1 \mid (n_1, n_2)) = \binom{n_1 + n_2}{k} \Big/ \binom{n_1 + n_2}{n_1} = n_1! \, n_2!/k! \, (n_1 + n_2 - k)!. $$

$$(8.14)$$

Average $P(B_1 \mid n_1, n_2)$ over the multinomial distribution of n_1, n_2 for $n_1 < k$, $n_2 < k$, and $n_1 + n_2 \geq k$. Rewrite the double sum over n_1 and n_2, as a double sum over $N - n_1 - n_2$ (denoted by e) and n_1 (denoted by c) to find

$$P(B_1) = \sum_{e=\zeta}^{N-k} \sum_{c=N-k-e+1}^{k-1} [N!/k! \, (N - k - e)! \, e!](1 - 2w)^e w^{N-e} V(e, L - 2)$$

$$= \sum_{e=\zeta}^{N-k} (2k + e - N - 1)[N!/k! \, (N - k - e)! \, e!]$$

$$\times (1 - 2w)^e w^{N-e} V(e, L - 2), \qquad (8.15)$$

where $\zeta = \max(0; N - 2k + 2)$, and

$$V(e, L - 2) = P\left(n_i < k, \ i = 3, \ldots, L \left| \sum_{i=3}^{L} n_i = e = N - n_1 - n_2\right.\right).$$

For $k \geq N/2$, $\zeta = 0$, $V(e, L - 2) = 1$, and (8.15) simplifies to

$$P(B_1) = \sum_{e=0}^{N-k} \sum_{c=N-k-e+1}^{k-1} [N!/k!\,(N - k - e)!\,e!](1 - 2w)^e w^{N-e}$$

$$= \{(2k - N - 1) + [(L - 2)(N - k)/(L - 1)]\}b(k; N, w). \quad (8.16)$$

Equation (8.16) is valid for $k > N/2$.

8.4.2 Finding $P(B_1 \cap B_2)$ for $k > N/2$

Naus (1965, pp. 536–537) gives a combinatorial argument for $P(B_1 \cap B_2)$ valid only for the case $k > N/2$. (It was not clear until later how to generalize this for other k.) This combinatorial argument conditions on n_1, n_2, n_3 the number of points in the first three intervals of length w. The approach lets $n_1 + n_2 + n_3 = M$, $n_1 = x + r$, $n_2 = k - x$, and $n_3 = x + j$. Note that if $n_1 < k$, $n_2 < k$, $n_3 < k$, $n_1 + n_2 \geq k$, $n_2 + n_3 \geq k$, $B_1 \cap B_2$ happens if x points in the first interval come later in that interval, than do $k - x$ second interval points (in their interval), and the latter come later than x third interval points (in their interval). If $k + x$ points satisfy this ordering, then no matter how the remaining r first interval and j third interval points mix into the arrangement of the $k + x$ points, then $B_1 \cap B_2$ happen. The positions in the arrangements for the $j + r$ points can be chosen in $M!/j!\,r!\,(M - j - r)!$ ways. It turns out that this is equal to the number of arrangements that correspond to given j, r, x values and satisfy $B_1 \cap B_2$. (The equivalence is not obvious; see footnote 4, p. 537, in Naus (1965a) for a more detailed discussion of this.) Averaging over the distribution of points gives

$$P(B_1 \cap B_2) = G_b(k + 1; N, W). \quad (8.17)$$

Substitute (8.16) and (8.17) into right-hand side of (8.13) and the result, and (8.12) into (8.11) to prove (8.8), for $w = 1/L$, for all integer $L \geq 2$. $P(k; N, w)$ is a polynomial in w for $k > N/2$, $w \leq 1/2$, and the order of the polynomial for given k and N is finite; therefore, the polynomial in $w = 1/L$ gives the polynomial for all $w \leq 1/2$. The proof of (8.9) follows in a similar way; Naus (1965a) gives the details.

8.5 A General Formula for $P(k; N, 1/L)$ for Integer L

For the case of $w \geq 1/2$, a combinatorial argument using the random path and reflection principle led to $P(k; N, w)$. For the case $w = 1/L$, L an integer,

$k > N/2$, the same approach gave $P(B_i)$. The key was the connection between the number of points in the scanning window of length w as it slides over $[0, 2w)$ and a random path reaching a certain level. To generalize the approach for all $w = 1/L$, L an integer, required some form of generalization of the path argument. The path argument had been used to derive results for the one-sided two-sample Kolmogorov–Smirnov statistic. We first explain the relation between the scan statistic probability $P(k; N, 1/L)$ and the distribution of the one-sided L-sample Kolmogorov–Smirnov statistic.

Divide the interval into L disjoint subintervals $[(i-1)/L, i/L)$ for $i = 1, 2, \ldots$, L. Let n_i denote the number, and $x_{1i}, x_{2i}, \ldots, x_{ni}$ the values of the points that fall into $[(i-1)/L, i/L)$. Let $v_i(t)$ denote the number of x_{ij} that fall in the subinterval $[(i-1)/L, \{(i-1)/L\} + t)$, where t is a given real number, $0 \le t \le 1/L$. Naus (1965a, 1966a) noted that

$$1 - P(k; N, 1/L)$$

$$= \Pr\left\{\sup_{i,t}[n_i - v_i(t) + v_{i+1}(t)] < k\right\}$$

$$= L^{-N} N! \sum_{\sigma} \Pr\left\{\sup_{i,t}[n_i - v_i(t) + v_{i+1}(t)] < k \mid \{n_i\}\right\} / \prod n_i! \quad (8.18)$$

where the sum is over the set σ of all partitions of N into L positive integers each less than k. Now view the L sets of x_{ij}'s as L samples, each rescaled to be over the interval $[0, 1/L)$. That is, set $x_{ij}^* = x_{ij} - (i-1)/L$.

Let $F_i(t)$ denote the empirical distribution function of the x_{ij}^*, namely the proportion of the sample of x_{ij}^* that are $\le t$, $F_i(t) = v_i(t)/n_i$. The one-sided L-sample Kolmogorov–Smirnov statistic is $\sup_{i,t}\{F_{i+1}(t) - F_i(t)\}$. For the case where the n_i's are equal, the distribution of this L-sample Kolmogorov–Smirnov statistic reduces to $\Pr\{\sup_{i,t}[y_{i+1}(t) - y_i(t)] \le C \mid \{n_i\}\}$ for some constant C. A comparison of this with (8.18) shows why the same types of combinatorial path arguments had proved useful for the two-sample Kolmogorov–Smirnov statistic, and $P(k; N, 1/2)$. Results on the L-sample Kolmogorov–Smirnov statistic might provide clues to $P(k; N, 1/L)$. Further, if we could find a general expression for (8.18) we would have a general formula for the L-sample one-sided Kolmogorov–Smirnov distribution for equal sample sizes.

Ozols (1956) had developed a path approach to generalize the path argument for the Kolmogorov–Smirnov test to the case of three samples. The approach could help find $P(k; N, 1/3)$, by counting the appropriate relative orders for the three intervals. Ozols viewed the path as an arrangement of three directions counterclockwise on an equilateral triangle in the plane. The directions of the first two sides give the ups and downs for the first and second intervals, and the second and third sides give the downs and ups corresponding to the second and third intervals. Ozols sought the number of paths that do not touch either of two *bisectral boundaries* parallel to directions one and three. H.T. David (1958) notes that this approach did not seem to offer great promise for further generalizations.

The random walk problem was also related to the classical ballot problem. Both problems deal with the relative order of votes (points) and the problems are connected. A generalization of the ballot problem to L candidates would provide the needed key. Barton and Mallows (1965) in a corollary to a theorem of Karlin and McGregor (1959) provided the ballot problem result.

Barton and Mallows' proof applies Karlin and McGregor's theorem, for the case of L independent Poisson processes $X_i(t)$ with common density λ, simultaneously starting at time 0 and ending at time T. Let the ith process start out at time 0 at α_i, and end at time T at $\alpha_i + a_i$, $i = 1, 2, \ldots, L$. Order the process by $\alpha_1 > \alpha_2 > \cdots > \alpha_L$, and assume that $\alpha_1 + a_1 > \alpha_2 + a_2 > \cdots > \alpha_L + a_L$. Let $X_i(t) + \alpha_i$ denote the accumulated number of votes for candidate i after t votes have been counted. Then Karlin and McGregor's theorem states that for the L simultaneous Poisson processes $X_i(t)$, starting out, respectively, at $X_i(0) = \alpha_i$, $i = 1, 2, \ldots, L$:

$$P\left\{\bigcap_i[(X_i(t) + \alpha_i > X_{i+1}(t) + \alpha_{i+1})] \cap \left[\bigcap_i(X_i(T) = \alpha_i + a_i)\right]\right\}$$

$$= \det\left|(\lambda T)^{c_{ij}} e^{-\lambda T}/c_{ij}!\right|, \tag{8.19}$$

where

$$c_{ij} = a_i + \alpha_i - \alpha_j.$$

Note that the Karlin and McGregor result (8.19) is not conditioned on (but is instead joint with) the ending values. To find the probability conditional on the endpoints, it is necessary to divide by the probability of achieving the end values, which is the product, $\prod_i c_{ii}!$. Once the problem is conditioned on the endpoints, all orders of increases in the paths are equally likely, and this yields

$$P\big(X_1(m) + \alpha_1 > X_2(m) + \alpha_2 > \cdots > X_L(m) + \alpha_L;$$
$$m = 1, 2, \ldots, N \mid \{a_i, \alpha_i\}\big) = \det|a_i!/(a_i + \alpha_i - \alpha_j)!|. \tag{8.20}$$

In Barton and Mallows' corollary (8.20) substitute $v_i(t)$ for $X_i(m)$, n_i for a_i, and $n_r - k$ for $\alpha_{r+1} - \alpha_r$. Sum in the resulting equation to find

$$P\left(\sup_{i,t}\{n_i - v_i(t) + v_{i+1}(t)\} < k \mid \{n_i\}\right) / \prod_i n_i! = \det|1/c_{ij}!|. \tag{8.21}$$

Substitute (8.21) into (8.18) to develop a formula for $P(k; N, 1/L)$. Naus (1966a) uses the above approach to prove the following theorem:

Theorem 8.1. *Let $2 \le k \le N$ and $L \ge 2$ be integers. Then*

$$P(k; N, 1/L) = 1 - N! \, L^{-N} \sum_{\sigma} \det|1/c_{ij}!|, \tag{8.22}$$

122

where

$$c_{ij} = (j - i)k - \left(\sum_{r=i}^{j-1} n_r\right) + n_i, \qquad i < j,$$

$$= (j - i)k + \sum_{r=j}^{i} n_r, \qquad i \geq j,$$

and where the sum is over the set σ of all partitions of N into L positive integers $n_i < k$, $i = 1, 2, \ldots, L$.

Equation (8.22) for $P(k; N, 1/L)$ is in terms of sums of $L \times L$ determinants. Wolf (1968) developed an algorithm to compute $P(k; N, 1/L)$, and tabulated these values for $N = 2(1)10$, $L = 3(1)10$, $2 \leq k \leq N/2$, and $N = 11(1)20$, $L = 3(1)7$, $2 \leq k \leq N/2$. Wolf found that (8.22) was not computationally practical beyond this range (given the computer power then). For large values of L (small w), the size of the determinants gets very large. For N large, and w small, the number of partitions to be summed over gets out of hand. Wolf (1968) points out that in order to compute $P(4; 10, .1)$, one needs 34,803 (10×10) determinants. For $w = .001$ one would need to sum many 1000×1000 determinants.

Research on the exact distribution of $P(k; N, w)$ proceeded in two complementary ways. Formulas generalizing Theorem 8.1 were found for $P(k; N, w)$ for all w. Procedures were developed to use these formulas to generate explicit polynomial formulas to efficiently compute special cases.

8.6   Simplifying Theorem 8.1 for the Special Case $P(k; N, 1/3)$

The reader can check that (8.22) agrees with (8.8) for $P(k; N, 1/L)$, $L = 2, 3$ and $k > N/2$. Equation (8.8) had given $P(k; N, 1/2)$ for all nontrivial cases of k and N. However, for $P(k; N, 1/3)$, (8.8) only gives the formula for $k > N/2$, but does not handle the remaining nontrivial case $(N/3) + 1 \leq k \leq N/2$. Applying Theorem 8.1, and expanding the 3×3 determinant, and summing gives the following result (Naus, 1966a):

Corollary 8.1. For $(N/3) + 1 \leq k \leq N/2$, $N \geq 6$:

$$P(k; N, 1/3) = 3G_b(k; N, 1/3) + 3G_b(2k; N, 2/3)$$

$$- 6 \sum_{t=2k}^{N} b(t; N, 2/3)G_b(k; t, 1/2)$$

$$+ (3k - N - 2)b(k; N, 1/3)\{1 - 2G_b(k; N - k, 1/2)\}$$

$$+ G_b(k + 1; N, 1/3) - G_b(4k - N - 1; N; 1/3)$$

$$-2 \sum_{i=2(N-2k+1)}^{N-k-1} b(N-i; N, 1/3)G_b(N-2k+1; i, 1/2)$$

$$+ b(2k; N, 2/3)\{(2k-N-1)G_b(N-2k+2; 2k, 1/2)$$

$$+ kG_b(N-2k+1; 2k-1; 1/2) - .5(3k-N-1)$$

$$- .5[k+(3k-N-1)^2]b(k; 2k, 1/2)\}. \tag{8.23}$$

In theory, we could apply Theorem 8.1 directly to find $P(k; N, 1/3)$ for any k and N. However, for large N the number of partitions of N is large, and it is not efficient to use (8.22). Equation (8.23) can be readily evaluated even for large N, using tables (or program) for the binomial and cumulative binomial distribution. A short table for $6 \le N \le 20$, and all $(N/3) + 1 \le k \le N/2$, is given in Naus (1966a, p. 1194).

8.7 General Formula for $P(k; N, w)$

Recall the reasoning underlying the combinatorial approach to (8.8). From the direct integration approach it can be shown that for given k, N, $P(k; N, w)$ is a polynomial in w, for $0 \le w \le 1/C$ for $C = C(k, N)$ sufficiently large. Given enough values of the polynomial for different w, we could fit the polynomial exactly. In particular, if we can find the polynomial expression for $P(k; N, w)$ for $w = 1/L$ for all integer $L \ge C(k, N)$, then this same polynomial will apply for $P(k; N, w)$ for all $0 \le w \le 1/C(k, N)$. For given k and N we could use Theorem 8.1 to find $P(k; N, 1/L)$ for enough L values ($L \ge C(k, N)$) to fit the polynomial in w for the tail range $0 \le w \le 1/C(k, N)$. (We call this a tail result.) Equations (8.1), (8.2), and (8.8) are all examples of tail results.

The other ranges for the piecewise polynomials are of the form $\{i/L, (i+1)/L\}$. To fit the polynomial for $i/L \le w \le (i + 1)/L$, we need a general formula that gives multiple values in the range. Wallenstein and Naus (1973) give a formula for $P(k; N, r/L)$ and r and L integers. View the unit interval divided into L disjoint equal-sized intervals, and let n_i denote the number of the N points in the ith interval. Let

$$J(a, b) = \sum_{i=a}^{b} n_i$$

and let V denote the set of $n_i \ge 0$, $i = 1, \ldots, L$, such that $J(1, L) = N$ and $J(i, i + r - 1) < k$ for $i \le L - r + 1$.

Theorem 8.2. *Given that r and L are positive integers with greatest common denominator of one, $0 < r/L < 1$, and given k and N are integers, with $2 \le k \le N$, then*

$$P(k; N, r/L) = 1 - N! \, L^{-N} \sum_V \prod_{s=1}^{r} \det D^s, \tag{8.24}$$

where D^s is a square matrix with elements $1/d_{a,b}(s)!$, where

$$
\begin{aligned}
d_{a,b}(s) &= (b-a)k - J(s+1+[a-1]r, s-1+[b-1]r), &\quad a < b, \\
&= (b-a)k - J(s+[b-1]r, s+[a-1]r), &\quad a \geq b,
\end{aligned}
$$

subject to convention that $1/x! = 0$ for $x < 0$.

Proof. Let B_i denote the event that no $\mathcal{A}_i$ occurs and that there exists an interval of length $1/L$, overlapping $([i-1]L, iL)$ and $(iL, (i+1)L)$ that contains at least k points. For general r and L, there are $(L-r)$ B_i's to consider, and these are grouped into r sets, $c(1), \dots, c(r)$, where $c(i) = \{s \mid s = i \pmod r, s \leq 1-r\}$. Let

$$
E_i = \bigcap_{s \in c(i)} B_s^c.
$$

Conditional on the $\{n_i\}$, the E_i's are mutually independent. The proof of Theorem 8.1 is used to find $P(E_1 \mid \{n_i\})$; the product of these probabilities are taken, and averaged over the multinomial distribution of $\{n_i\}$, to find (8.24).

Theorem 8.2 gives the formula for $P(k; N, r/L)$ in terms of the sums of products of several determinants. Huntington and Naus (1975) give a simpler expression for $P(k; N, w)$ for any w, in terms of the sum of products of two determinants. Let H denote the largest integer in $1/w$, and let $d = 1 - wH$.

Theorem 8.3. *Given k, N integers, $2 \leq k \leq N$, and $0 < w < 1$, let*

$$
M = \sum_{j=0}^{H} m_{2j+1},
$$

and

$$
R = N!\, d^M (w-d)^{N-M}.
$$

Then,

$$
P(k; N, w) = 1 - \sum_Q R \det|1/h_{ij}!| \det|1/v_{ij}!|, \tag{8.25}
$$

where the summation is over the set Q of all partitions of N into $(2H+1)$ integers m_i satisfying $m_i + m_{i+1} < k$, $i = 1, 2, \dots, 2H$, and where

$$h_{ij} = \sum_{s=2j-1}^{2i-1} m_s - (i - j)k \qquad 1 \le j \le i \le H + 1,$$

$$= - \sum_{s=2i}^{2j-2} m_s + (j - i)k, \qquad 1 \le i < j \le H + 1,$$

$$v_{ij} = \sum_{s=2j}^{2i} m_s - (i - j)k, \qquad 1 \le j \le i \le H,$$

$$= - \sum_{s=2i+1}^{2j-1} m_s - (j - i)k, \qquad 1 \le i < j \le H.$$

Proof. Let the points iw and $d + iw$, $i = 0, \ldots, L$, partition the unit interval into $2H + 1$ disjoint intervals, where the $H + 1$ odd intervals are of length d, and the remaining H intervals are of length $w - d$. Condition on the occuppany numbers $\{m_s\}$, $s = 1, \ldots, 2H + 1$. When the scanning interval of length w slides so that its left-most point is within the first odd interval $[0, d)$, it will always contain the m_2 points in $[d, w)$. The m_1 points in $[0, d)$ will drop out, and the m_3 points in $[w, w + d)$ come in. View the scanning of the unit interval in two stages. First let the left-most point of the scanning window of length w slide over all the odd intervals, then let it slide over the even intervals. Conditional on the $\{m_s\}$, the probability the scanning interval contains k or more points is the product of two probabilities. These probabilities can be evaluated by the procedure leading to Theorem 8.1, and the resulting product can be averaged over the multinomial distribution of the m_s. As a check, we note that if $d = 0$, then Theorem 8.3 reduces to Theorem 8.1.

Huntington (1974a) used Theorem 8.3 to compute $P(k; N, w)$ for $\{N = 3(1)15, k = 2(1)N, w = .21(.01).50\}$ and for $\{N = 16(1)30, k = 2(1)N, w = .26(.01).50\}$. Even within this range, direct use of the formula was sometimes complex, and certain of Huntington's values were corrected in Neff (1978). For larger N and smaller w, direct use of the formula was too complex.

Hwang (1977) derives an alternate general formula for $P(k; N, w)$ that extended somewhat the range of direct computation. Hwang's result is based on a generalized version of the Karlin–McGregor theorem that led (through the Barton and Mallows' corollary) to the proof of Theorem 8.1.

Theorem 8.4. *Given k, N integers, $2 \le k \le N$, and $0 < w < 1$, let $L = [1/w]$, $v = 1 - wL$, then*

$$P(k; N, w) = 1 - N! \sum_{\Phi} \det|g_{ij}/(\beta_j - \alpha_i)!| \qquad (8.26)$$

where for $\zeta = \max\{0, (\beta_{L+1} + 1 - \alpha_i)\}$:

$$g_{ij} = w^{(\beta_j - \alpha_i)} \sum_{s=\zeta}^{\beta_j - \alpha_i} b(s; \beta_j - \alpha_i, v/w), \qquad j \le L, \quad \beta_j - \alpha_i \ge 0,$$

$$= v^{(\beta_j - \alpha_i)}, \qquad\qquad\qquad\qquad j = L+1, \quad (\beta_j - \alpha_i) \ge 0,$$

$$= 0, \qquad\qquad\qquad\qquad\qquad\quad (\beta_j - \alpha_i) < 0,$$

and where the sum of over the set Φ *of all partitions of* N *into* $L+1$ *integers each of which is less than* k.

Neff (1978, pp. 94–97) notes that the correct value for ζ is as given in (8.26), and shows how to use the Hwang formula to derive the conditional probability $P(k; N, w)$ for the case $w > 1/2$, and also the corresponding unconditional (on N) probability. For the conditional case this is (8.9). Hwang's formula extends the range of computation somewhat over Theorem 8.3; however, neither method is practical for the case where w is very small.

8.8   Simplifying the General Formula for $P(k; N, w)$ for Broad Classes of Cases

One way around the difficulty of computing $P(k; N, w)$ for small w, is to use the general formula to derive the piecewise polynomial expressions for specific k, N values (or ranges of k, N values), and use these expressions for computation. For example, (8.8) gives a polynomial expression for $k > (N + 1)/2$ for all $0 \le w \le 1/2$. Such an expression allows us to compute $P(k; N, w)$ within this range for very small w values. We would like to derive similar expressions for other ranges of k and N. Wallenstein and Naus (1974) show a procedure to do this, and implement the procedure for the range $N/3 < k \le N/2$. Wallenstein (1971) tabulates $P(k; N, 1/L)$ for $\{N = 6(1)20, L = 3(1)10(5)50, N/3 < k \le N/2\}$ and for $\{N = 20(1)100, L = 3(1)10, N/3 < k \le N/2\}$. Wallenstein and Naus (1974) give a table for $P(k; N, 1/L)$ for

$$\{N = 6(1)10(2)20(10)60(20)100, \ L = 3(1)10(5)50, \ N/3 < k \le N/2\}.$$

We describe in detail this approach.

Wallenstein (1971) generalizes the combinatorial approach for $P(k; N, 1/L)$, $k \le (N + 1)/2, L \ge 2$. Divide the unit interval into L disjoint intervals, $\{(i - 1)/L, i/L\}$, $i = 1, 2, \ldots, L$. Let $\mathcal{A}_i$ denote the event that there are at least k points in the ith interval. Let B_i denote the event that no $\mathcal{A}_i$ occurs, and that there exists an interval of length $1/L$ overlapping the ith and $(i + 1)$st intervals that contains at least k points. Let $\mathcal{A} = \bigcup \mathcal{A}_i$ and $B = \bigcup B_i$, $\mathcal{A}$ and B are mutually exclusive events, and (8.11) holds

$$P(k; N, 1/L) = P(\mathcal{A} \cup B) = P(\mathcal{A}) + P(B). \qquad (8.27)$$

8.8.1 Finding $P(\mathcal{A})$

To calculate $P(\mathcal{A})$ we can sum the multinomial probability $(L^{-N}N!/\prod n_i!)$ of the number of points in the L intervals (cells). Summing the probability over the set where all cell numbers are less than k gives $1 - P(\mathcal{A})$. Alternatively, we can apply the principle of exclusion and inclusion to $P(\mathcal{A}) = P(\bigcup \mathcal{A}_i)$, and evaluate only the necessary terms. For example, for $N/3 < k \leq N/2$, the $\mathcal{A}_i$ are not mutually exclusive events. Apply the principle of exclusion and inclusion to find

$$P(\mathcal{A}) = LP(\mathcal{A}_i) - [L(L-1)/2]P(\mathcal{A}_1 \cap \mathcal{A}_2)$$

and

$$P(\mathcal{A}_i) = LG_b(k; N, 1/L).$$

To find $P(\mathcal{A}_1 \cap \mathcal{A}_2)$ sum over the trinomial distribution for the points in cell 1, cell 2, and the rest of the unit interval. For the general case, one can use a recursion formula to find $P(\mathcal{A})$. Let $h_k(N, L)$ denote the number of ways of distributing N distinguishable balls (points) into L distinguishable cells (intervals) in such a way that every cell has less than k balls. Here the points (balls) are distinguished by their relative nearness to the beginning of their cell interval, $P(\mathcal{A}) = 1 - L^{-N}h_k(N, L)$. Riordan (1958, p. 102) gives the recursion formula

$$h_k(N+1, L) = Lh_k(N, L) - Lh_k(N-k+1, L-1)\binom{N}{k-1}, \qquad (8.28)$$

where $h_k(0, L) = 1$, $L \geq 0$. See Kozelka (1980) for some other references to compute the distribution of the maximum of a multinomial sample.

8.8.2 Finding $P(B)$

To compute $P(B) = P(\bigcup B_l)$, apply the principle of exclusion and inclusion, and use the exchangeability of certain combinations of B_i's. For any given ratio of N to k, there are a given number of combinations of B_i's to evaluate.

For example, for $k > (N+1)/2$, B_i and B_{i+1} can simultaneously happen. We only need $P(B_i)$ and $P(B_i \cap B_{i+1})$. By symmetry, $P(B_i) = P(B_1)$ and $P(B_i \cap B_{i+1}) = P(B_1 \cap B_2)$. Applying the principle of exclusion and inclusion gives, $P(B) = (L-1)P(B_1) - (L-2)P(B_1 \cap B_2)$. For this case, we only have to compute the probability for the two canonical symmetry types, B_1 and $B_1 \cap B_2$.

For $N/3 < k \leq N/2$, there are seven symmetry types of intersections of B_i's. We can list these, and group them in terms of the number of runs of consecutive subscript B's, as follows:

one run:	B_1,	$B_1 \cap B_2$,	$B_1 \cap B_2 \cap B_3$,	$B_1 \cap B_2 \cap B_3 \cap B_4$,
two runs:	$B_1 \cap B_3$,	$B_1 \cap B_3 \cap B_4$,	$B_1 \cap B_2 \cap B_4 \cap B_5$.	

(Note, for example, that $B_1 \cap B_3 \cap B_4$ and $B_1 \cap B_2 \cap B_4$ have equal probabilities.) We can denote the symmetry types in terms of the length of the runs of consecutive

B's in the combination type. Thus, $B_1 \cap B_3 \cap B_4$ is a $(1, 2)$ type. For $N/3 < k \le N/2$, the canonical symmetry types are: one run: $1, 2, 3, 4$; two runs: $(1, 1)$, $(1, 2)$, $(2, 2)$.

Note that different runs of B's depend on nonoverlapping sets of intervals. For example, $B_1 \cap B_2 \cap B_4 \cap B_5$ are two runs of B's and $B_1 \cap B_2$ depends on the first three intervals, while $B_4 \cap B_5$ depends on the fourth through sixth intervals. This implies that each run of B's requires at least k points, and the number of runs cannot exceed N/k. It further implies that, conditional on the cell occupancy numbers, the occurrence of one run of B's is independent of the occurrence of another run. Thus, $P(B_1 \cap B_2 \cap B_4 \cap B_5) \mid \{n_i\}) = P(B_1 \cap B_2 \mid \{n_i\}) P(B_4 \cap B_5 \mid \{n_i\})$. We explain below how to find these conditional probabilities, and use them to find the probability of a particular combination of B_i's. To find $P(B)$, we apply the principle of exclusion and inclusion over the set of possible combinations of B_i's. We first consider the general types of combinations of B_i's that are of interest, taking into account the symmetry conditions of the problem and the types of combinations that can occur for given N and k.

In general, any intersection of B_i's can be denoted in terms of I, the number of runs; $S = (s_1, s_2, \ldots, s_I)$ where s_i is the starting index of the ith run; and $R = (r_1, r_2, \ldots, r_I)$ where r_i is the number of B_j's in the ith run. The tth run of B_i's is the intersection of B_j, $s_t \le j \le s_t + r_t - 1$. Denote the general intersection of I runs of B_i's by $B(S, R, I)$. The event

$$B(S, R, I) = \bigcap_{t=1}^{I} \bigcap_{j=s_t}^{s_t + r_t - 1} B_j.$$

The runs must be separated in the sense that the last index in one run must be at least two less than the index starting the next run; this requires $s_{i+1} > s_i + r_i$. Since each run must have at least one B_i, $r_i \ge 1$.

For a given ratio of N to k, only certain combinations of B_i's can occur. A run of four B's, $B_1 \cap B_2 \cap B_3 \cap B_4$ requires at least $2k + 1$ points, the lower limit requiring the number of points in the first five cells to be $(1, k - 1, 1, k - 1, 1)$. A run of J B's requires at least $V(J)$ points where $V(J) = [(J + 1)/2]k$ for J odd and $([J/2]k) + 1$ for J even. For a given N and k, the set of all possible intersections of the B_i's is contained in the set of all $B(S, R, I)$ where (S, R, I) satisfy the constraints

$$s_{i+1} > s_i + r_i, \qquad s_I + r_I \le L, \qquad s_i > 0, \quad r_i \ge 1, \quad I \le [L/2], \quad (8.29)$$

$$\sum_{r_i=1}^{I} V(r_i) \le N, \qquad \sum_{i=1}^{I} (r_i + 1) \le L.$$

The symmetry conditions of the problem imply that for (S, R, I) that satisfy (8.29), that the probability of $B(S, R, I)$ does not depend on the starting numbers S, nor on the order of the r_i's in R. For example, $P(B_1 \cap B_2 \cap B_4 \cap B_5 \cap B_6) =$

$P(B_5 \cap B_6 \cap B_7 \cap B_9 \cap B_{10})$. We can thus concentrate on a smaller set of intersections of B's of the form $B(S, R, I)$ where (S, R, I) satisfy (8.29) and

$$s_i = 1, \qquad s_{i+1} = s_i + r_i + 1 \qquad \text{and} \qquad r_1 \leq r_2 \leq \cdots \leq r_I. \qquad (8.30)$$

Let $V(L, k, N)$ denote the set of all (S, R, I) that simultaneously satisfy (8.29) and (8.30).

Recall our view of the sample space. We divide the unit interval into L disjoint intervals, $([i-1]/L, iL), i = 1, 2, \ldots, L$. To compute the probabilities we seek, view the sample space as consisting of L^N equally likely ways to distribute the N distinguishable points over the L distinct intervals. View the points as distinguished by their relative nearness to the beginning of whichever interval they fall into. Let $N(S, R, I \mid L, k, N)$ denote the number of the L^N equally likely ways that leads to the event $B(S, R, I)$. Abbreviate $N(S, R, I \mid L, k, N)$ to $N(S, R, I)$ when L, k, N are clear from context. Theorem 8.5 derives a general formula for $P(B)$ in terms of the $N(S, R, I)$ and gives a recursion formula for $N(S, R, I)$. Theorem 8.6 derives a direct formula for $N(S, R, I)$.

Theorem 8.5. *For k, N, L integers, $2 \leq k \leq N, L \geq 2$:*

$$P(B) = L^{-N} \sum_{V(L, k, N)} (-1)^{r(I)+1} [L - r(i)]! \, N(S, R, I)/(L - r(I) - I)! \prod_i d_i!,$$
$$(8.31)$$

where $r(I) = \sum_{1 \leq i \leq I} r_i$ and where d_i is the number of values in the set $r_1, \ldots, r_I$ such that $r_j = i, j \leq I, \sum d_i = I$. Further, for S, R, I in $V(L, k, N)$:

$$N(S, R, I) = \sum [N!/(N - M)!] h_k(N - M, L - r(I) - I)$$
$$\times \left\{ \prod_{i=1}^{I} N(1, r_i, 1 \mid r_i + 1, k, M_i)/M_i! \right\}, \qquad (8.32)$$

where the sum is over all values of M_i such that $\sum_{1 \leq i \leq I} M_i \leq N$, and $V(r_i) \leq M_i \leq (r_i + 1)(k - 1)$ for $i = 1, 2, \ldots, I$, and $h_k(N, L)$ is defined prior to (8.28).

Proof. We outline the proof and leave the details to the reader. A more detailed proof appears in Wallenstein and Naus (1974). The proof of (8.31) applies the principle of exclusion and inclusion to $P(B) = P(\bigcup B_i)$, and uses the symmetry conditions embodied in $V(L, k, N)$.

Equation (8.32) introduces the quantities M_i, which denote the number of points in the intervals involved in the ith run of B's. The ith run of B's involves $r_i + 1$ intervals. I sets of runs involve M points spread over $r(I) + I$ intervals. The remaining $N - M$ points are distributed in the remaining $L - r(I) - I$ intervals. Conditional on the number of points $\{n_i\}$ in the L intervals, and given S, R, I in $V(L, k, N)$, the number of arrangements of N points in L intervals that leads to $B(S, R, I)$ is the product of three terms. The first term is the product (over i, $1 \leq i \leq I$) of the arrangements of the M_i points in $r_i + 1$ cells leading to the ith run. The second term is the number of unrestricted arrangements of the remaining $N - M$ points in $L - r(I) - I$ remaining cells. The third term is the number of ways to mix the first two mentioned sets of arrangements. We sum the product of the three terms to complete the proof.

Note that Theorem 8.5 gives a practical way to construct tables of $P(B)$, and thus $P(k; N, 1/L)$. Formula (8.32) uses quantities of the form $N(1, r, 1 \mid r + 1, k, M) = (r + 1)^M P(\bigcap_{j=1}^r B_j)$. In the proof of Theorem 8.1, let $L = r$. This allows us to find $P(\bigcap_{j=1}^r B_j^c)$, where B_j^c denotes the complement of B_j. Write

$$P\left(\bigcap_{j=1}^r B_j\right) = 1 - P\left(\bigcup_{j=1}^r B_j^c\right), \qquad (8.33)$$

and apply the principle of exclusion and inclusion to the latter term. Apply the proof of Theorem 8.1 directly to find the probability of the intersection of consecutively indexed B's, $P(\bigcap_{j=1}^r B_j^c)$. For the case of nonconsecutive B's, use the conditional (on $\{n_i\}$) argument.

Theorem 8.6 gives a direct expression for $P(\bigcap_{j=1}^{L-1} B_j)$. Let $R^*(L)$ denote the set of all permutations of the integers $1, 2, \ldots, L$. Let $j_1, j_2, \ldots, j_L$ denote a typical permutation of the first L integers. Let d denote the number of inversions in $j_1, j_2, \ldots, j_L$. Let $H_i = \{j_i, j_i + 1, \ldots, i - 1\}$ if $i > j$, and equal the null set if $i \leq j$. Let $R(L)$ denote the subset of $R^*(L)$ such that $\bigcup_{1 \leq i \leq L} H_i = \{1, 2, \ldots, L - 1\}$. For example, $R^*(3) = (2, 3, 1); (3, 1, 2); (3, 2, 1)$.

Theorem 8.6. *Given $2 \leq k \leq N, 2 \leq L$:*

$$P\left(\bigcap_{j=1}^{L-1} B_j\right) = N! \, L^{-N} \sum_\sigma \sum_{R(L)} (-1)^{d+L-1} \prod_{a=1}^L (1/c_{aj_a}!), \qquad (8.34)$$

where

$$c_{ij} = (j - i)k - \left(\sum_{r=i}^{j-1} n_r\right) + n_i \qquad i < j,$$

$$= (j - i)k + \sum_{r=j}^i n_r, \qquad\qquad i \geq j,$$

and where σ is the set of all partitions of N into L positive integers $n_i < k$, $i = 1, 2, \ldots, L$; d is the number of inversions in $j_1, j_2, \ldots, j_L$, and $1/x! = 0$ for $x < 0$.

Proof. Note that c_{ij} is as defined in Theorem 8.1, (8.22). It is sufficient to prove that for all $(n_1, n_2, \ldots, n_L)$ in σ, that conditional on $(n_1, n_2, \ldots, n_L)$, the number of arrangements that lead to $\bigcap_{j=1}^{L-1} B_j$ satisfy

$$N\left(\bigcap_{j=1}^{L-1} B_j \mid n_1, n_2, \ldots, n_L\right) = N! \, L^{-N} \sum_{R(L)} (-1)^{d+L-1} \prod_{a=1}^L (1/c_{aj_a}!). \quad (8.35)$$

For $L = 2$, (8.35) holds. From (8.14):

$$N(B_1 \mid n_1, n_2) = (n_1 + n_2)!/k! \, (n_1 + n_2 - k)! = (n_1 + n_2)! \, c_{12!}c_{21!}.$$

In the 2×2 determinant C (Theorem 8.1, for $L = 2$), there are only two products, namely, $c_{11!}c_{22!}$ and $c_{12!}c_{21!}$. The indices of $c_{12!}c_{21!}$ belong to $R(2)$, while the indices of $c_{11!}c_{22!}$ do not. This proves that (8.35) holds for $L = 2$. The rest of the proof is by induction. (For details, see Wallenstein and Naus (1974, Proof of Theorem 2).) The reader can better interpret the result by expanding the determinant of the matrix $(1/c_{ij}!)$ in (8.22) for the case $L = 3$. The terms will fall into sets corresponding to the events B_1, B_2, and $B_1 \cap B_2$. $N(B_1 \mid n_1, n_2, n_3) = N!$ $c_{12!}c_{21!}c_{33!}$. $N(B_2 \mid n_1, n_2, n_3) = N! \, c_{11!}c_{23!}c_{32!}$. $N(B_1 \cap B_2 \mid n_1, n_2, n_3)$ can be computed from the rest of the terms using relation (8.33):

$$N(B_1 \cap B_2 \mid n_1, n_2, n_3)$$
$$= N! \, (c_{12!}c_{23!}c_{31!} + c_{13!}c_{21!}c_{32!} - c_{13!}c_{22!}c_{31!})$$
$$= [N!/k!\,k!\,(N - 2k)!] + [N!/(2k - n_2)! \, (n_1 + n_2 - k)! \, (n_2 + n_3 - k)!]$$
$$- [N!/(2k - n_2)! \, n_2! \, (N - 2k)!]. \tag{8.36}$$

For $k > N/2$, the first and third terms vanish, and this leads to the conditional result preceding (8.16) for $P(B_1 \cap B_2 \mid n_1, n_2, n_3)$. Equation (8.36) gives the result for general k and N, conditional on the occupancy numbers n_1, n_2, n_3 in the first three cells. To find the number of arrangements over all L cells leading to $B_1 \cap B_2$, conditional on all L cell occupancy numbers, write:

$$N(B_1 \cap B_2) = \sum N(B_1 \cap B_2 \mid n_1, n_2, n_3) N!/(n_1 + n_2 + n_3)! \, n_3! \, n_4! \dots n_L!, \tag{8.37}$$

where the sum is over $n_i < k$ for $i = 3, \dots, L$. This example illustrates the basic idea behind Theorem 8.6.

8.9 Generating the Piecewise Polynomials from the General Formulas

We saw that one way around the difficulty of computing $P(k; N, w)$ for small w, is to use the general formula to derive the piecewise polynomial expressions for specific k, N values (or ranges of k, N values), and use these expressions for computation. For example, (8.8) gives a polynomial expression for $k > (N+1)/2$ for all $0 \le w \le 1/2$. Such an expression allows us to compute $P(k; N, w)$ within this range for very small w values. Wallenstein and Naus (1974) show a procedure for doing this, and implement the procedure for the range $N/3 < k \le N/2$. Given a general formula for $P(k; N, w)$ there are different ways to use the information in the formula to find computationally efficient forms. Theorem 8.3, (8.25), used a particular partition of the unit interval into $2H + 1$ parts, to find a general formula for $P(k; N, w)$ as the sum of products of two determinants. Neff (1978) uses the results of such general formulas in a systematic way to derive the piecewise polynomials for $P(k; N, w)$ for specific k and N values. To illustrate Neff's approach recall formula (8.5) for $P(3; 8, w)$, and see how it might be derived by this approach,

$$
\begin{aligned}
1 - P(3; 8, w) &= 14(1 - 3w)^8 - (1 - 4w)^6(13 - 24w), & 0 \le w \le 1/4, \\
&= 14(1 - 3w)^8, & 1/4 \le w \le 1/3, \\
&= 0, & 1/3 \le w \le 1.
\end{aligned}
$$

Suppose that Elteren and Gerritis (1961) had not done the direct integration to find formula (8.5), and that we sought the probability $P(3; 8, 1/100)$. To apply Theorem 8.1 would involve summing 100×100 determinants. Not practical! Direct application of Theorem 8.3 appears useless. It would have been easy to use Theorem 8.1 to find $P(3; 8, 1/4)$ since that only involves summing 4×4 determinants. We could even use Theorem 8.3 to find $P(3; 8, w)$ for some w in the range $1/5 < w \le 1/4$ since that would only involve summing the product of two determinants, one 4×4, and the other 5×5. We could use Theorem 8.3 to compute $P(3; 8, w)$ for as many w as we like in the range $1/5 < w \le 1/4$. If we know that $P(3; 8, w)$ is a polynomial in w for $0 \le w \le 1/4$, we could use enough of the computed values (for the range $1/5 < w \le 1/4$) to fit the polynomial. Neff (1978) proved

Theorem 8.7. $P(k; N, w)$ *is a polynomial in w on the domain* $0 \le w \le 1/\{[N/k]+ [(N - 1)/k]\}$, *where $[x]$ denotes the largest integer in x.*

For the example, $P(3; 8, w)$, Theorem 8.7 states that it is a polynomial in w for $0 \le w \le 1/\{[8/3] + [7/3]\} = 1/4$. We can thus use Theorem 8.3 to find the polynomial for $P(3; 8, w)$ for $0 < w \le 1/4$. Neff (1978) notes this can be done directly, by modifying the definition of H in Theorem 8.3. Immediately prior to Theorem 8.3, H is defined as the largest integer in $1/w$, and $d = 1 - wH$. Instead let H be defined as the minimum of the quantities $[1/w]$ and $\{[N/k]+[(N-1)/k]\}$. Even with this modification, the computation of the pieces of the polynomials $P(k; N, w)$ can be computationally intensive. Neff (1978) rearranges the formula in Theorem 8.3, and develops a variety of approaches to allow for more efficient generation of the piecewise polynomials. This is detailed in Neff and Naus (1980), and the full set of piecewise polynomials are given in Table 3 of that book, for $\{k = 3, 4; N = k(1)16\}$, $\{k = 5; N = k(1)17\}$, $\{k = 6; N = 6(1)18\}$, $\{k = 7; N = k(1)19\}$, $\{k = 8, 9, N = k(1)20\}$. These polynomials together with (8.2) for $k = 2$, and (8.8) and (8.9) for $k > N/2$, $w \le 1/2$, and for the case $w > 1/2$ give all the piecewise polynomials for $N < 20$. (For $N = 20$, the piecewise polynomials are given for all k except 10; the program then being used was reaching the limits of the quadruple precision.) Tables of exact values of $P(k; N, w)$ are also given in Neff and Naus (1980).

8.10 The Approach of Huffer and Lin

The r-scan statistic can be viewed as the maximum of a sum of r consecutive spacings. Formally, let $X_1, X_2, \ldots, X_N$, be i.i.d. uniform random variables. Let $X_{(1)} \leq X_{(2)} \leq \cdots \leq X_{(N)}$ denote the ordered values of the X's. The quantities $X_{(i+1)} - X_{(i)}$ are called the *spacings*, between the ith and $(i+1)$st point. The scan statistic W_k can be viewed as the minimum of the sum of k consecutive spacings:

$$W_k = \min_{1 \leq i \leq N-k+1} \{X_{(i+k-1)} - X_{(i)}\} = \min_{1 \leq i \leq N-k+1} \left\{ \sum_{j=1}^{k-1} (X_{(j+i)} - X_{(j+i-1)}) \right\}.$$

Lin (1993) and Huffer and Lin (1997b) develop a general approach to find the distribution of the minimum (or maximum) of sums of adjacent spacings. They apply their approach to find the distribution of the scan statistic. Their approach uses a recursion to rewrite the joint distribution of linear combinations of spacings as the sum of simple explicit components. Their results give the piecewise polynomial expressions for the distribution of the scan statistic.

We first illustrate their approach for the simple example of deriving the piecewise polynomial for $P(3; 4, w)$. Given X_1, X_2, X_3, X_4, i.i.d. uniform $[0, 1)$ random variables, let $X_{(1)} \leq X_{(2)} \leq X_{(3)} \leq X_{(4)}$ denote the ordered values of the X's. Let

$$S_1 = X_{(1)}, \quad S_2 = X_{(2)} - X_{(1)}, \quad S_3 = X_{(3)} - X_{(2)},$$
$$S_4 = X_{(4)} - X_{(3)}, \quad S_5 = 1 - X_{(4)},$$

$$1 - P(3, 4; w) = P\{(X_{(3)} - X_{(1)} > w) \cap (X_{(4)} - X_{(2)} > w)\}$$
$$= P\{(S_2 + S_3 > w) \cap (S_3 + S_4 > w)\}.$$

Lin (1993) writes this last term in matrix notation. Let S denote the 5×1 vector $(S_1, S_2, S_3, S_4, S_5)'$, let w denote the 2×1 vector $(w, w)'$, and let Γ denote the 2×5 matrix:

$$\begin{pmatrix} 0 & 1 & 1 & 0 & 0 \\ 0 & 0 & 1 & 1 & 0 \end{pmatrix}.$$

Then $1 - P(3; 4, w)$ can be written in the matrix notation $P(\Gamma S > w)$. Lin uses an approach of Huffer (1988) to simplify the computation of this probability by using the following recursion which applies to the (in general, $n + 1$) uniform spacings. (Lin also proves the result for exponential spacings.)

Theorem 8.8 (Theorem 4.1 in Lin (1993)). *Let S denote an $(n + 1) \times 1$ vector $(S_1, S_2, \ldots, S_{n+1})'$ of uniform spacings, let w denote a $k \times 1$ vector of constants, and let Γ denote a $k \times (n + 1)$ real matrix. Let $d = (d_1, d_2, \ldots, d_{n+1})'$ be a $(n + 1) \times 1$ vector of constants that sum to 1. (The individual d_i's can be positive, negative, or zero.) Let $\xi = \Gamma d$, be a $k \times 1$ vector. Let $\Gamma_{i,\xi}$ be the $k \times (n + 1)$*

matrix obtained by replacing the ith column of Γ by ξ. Then

$$P(\Gamma S > w) = \sum_{1 \leq i \leq n+1} d_i P(\Gamma_{i,\xi} S > w).$$

Applying this theorem to our example, let $d = (0, 1, -1, 1, 0)$. Then $\xi = \Gamma d$ is the 2×1 column vector $(0, 0)'$, and $P(\Gamma S > w) = 0P(\Gamma_{1,\xi} S > w) + 1P(\Gamma_{2,\xi} S > w) - 1P(\Gamma_{3,\xi} S > w) + 1P(\Gamma_{4,\xi} S > w) + 0P(\Gamma_{5,\xi} S > w)$. Here

$$\Gamma_{2,\xi} = \begin{pmatrix} 0 & 0 & 1 & 0 & 0 \\ 0 & 0 & 1 & 1 & 0 \end{pmatrix}, \qquad \Gamma_{3,\xi} = \begin{pmatrix} 0 & 1 & 0 & 0 & 0 \\ 0 & 0 & 0 & 1 & 0 \end{pmatrix},$$

$$\Gamma_{4,\xi} = \begin{pmatrix} 0 & 1 & 1 & 0 & 0 \\ 0 & 0 & 1 & 0 & 0 \end{pmatrix}.$$

Note that $P(\Gamma_{2,\xi} S > w) = P\{(S_3 > w) \cap (S_3 + S_4 > w)\} = P(S_3 > w)$, since spacings are nonnegative. $P(\Gamma_{3,\xi} S > w) = P\{(S_2 > w) \cap (S_4 > w)\}$ and $P(\Gamma_{4,\xi} X > w) = P(S_3 > w)$. Thus, all the terms are simple in the sense that they involve the distribution of individual spacings, or the joint distribution of nonoverlapping sets of spacings. The probabilities are then simply computed from applying the following well-known result for uniform spacings (see (2.3) in Lin (1993)).

For constants $c_i \geq 0$:

$$P\left\{\bigcap_{i=1}^{n+1} (S_i > c_i)\right\} = \left(\left(1 - \sum_{i=1}^{n+1} c_i\right)_+\right)^n,$$

where $(y)_+ = \max(y, 0)$. Thus,

$$P(S_3 > w) = (1 - w)^4$$

and

$$P\{(S_2 > w) \cap (S_4 > w)\} = ((1 - 2w)_+)^4.$$

Lin's method yields:

$$1 - P(3; 4, w) = 2(1 - w)^4 - ((1 - 2w)_+)^4. \tag{8.38}$$

Expanding the terms in (8.38) gives the result (8.7) found earlier by direct integration

$$\begin{aligned} P(3; 4, w) &= 12w^2 - 24w^3 + 14w^4, & w \leq 1/2, \\ &= -1 + 8w - 12w^2 + 8w^3 - 2w^4, & w \geq 1/2. \end{aligned}$$

Formula (8.38) is more compact than formula (8.7), and this is a nice feature of Lin's method.

Lin describes the simplifications in terms of the Γ matrices. Columns of zeros can be eliminated. Rows that dominate another row (everywhere at least equal, and somewhere greater) are eliminated. Thus in $\Gamma_{2,\xi}$, the row 00110 is eliminated because of the row above it. Symmetries due to exchangeability of spacings mean that rows (or columns) can be exchanged. In terms of this symbolic approach, the original matrix Γ is simplified as follows: First drop the first and last columns of zeros. Then apply Theorem 8.8 to *expand* Γ, as

$$\begin{pmatrix} 1 & 1 & 0 \\ 0 & 1 & 1 \end{pmatrix} = 1 \begin{pmatrix} 0 & 1 & 0 \\ 0 & 1 & 1 \end{pmatrix} - 1 \begin{pmatrix} 1 & 0 & 0 \\ 0 & 0 & 1 \end{pmatrix} + 1 \begin{pmatrix} 1 & 1 & 0 \\ 0 & 1 & 0 \end{pmatrix} = 2(1) - 1 \begin{pmatrix} 1 & 0 \\ 0 & 1 \end{pmatrix}.$$

As a second illustration of their method and matrix notation, the following is the derivation of the piecewise polynomial for $P(3; 5, w)$. Let $S_i, i = 1, 2, \ldots, 6$, denote the six sample spacings. Dropping off the first and last column of zeros, gives the 3×4 Γ matrix, with rows (1100; 0110; 0011). (The matrix refers to spacings $S_i, i = 2, \ldots, 5$.) Let $d = (1 \ -1 \ 1 \ 0)$ and $\xi = \Gamma d = (0 \ 0 \ 1)'$. Then we apply Theorem 8.8 to expand Γ, as

$$\Gamma = 1 \begin{pmatrix} 0100 \\ 0110 \\ 1011 \end{pmatrix} - 1 \begin{pmatrix} 1000 \\ 0010 \\ 0111 \end{pmatrix} + 1 \begin{pmatrix} 1100 \\ 0100 \\ 0011 \end{pmatrix} + 0 \begin{pmatrix} 1100 \\ 0110 \\ 0011 \end{pmatrix}.$$

Eliminate *dominating* rows, and then any columns of zeros in the resulting reduced matrices to find

$$\Gamma = 1 \begin{pmatrix} 1000 \\ 0111 \end{pmatrix} - 1 \begin{pmatrix} 10 \\ 01 \end{pmatrix} + 1 \begin{pmatrix} 100 \\ 011 \end{pmatrix}.$$

$$1 - P(3; 5, w) = P\{(S_2 > w) \cap (S_3 + S_4 + S_5 > w)\}$$
$$- P\{(S_2 > w) \cap (S_4 > w)\}$$
$$+ P\{(S_3 > w) \cap (S_4 + S_5 > w)\},$$

and by exchangeability of the S_i's, we can write this as

$$1 - P(3; 5, w) = P\{(S_1 > w) \cap (S_2 + S_3 + S_4 > w)\}$$
$$- P\{(S_1 > w) \cap (S_2 > w)\}$$
$$+ P\{(S_1 > w) \cap (S_2 + S_3 > w)\}.$$

As before, using Lin (1993, equation (2.3)):

$$P\{(S_1 > w) \cap (S_2 > w)\} = (1 - 2w)_+^5.$$

To find the other terms we use formula (2.4) in Lin (1993) (or equation (11) in Huffer and Lin, (1997b) which they note is a special case of a general result of Khatri and Mitra (1969). These other terms involve the intersection of disjoint sets of S_i's. Let $\delta_i, i = 1, 2, \ldots, r$, denote r disjoint (nonempty) sets of the integers $\{1, 2, \ldots, n + 1\}$, with cardinalities $1 + m_i, i = 1, 2, \ldots, r$. Let $\kappa =$

$(k_1, k_2, \ldots, k_r)$ denote an r-tuple of integers. Let $K = \sum k_i$. Let σ denote the set of values for $(k_1, k_2, \ldots, k_r)$, such that $0 \le k_i \le m_i$ for all $i = 1, 2, \ldots, r$:

$$P\left(\bigcap_{i=1}^{r}\{S(\delta_i) > w\}\right) = \sum_{\sigma}\binom{K}{k} R(K, r), \qquad (8.39)$$

where

$$R(j, r \mid n, w) = r^{-j} b(j; n, rw) = \binom{n}{j} w^j (1 - rw)^{n-j}, \quad rw < 1,$$

$$= 0, \quad \text{otherwise.}$$

Applying this result here to evaluate $P\{(S_1 > w) \cap (S_2 + S_3 > w)\}$, $r = 2$ sets, $m_1 = 0, m_2 = 1, \sigma = \{(0, 0); (0, 1)\}$:

$$P\{(S_1 > w) \cap (S_2 + S_3 > w)\} = R(0, 2) + R(1, 2).$$

Similarly,

$$P\{(S_1 > w) \cap (S_2 + S_3 + S_4 > w)\} = R(0, 2) + R(1, 2) + R(2, 2),$$

$$1 - P(3; 5, w) = 2R(0, 2) + 2R(1, 2) + R(2, 2) - (1 - 2w)^5, \quad w \le .5,$$

or

$$1 - P(3; 5, w) = 1 - 30w^2 + 100w^3 - 120w^4 + 48w^5, \qquad w \le .5.$$

This agrees with the polynomial for $P(3; 5, w)$ in Neff and Naus (1980).

Lin's method expands the range of values of N and k for which the polynomials for $P(k; N, w)$ can be computed, but there is still difficulty when k is small and N is large. They can go up to $N = 61$, but at that level only for k values fairly close to $N/2$. They note, for example, that they can compute $P(31; 61, w)$ using a Sparc 20 workstation in 21 seconds; and that they could get the polynomials for $P(19; 41, w)$, but not for $P(18; 41, w)$. The problem with the latter is due to high-memory requirement for storing of terms.

8.11 The Expectation and Variance of W_k, the Size of the Smallest Interval

The continuous random variable, W_k, has cumulative distribution function $P(W_k \le w) = F(w) = P(k; N, w)$. The sth moment of W_k can be evaluated by integrating over the appropriate densities. For example, for $k > (N + 1)/2$, (8.8) and (8.9) give

$$P(k; N, w) = C(k; N, w) \qquad\qquad w \le 1/2, \quad k > N/2,$$

$$= C(k; N, w) - R(k; N, w), \quad w \ge 1/2, \quad k > (N + 1)/2,$$

where $C(\ )$ and $R(\ )$ are defined following (8.9). For $k > (N+1)/2$:

$$E(\{W_k\}^s) = \int_0^1 w^s (\partial C(k; N, w)/\partial w)\, dw - \int_{.5}^1 w^s (\partial R(k; N, w)/\partial w)\, dw.$$

(8.40)

To evaluate the integrals in (8.40), use the following identity established by integration by parts,

$$\int_a^b w^s (\partial H(w)/\partial w)\, dw = b^s H(b) - a^s H(a) - s \int_a^b w^{s-1} H(w)\, dw. \quad (8.41)$$

Apply some identities—see Naus (1966a, p. 1198) for details—to prove for $(N+1)/2 < k \le N$:

$$E(W_k) = \{k - 2(N - k + 1)b\}(N + 1)$$
$$\text{where} \quad b = b(N - k + 1, 2(N - k + 1); .5)$$

and

$$\mathrm{Var}(W_k) = (N - k + 1)\{(N + k + 1) + 2(2k - N - 1)b$$
$$- 4(N + 2)(N - k + 1)b^2\}/(N + 1)^2(N + 2). \quad (8.42)$$

Neff and Naus (1980) generate tables for the expectation and variance of W_k for $\{k = 3, 4, 5; N = k(1)19\}$; $\{k = 6; n = 6(1)17\}$; $\{k = 7; N = 7(1)20\}$; $\{k = 8; N = 8(1)23\}$; $\{k = 9; N = 9(1)25\}$.

8.12   The Scan Statistic on the Circle

For certain applications it is reasonable to view the N points as being uniformly distributed over a circle rather than a line. In one application, a researcher may ask whether events (birthdays, or cases of a disease) tend to cluster during certain times of the year. In this case, the year is viewed as a circle, with December 31 adjacent to January 1. In another application, a molecular biologists might be looking at the clustering of certain genetic markers on a DNA strand. In some cases the strands are lines, but in other cases, such as E. coli, the strand is circular.

Let N points be independently drawn from the uniform distribution on the unit circle. Define S_w as the size of the maximum number of the N points in any arc of length w on the unit circle. Define W_k as the size of the smallest subarc of the unit circle that contains k points. The distributions of the scan statistics S_w and W_k are related, $P(S_w \ge k) = P(W_k \le w)$. We denote the common probability as $P_c(k; N, w)$.

Ajne (1968) derives $P_c(k, N, 1/2)$ as possibly an infinite series. Takacs (1996) derives $P_c(k, N, 1/3)$. Rothman (1972) computes $P_c(k, N, w)$ for $k > (N+1)/2$,

$w = 1/L$, $L > 4$. Wallenstein (1971) gives an algorithm (modified slightly and described below) for computing $P_c(K, N, 1/L)$ for $k > 2N/L$. Weinberg (1980) finds $P_c(k, N, r/L)$ for r and L relatively prime integers and $k \geq (r + 1)N/L$. Cressie (1977a,b,c) derives some interesting asymptotic results, but as will be elaborated below, his result is not sufficiently accurate. This chapter focuses on exact results for $P_c(k, N, 1/L)$; bounds and approximations are given, respectively, in Chapters 9 and 10.

8.12.1 Derivation of Exact Results

Results concerning the scan statistic on the topologically different circle do not arise as direct corollaries to the results for the line segment. Burnside (1928, p. 72) finds

$$P_c(N; N, w) = \sum_{r=1}^{m}(-1)^{r+1}\binom{N}{r}[1 - r(1 - w)]^{N-1},$$

$$1/(m + 1) < 1 - w < 1/m. \qquad (8.43)$$

$P_c(N; N, w)$ is piecewise polynomial in $(1 - w)$ even for this simple case. By contrast, the linear case has $P(N; N, w) = Nw^{N-1} - (N - 1)w^N$. Note that for $0 < w < 1/2$, the right-hand side of (8.43) reduces to Nw^{N-1}, and thus the complexity of the circular case occurs for $w \geq 1/2$.

Ajne (1968) finds the exact and asymptotic distribution of $P_c(k; N, 1/2)$. Takacs (1996) uses a combinatorial approach to find $P_c(k; N, 1/L)$ for $L = 2, 3$. For $k \leq (N + 1)/2$, $P_c(k; N, 1/2) = 1$. Takacs notes that use of the reflection principle (see Chapter 7) gives, for the nontrivial case, $(N + 1)/2 < k \leq N$:

$$P_c(k; N, 1/2) = (2k - N)(.5)^{2N-1} \sum_{r=0}^{[(N-k)/(2k-N)]}\binom{N}{k + (2k - N)r}, \qquad (8.44)$$

or, alternatively,

$$P_c(k; N, 1/2) = 1 - 2\sum_{r=1}^{[(2k-N)/2]}(-1)^{r-1}\left(\cos\{r\pi/(2k - N)\}\right)^N. \qquad (8.45)$$

For $w = 1/3$, $P_c(k; N, 1/3) = 1$ for $k \leq (N + 2)/3$. For $k > (N + 2)/3$, there are two nontrivial ranges to consider. Takacs (1996, Theorem 3) combines these

$$P_c(k; N, 1/3) = (9k - 3N)3^{-N}\sum_{r=k \bmod(3k-n)}\binom{N}{r}2^{N-r-1}$$

$$- .5\zeta(k, k, N - 2k)3^{-N}, \qquad (N/3) + 1 \leq k \leq N. (8.46)$$

where,

$$\zeta(k, k, N - 2k) = \sum_{x=0}^{3k-N-1}\sum_{y=0}^{3k-N-1}(1 + w^x + w^y)^N w^{-kx-ky}, \qquad (8.47)$$

where $w = \exp(2\pi i/(3k - N))$. This simplifies for a special part of the range to

$$P_c(k; N, 1/3) = (9k - 3N)\binom{N}{k}2^{N-k-1}3^{-N}, \qquad N/2 < k \le N. \qquad (8.48)$$

To derive exact results for $P_c(k; N, w)$, for general w, the overall ballot problem is not easily applicable since such problems are not traditionally formulated in a circular manner. However, we can use the results from the line to solve almost all problems of practical interest.

Take any arbitrary point on the circle as the origin. Let Y_t be the number of points in $[t, (t + w) \bmod 1)$. Define $\mathcal{A}$ and B_i, $i = 1, \ldots, L - 1$, as in Section 8.8. Define a new event $B_L = \{\mathcal{A}^c \cap (Y_t \ge k, \text{for some } t \text{ with } (L-1)/L < t < 1)\}$, and let $B = \bigcup_{i=1}^{L} B_i$. It then follows that $P_c(k, N, 1/L) = P(\mathcal{A}) + P_c(B)$.

We can still use the representation given by Theorem 8.5 with minor modifications. Let $B_c^*(I; R, S)$ be defined as in Section 8.8 except we relax the condition $s_i + r_i \le L$ to $s_i + r_i \le L + 1$. Similarly, define $B_c(I; R)$ as the *canonical form* with the change in the definition above implying that $S(r_i + 1) \le L + 1$, but being careful to note that, say for $L = 4$, $B_1 B_2 B_4$ maps into $B_1 B_2 B_3$. It will then follow for $w = 1/L$:

$$B_c(I; R) = B_c(I; R) \cup \{1, L\}. \qquad (8.49)$$

Let $M_c(I, R)$ be the number of elements of $B_c^*(I; R, S)$ that map to $B_c(I; R)$. Note that $M_c(1, r) = L$. For given k and N, let $V_c(L, k, N)$ contain all values of $\{I; R\}$ such that $P_c\{B(I; R)\} > 0$:

$$V_c(L, k, N) = V(L, k, N) \cup \{1, L\}, \qquad N > D(L, k),$$
$$V_c(L, k, N) = V(L, k, N), \qquad\qquad \text{otherwise,}$$

where

$$D(L, k) = k\left[\frac{L+1}{2}\right], \qquad L \text{ odd},$$
$$= kL/2 + 1, \qquad L \text{ even}.$$

Apply the same results used to derive Theorem 8.5, to find

$$P_c(B) = L^{-N}\sum_{V_c(L,k,N)}(-1)^{S(I;R)-1}M_c(1, r)$$

$$\times \sum_{M_1,\ldots,MI_I}\binom{N}{N - M\ M_1\ M_2\ldots M_I}$$

$$\times h_k(N - M, L - S(I; R) - I)\prod_{i=1}^{I}N(r_i \mid k, M_i). \qquad (8.50)$$

For $k < D^{-1}(N, L)$, the expression for the probability on the circle is the same as for the line except that $M_c(I; R)$ replaces $M(I; R)$. Wallenstein (1971) uses (8.50) to calculate $P_c(k, N, 1/L)$ for $L = 5(1)10$, $N = 10(1)60$, $[N/3] + 1 \le k \le [N/2]$, $k < 2N/L$.

8.12.2   Relation of Scan Statistic on Circle and Coverage Problems

Various formula for $P_c(k; N, w)$ have been derived under the topic of coverage problems. In the classical coverage problem on the circle, arcs of length V are dropped at random on the unit circle. By *random* is meant that the centers of the arcs are i.i.d. uniform over the unit circle. A position x on the circle is said to be covered by an arc centered at y, iff $y-.5V \le x \le y+.5V$. The circle is said to be covered if all positions $0 \le x \le 1$ are covered. In the simplest coverage problem we seek the probability that the N arcs completely cover the circle (at least once). A generalization seeks the probability, $P_{m,N}(V)$, that the N arcs completely cover the circle at least m times.

The scan cluster and coverage problems are related. For the event corresponding to $P_c(k; N, w)$, scan the circle with a window of size w, and ask if this scanning window ever contains k or more points. For the event corresponding to $P_{m,N}(1-w)$, scan the circle with a window of size $1-w$, and ask if this scanning window always contains m or more points. When the circle is scanned with a window of size w, it is simultaneously being scanned with the complementary window of size $1-w$. Whenever there are k of the N points in the window of size w, there must be $N-k$ points in the complementary window of size $1-w$.

The m-coverage and cluster probabilities are related by the identity

$$P_c(k; N, w) = 1 - P_{N-k+1,N}(1 - w). \qquad (8.51)$$

To prove this point, view the N random points as centers of N random subarcs of length $V = 1 - w$. Let $N_V(t)$ denote the number of random points that fall in $(t, t+V)$. If $N_V(t) \ge N-k+1$ then the position $(t+.5V)$ will be covered at least $N-k+1$ times. If, for all coordinates t on the unit circle, $N_V(t) \ge N-k+1$, then the circle is covered at least $N-k+1$ times. Alternatively, if for some t, $N_V(t) < N-k+1$, then in the arc of length $w = 1-V$, that is the complement of $(t, t+V)$, there would be at least k points.

Various exact and asymptotic results have been derived for the coverage problem. The probability of covering the circle at least once is $P_{1,N}(V)$, and from (8.51) for $N-k+1 = 1$ or $k = N$, $P_{1,N}(V) = 1 - P_c(N; N, 1-V)$. Equation (8.43), with $w = 1 - V$, gives the probability of coverage at least once. Kaplan (1977) gives asymptotic results. For related multiple coverage problems, see Glaz and Naus (1979).

9
Scanning N Uniform Distributed Points: Bounds

In the study of bounds for scan statistic probabilities two methods have been employed. The first method utilizes the scanning process representation of the scan statistic that has been discussed in Naus (1982), Wallenstein (1980), and Wallenstein and Neff (1987). The second method is based on the order statistics representation of the scan statistics investigated in Berman and Eagleson (1985), Gates and Westcott (1984), Glaz (1989, 1992), and Krauth (1988). The class of inequalities that we will present here is known in the statistical literature as Bonferroni-type inequalities. For a thorough treatment of these inequalities and many interesting references and applications, see a recent book by Galambos and Simonelli (1996). The Bonferroni-type inequalities that we will use for developing bounds for scan statistic probabilities are usually tigher than the classical Bonferroni inequalities introduced in Bonferroni (1936). Therefore, the classical Bonferroni inequalities will not be discussed here.

9.1 Bounds Based on the Scanning Process Representation

Suppose that N points are uniformly distributed in the interval $[0, 1)$. First assume that $w = 1/L$ where $L \geq 4$ is an integer. Divide the interval $[0, 1)$ into L subintervals of length w. Then, $P(k; N, w)$, the probability of observing at least one interval of length w containing k or more points is given by

$$P(k; N, w) = P\left(\bigcup_{i=1}^{L-1} E_i^c\right),\qquad(9.1)$$

where for $1 \leq i \leq L - 1$ and $0 \leq t \leq 1 - w$ the events E_i are given by

$$E_i = \left(\left[\max_{(i-1)w \leq t < iw} Y_t(w)\right] \leq k - 1\right)\qquad(9.2)$$

and $Y_t(w)$ is the number of points in the interval $[t, t + w)$.

A second-order Bonferroni-type upper bound for $P(k; N, w)$ is derived below based on the approach in Hunter (1976). For the problem at hand, we have

$$\bigcup_{i=1}^{L-1} E_i^c = E_1^c \cup \left\{\bigcup_{i=2}^{L-1}\left(E_i^c \cap \left[\bigcap_{j=1}^{i-1} E_j\right]\right)\right\}.$$

Since the events E_1^c, $\{E_i^c \cap [\bigcap_{j=1}^{i-1} E_j]\}_{i=2}^{L-1}$ are mutually disjoint and

$$\left(E_i^c \cap \left[\bigcap_{j=1}^{i-1} E_j\right]\right) \subset (E_i^c \cap E_{i-1})$$

we get that

$$P(k; N, w) \leq P(E_1^c) + \sum_{i=2}^{L-1} P\left(E_i^c \cap E_{i-1}\right)$$

$$= \sum_{i=1}^{L-1} P(E_i^c) - \sum_{i=2}^{L-1} P\left(E_i^c \cap E_{i-1}^c\right)$$

$$= (L-1)P(E_1^c) - (L-2)P\left(E_1^c \cap E_2^c\right)$$

$$= 1 + (L-3)Q_2 - (L-2)Q_3,\qquad(9.3)$$

where $Q_2 = P(E_1)$ and $Q_3 = P(E_1 \cap E_2)$. The reason that we have expressed the upper bound for $P(k; N, w)$ in terms of Q_2 and Q_3 is that they are relatively easy to evaluate based on existing algorithms. To evaluate Q_i, $i = 2, 3$, we condition on the number of points in the interval $[0, iw)$ being equal to j to get that

$$Q_i = \sum_{j=0}^{i(k-1)} Q(k; j, 1/i)b(j; N, iw),\qquad(9.4)$$

where $Q(k; j, 1/i) = 1 - P(k; j, 1/i)$ and

$$b(j; N, w) = \binom{N}{j}w^j(1-w)^{N-j}\qquad(9.5)$$

is the binomial probability function. Explicit formulas for $Q(k; j, 1/i), i = 2, 3$, in terms of binomial and cumulative binomial probabilities are given in Section 8.3, (8.8)–(8.9), and Section 8.6, (8.23). Numerical results to evaluate the performance of the Bonferroni-type upper bound in (9.3) for selected values of k, N, and w are given in Tables 9.1 and 9.2.

To derive a second-order Bonferroni-type lower bound for $P(k; N, w)$ we employ the approach in Kwerel (1975). Let

$$t_1 = \sum_{i=1}^{L-1} P(E_i^c) = (L - 1)(1 - Q_2) \tag{9.6}$$

and

$$t_2 = \sum_{j=2}^{L-1} \sum_{i=1}^{j-1} P(E_i^c \cap E_j^c)$$

$$= .5(L - 1)(L - 2)(1 - 2Q_2) + (L - 2)Q_3 + \sum_{j=3}^{L-1} \sum_{i=1}^{j-2} P(E_i \cap E_j). \tag{9.7}$$

It follows from Kwerel (1975) that the best second-order Bonferroni-type lower bound for $P(k; N, w)$ based on a linear combination of t_1 and t_2 is given by

$$P(k; N, w) \geq 2t_1/a - 2t_2/(a(a - 1)), \tag{9.8}$$

where $a = [2t_2/t_1 + 2]$ and $[x]$ denotes the integer part of x. To evaluate the lower bound in (9.8), we first show that for $j - i \geq 2$:

$$Q_{2,2} = P(E_1 \cap E_3) = P(E_i \cap E_j). \tag{9.9}$$

Let V_i and V_j be the number of points in the intervals $[(i - 1)w, (i + 1)w)$ and $[(j - 1)w, (j + 1)w)$, respectively. Since, $j - i \geq 2$, these intervals are disjoint. Condition on $V_i = a$ and $V_j = b$ to get that for $j - i \geq 2$:

$$P(E_i \cap E_j) = \sum_{a=0}^{2k-2} \sum_{b=0}^{2k-2} P(E_i \cap E_j \mid V_i = a, V_j = b) P(V_i = a, V_j = b)$$

$$= \sum_{a=0}^{2k-2} \sum_{b=0}^{2k-2} P(E_i \mid V_i = a) P(E_j \mid V_j = b) P(V_i = a, V_j = b)$$

$$= \sum_{a=0}^{2k-2} \sum_{b=0}^{2k-2} Q(k \mid a, 1/2) Q(k \mid b, 1/2) P(V_i = a, V_j = b), \tag{9.10}$$

where (V_i, V_j) has a trinomial distribution with cell probabilities $2/L$, $2/L$ and $1 - 4/L$ and $a + b \leq n$. It follows from (9.9) and (9.10) that

$$t_2 = .5(L - 1)(L - 2)(1 - 2Q_2) + (L - 2)Q_3 + .5(L - 2)(L - 3)Q_{2,2}. \tag{9.11}$$

Numerical results for the lower bound in (9.8) are given in Tables 9.1 and 9.2.

If $1/w > 4$ is not an integer let $L = [1/w] + 1$. In this case, we have $L - 1$ intervals of length w and one interval at the right end of length less than w. In this case, the upper bound for $P(k; N, w)$ is given by

$$P(k; N, w) \le 1 + (L - 4)Q_2 - (L - 3)Q_3 + P(E_{L-1}) - P(E_{L-2} \cap E_{L-1}).$$

To evaluate $P(E_{L-1})$ one has to divide the interval $[(L-2)w, 1)$ into three subintervals: $[(L - 2)w, 1 - w)$, $[1 - w, (L - 1)w)$, and $[(L - 1)w, 1)$. Condition on the number of points that fall into these intervals to be a, b, and c, respectively. When we scan the interval $[(L - 2)w, 1)$ with an interval of length w, the interval $[1 - w, (L - 1)w)$ and the b points remain within that interval of length w. Therefore,

$$P(E_{L-1}) = \sum_{j=0}^{2(k-1)} Q(k - b; j - b, 1/2)m(b, j - b; N, w_1, w_2),$$

where

$$m(i, j; N, w_1, w_2) = \frac{N!}{i! \, j! \, (N - i - j)!} w_1^i w_2^j (1 - w_1 - w_2)^{N-i-j} \quad (9.12)$$

is a trinomial probability function, $w_1 = Lw - 1$ and $w_2 = 2(1 - (L - 1)w)$. An explicit formula for $Q(k - b; j - b, 1/2)$ is given in Section 8.3. If $k - b \le 0$, $Q(k-b; j-b, 1/2)$ is set to be equal to 0. To evaluate $P(E_{L-2} \cap E_{L-1})$ a method developed in Huntington and Naus (1975) can be employed. Since in applications usually $1/w$ is an integer we will not present the details for evaluating $P(E_{L-2} \cap E_{L-1})$. Moreover, in Chapter 10, accurate approximations will be derived that will not require the evaluation of this event. Similarly, the lower bound given in (9.8) can be extended to the case when $1/w > 4$ is not an integer. We do not present these details here.

A different method to derive inequalities for $P(k; N, w)$ has its roots in Wallenstein (1980). Let the events E_i be defined as in (9.2), namely that any interval of length w in $[(i - 1)w, (i + 1)w)$ has at most $k - 1$ points. For $1 \le i \le L$, define the event that the number of points in the interval $[(i - 1)w, iw)$ is at least k, denoted by

$$\mathcal{A}_i = \left(Y_{(i-1)w}(w) \ge k\right)$$

and let $\mathcal{A} = \bigcup_{i=1}^{L} \mathcal{A}_i$. Let

$$B_i = E_i^c \cap \mathcal{A}^c$$

and let $B = \bigcup_{i=1}^{L-1} B_i$. It follows that

$$P(k; N, w) = P(\mathcal{A}) + P(B). \quad (9.13)$$

We propose to evaluate $P(\mathcal{A})$ exactly, using a recursive formula given below, and to bound $P(B)$ by an upper Hunter (1976) inequality and a Kwerel (1975) lower inequality.

Let $h(m, l)$ be the number of ways of placing m distinguishable balls in l distinguishable urns, such that each urn will have at most $k - 1$ balls. Define

$$H(m, l) = \frac{h(m, l)}{l^m}. \tag{9.14}$$

Note that $H(m, l)$ is the cumulative distribution function (c.d.f.) of the largest-order statistic of an l-dimensional multinomial vector with parameter m and cell probabilities equal to $1/l$, evaluated at $k - 1$. $H(m, l)$ can be evaluated recursively as follows:

$$H(m, l) = \sum_{j=0}^{\min(m, k-1)} b(j; m, w) H(m - j, l - 1), \tag{9.15}$$

with the initial conditions $H(m, l) = 1$, for $m < k$ and $H(m, l) = 0$, for $m \geq k$. For computational purposes in the sequel, set $H(m, l) = 0$ if $m > 0$ and $t \leq 0$, and set $H(0, 0) = 1$. It follows that

$$P(\mathcal{A}) = 1 - H(N, L). \tag{9.16}$$

To get accurate results the use of quadruple precision is advisable. For very large values of N and L, if $H(N, L)$ cannot be evaluated exactly using the above algorithm, one can always employ Bonferroni-type inequalities (Galambos and Simonelli, 1996) to bound $P(\mathcal{A})$. We would like to mention that in Riordan (1958, p. 102) a similar recursive formula is given for $h(m, l)$.

The second-order Bonferroni-type upper inequality in Hunter (1976) for $P(B)$ is given by

$$P(B) \leq \sum_{i=1}^{L-1} P(B_i) - \sum_{i=1}^{L-2} P(B_i \cap B_{i+1}) \tag{9.17}$$

and the second-order Bonferroni-type lower inequality in Kwerel (1975) is given by

$$P(B) \geq 2t_1^*/a^* - 2t_2^*/(a^*(a^* - 1)), \tag{9.18}$$

where $a^* = [2t_2^*/t_1^* + 2]$:

$$t_1^* = \sum_{i=1}^{L-1} P(B_i)$$

and

$$t_2^* = \sum_{j=2}^{L-1} \sum_{i=1}^{j-1} P(B_i \cap B_j) = (L - 2)P(B_1 \cap B_2) + .5(L - 2)(L - 3)P(B_1 \cap B_3).$$

To evaluate $P(B_1)$, $P(B_1 \cap B_2)$, and $P(B_1 \cap B_3)$ condition on the number of observations in the intervals $[(i - 1)w, iw)$ for $i = 2, 3, 4$, respectively, to get from Section 8.7 that

$$
\begin{aligned}
P(B_1) &= \sum_{j=k}^{\min(N,2k-2)} P(E_1^c \cap \mathcal{A}_1^c \cap \mathcal{A}_2^c \mid Y_0(2w) = j) \\
&\quad \times b(j; N, 2w) H(N - j, L - 2) \\
&= \sum_{j=k}^{\min(N,2k-2)} \frac{2k - 1 - j}{2^j} \binom{j}{k} b(j; N, 2w) H(N - j, L - 2),
\end{aligned} \tag{9.19}
$$

$$
\begin{aligned}
P(B_1 \cap B_2) &= \sum_{j=k+1}^{\min(N,3k-3)} P\left(E_1^c \cap E_2^c \cap \left(\bigcap_{m=1}^{3} \mathcal{A}_m^c \right) \mid Y_0(2w) = j \right) \\
&\quad \times b(j; N, 2w) H(N - j, L - 3) \\
&= \sum_{j=k+1}^{\min(N,3k-3)} b(j; N, 3w) H(N - j, L - 3) \\
&\quad \times (1/3)^j \sum_{x=1}^{k-1} \sum_{y=1}^{\min(k-1,j-1-x)} B(x, y),
\end{aligned} \tag{9.20}
$$

where

$$
\begin{aligned}
B(x, y) &= \frac{j!}{k!\,k!\,(j - 2k)!} + \frac{j!}{(2k - y)!\,(x + y - k)!\,(j - x - k)!} \\
&\quad - \frac{j!}{(2k - y)!\,y!\,(j - 2k)!}
\end{aligned} \tag{9.21}
$$

and

$$
\begin{aligned}
P(B_1 \cap B_3) &= \sum_{a=k}^{2k-2} \sum_{b=k}^{2k-2} P\left(E_1^c \cap E_3^c \cap \left(\bigcap_{m=1}^{4} \mathcal{A}_m^c \right) \mid Y_0(2w) = a, Y_{2w}(2w) = b \right) \\
&\quad \times P(V_1 = a, V_2 = b) H(N - a - b, L - 4) \\
&= \sum_{a=k}^{2k-2} \sum_{b=k}^{\min(2k-2,N-a)} \frac{(2k - 1 - a)(2k - 1 - b)}{2^{a+b}} \binom{b}{k} \binom{a}{k} \\
&\quad \times P(V_1 = a, V_2 = b) H(N - a - b, L - 4),
\end{aligned} \tag{9.22}
$$

where V_1 and V_2 have a trinomial distribution with cell probabilities $2w$, $2w$ and $1 - 4w$ and $a + b \leq N$. Numerical results for the lower and upper bounds in (9.16)–(9.18) are given in Tables 9.1 and 9.2.

9.2 Bounds Based on Spacings

We now turn to derive lower and upper Bonferroni-type bounds for $P(k; N, w)$ using the order statistic representation of the scan statistic. Let $X_1, \ldots, X_N$ be independent and identically distributed (i.i.d.) observations from a uniform distribution on the interval $[0, 1)$. Denote by $X_{(1)} < \cdots < X_{(N)}$ the order statistics. For $3 \le k \le N, 0 \le i \le N - k + 1$, and $0 < w < .5$ define the events

$$A_i = \left(X_{(i+k-1)} - X_{(i)} \le w\right), \tag{9.23}$$

where $X_{(0)} = 0$. It follows that

$$P(k; N, w) = P\left(\bigcup_{i=1}^{N-k+1} A_i\right). \tag{9.24}$$

Using the approach that lead to the upper bound given in (9.3), a second-order Bonferroni-type upper bound for $P(k; N, w)$ has been derived in Berman and Eagleson (1985):

$$P(k; N, w) \le \sum_{i=1}^{N-k+1} p_i - \sum_{i=2}^{N-k+1} p_{i-1,i}$$
$$= (N - k + 1)p_0 - (N - k)p_{01}, \tag{9.25}$$

where

$$p_i = P(A_i), \qquad p_{ij} = P(A_i \cap A_j), \qquad 0 \le i < j \le N - k + 1.$$

To evaluate the upper bound in (9.25) one uses the well-known results about the uniform spacings (Arnold, Balakrishnan, and Nagaraja (1992, Chap. 2)) to get that

$$p_0 = P(X_{(k-1)} < w) = \sum_{j=k-1}^{N} b(j; N, w) \tag{9.26}$$

and

$$p_{01} = \sum_{j=k-1}^{N} (-1)^{j+k-1} b(j; N, w), \tag{9.27}$$

where $b(j; N, w)$ is the binomial probability function given in (9.5).

Using the approach that led to the lower bound given in (9.8), a second-order Bonferroni-type lower bound for $P(k; N, w)$ has been derived in Glaz (1989):

$$P(k; N, w) \geq \frac{2}{a_2} \sum_{i=1}^{N-k+1} P(A_i) - \frac{2}{a_2(a_2 - 1)} \sum_{j=2}^{N-k+1} \sum_{i=1}^{j-1} P(A_i \cap A_j)$$

$$= \frac{2}{a_2}(N - k + 1)p_0$$

$$- \frac{2}{a_2(a_2 - 1)} \sum_{j=0}^{N-k+1} (N - k + 1)p_{1,j+2}, \qquad (9.28)$$

where

$$a_2 = \left[\frac{2 \sum_{j=0}^{N-k+1}(N - k + 1)p_{1,j+2}}{(N - k + 1)p_0} + 2 \right],$$

$$p_{1,j+2} = \begin{cases} G(k + j; N, w) + \displaystyle\sum_{i=0}^{N-k-j} R(j, i), & 0 \leq j \leq k - 2, \\[2ex] G(k + j; N, w) + \displaystyle\sum_{i=0}^{N-k-j} R(j, i) \\[1ex] \qquad + \displaystyle\sum_{r=0}^{j-k+1} \sum_{s=k-1}^{j-r} T(r, s), & k - 1 \leq j \leq N - k - 1, \end{cases}$$

$$G(j; N, w) = \sum_{i=j}^{N} b(i; N, w), \qquad (9.29)$$

$$R(j, i) = (-1)^i b(k + j + i; N, w) \sum_{r=0}^{j} \sum_{s=0}^{h(j,r)} \binom{r + s + i}{r}\binom{s + i}{s},$$

$$T(r, s) = m(s, k + j - r - s - 1; N, w, w),$$

is the trinomial probability function given in (9.12) and

$$h(j, r) = \begin{cases} j, & 0 \leq j \leq k - 2, \\ \min(j, k + j - r - 1), & j \geq k - 1. \end{cases}$$

These formulas for $p_{1,j+2}$ have been derived in Glaz and Naus (1983) based on the well-known results for the uniform spacings and will not be presented here. Numerical results for the upper bound in (9.25) are presented in Tables 9.1 and 9.2, for selected values of k, N, and w. Numerical results for the lower bound (9.28) are given in Glaz (1989). We do not present it here since the performance of the other lower bounds is by far superior.

Using the scan statistic for testing the null hypothesis of uniformity against a clustering alternative requires accurate approximations for $P(k; N, w)$ for values that are less than or equal to .20. From the numerical results in Table 9.1 it is evident that the second-order Bonferroni-type inequalities based on the scanning process are tight. Therefore there is no need to evaluate higher-order Bonferroni-type inequalities for values less than .20. On the other hand, it was noted in Glaz (1989, 1992) that the second-order Bonferroni-type inequalities based on the order statistics representation of the scan statistics can be too conservative. We now proceed to derive higher-order Bonferroni-type upper bounds for $P(k; N, w)$ based on the approach in Glaz (1992). From the identity for a finite union of sets (Hunter, 1976) we get

$$\bigcup_{i=1}^{N-k+1} A_i = A_1 \cup \left\{ \bigcup_{i=2}^{N-k+1} \left(A_i \cap \left[\bigcap_{j=1}^{i-1} A_j^c \right] \right) \right\}.$$

Therefore,

$$P\left(\bigcup_{i=1}^{N-k+1} A_i \right) = P(A_1) + \sum_{i=2}^{N-k+1} P\left(A_i \cap \left[\bigcap_{j=1}^{i-1} A_j^c \right] \right). \qquad (9.30)$$

Since for $i \geq m$, $\left(A_i \cap \left[\bigcap_{j=1}^{i-1} A_j^c \right] \right) \subset \left(A_i \cap \left[\bigcap_{j=i-m+1}^{i-1} A_j^c \right] \right)$, it follows from (9.30) that a Bonferroni-type upper bound of order $m \geq 3$ is given by

$$P\left(\bigcup_{i=1}^{N-k+1} A_i \right) \leq P(A_1) + \sum_{i=2}^{m} P\left(A_i \cap \left[\bigcap_{j=1}^{i-1} A_j^c \right] \right)$$

$$+ \sum_{i=m+1}^{N-k+1} P\left(A_i \cap \left[\bigcap_{j=i-m+1}^{i-1} A_j^c \right] \right)$$

$$= \sum_{i=1}^{N-k+1} P(A_i) - \sum_{i=2}^{N-k+1} P(A_i \cap A_{i-1})$$

$$- \sum_{j=2}^{m-1} \sum_{i=1}^{N-k+1-j} P\left(A_i \cap \left[\bigcap_{v=i+1}^{i+j-1} A_v^c \right] \cap A_{i+j} \right)$$

$$= (N - k + 1)p_0 - (N - k)p_{01}$$

$$- \sum_{j=2}^{m-1} (N - k + 1 - j)p_{1,\ldots,j+1}^*, \qquad (9.31)$$

where p_0 and p_{01} are given in (9.26) and (9.27), respectively, and

$$p_{1,\ldots,j+1}^* = P\left(A_1 \cap \left[\bigcap_{v=2}^{j} A_v^c \right] \cap A_{j+1} \right). \qquad (9.32)$$

For $2 \leq m \leq k \leq N/2$, let

$$\alpha_1^* = P(A_0), \qquad \alpha_m^* = P\left(A_0 \cap \left[\bigcap_{j=1}^{m-1} A_j^c \right] \right) \qquad (9.33)$$

and

$$\alpha_1 = P(A_0^c), \qquad \alpha_m = P\left(\bigcap_{j=0}^{m-1} A_j^c\right). \qquad (9.34)$$

For $1 \le j \le k - 1$, it follows from (9.32) that $p_{1,\dots,j+1}^* = \alpha_j^* - \alpha_{j+1}^*$. For $1 \le i \le N - k$, it follows from (9.33) and (9.34) that $\alpha_{i+1} = \alpha_i - \alpha_{i+1}^*$ and therefore, for $2 \le i \le N - k$:

$$\alpha_i = \alpha_1 - \sum_{j=2}^{i} \alpha_j^*.$$

Therefore, it follows from (9.31) that for $3 \le m \le k$, an mth-order upper bound for $P(k; N, w)$ is given by

$$P(k; N, w) \le 1 - \alpha_m + (N - k + 1 - m)\alpha_m^*. \qquad (9.35)$$

The best upper bound is given for $m = k$. The terms α_m and α_m^* can be evaluated from Theorem 9.1 below. Numerical results for the upper bound given in (9.35), for $m = k$, for selected values of the parameters, are presented in Table 9.1.

Remark. The mth-order upper bounds given in (9.35) provide significant improvement over the second-order upper bound given in (9.25), and they are members of a more general class of Bonferroni-type upper bounds investigated in Hoover (1990). The members of this class of upper bounds decrease as the order of the bound increases, which is not necessarily true for the classical Bonferroni upper bounds (Schwager, 1984). General methods for constructing improved Bonferroni-type bounds are discussed in Galambos and Simonelli (1996), Hoppe and Seneta (1990), Prekopa (1988), Seneta (1988), and Tomescu (1986).

The following result, presented in Theorem 9.1 below, is fundamental to the implementation of the upper bounds given in (9.35) and the product-type approximations for $P(k; N, w)$, based on the order statistics representation, presented in Chapter 10. The following two technical results are needed in the proof of Theorem 9.1.

Lemma 1 (Lemma A.1 in Glaz (1992)); *For* $0 \le j \le m - 2$:

$$I_j = a_j \int_0^w \int_0^{t_{m-1}} \cdots \int_0^{t_2} (w - t_{m-1})^{k-m} (1 - w - t_{m-1})^{N-k+1-j}$$

$$\times (t_{m-1} - t_{m-2})^j \prod_{r=1}^{m-1} dt_r$$

$$= \sum_{h=j}^{N-k+1} \frac{(-1)^{h-j}}{(m-2+j)!} \left[\prod_{i=1}^{m-2+j} (h + i - j)\right] b(k + h - 1; N, w),$$

where

$$a_j = \frac{N!}{(N-m+1)!}\binom{N-m+1}{k-m}\binom{N-k+1}{j}, \quad 0 < t_1 < \cdots < t_{m-1} < w,$$

and $b(j; N, w)$ is defined in (9.5).

Proof. Integrating with respect to $t_1, \ldots, t_{m-3}$ yields

$$I_j = \frac{a_j}{(m-3)!}\int_0^w (w-t_{m-1})^{k-m}(1-w-t_{m-1})^{N-k+1-j}$$

$$\times \int_0^{t_{m-1}}(t_{m-1}-t_{m-2})^j t_{m-2}^{m-3}\, dt_{m-2}\, dt_{m-1}.$$

To evaluate the inner integral we employ the substitution $v = t_{m-2}/t_{m-1}$ to get

$$\int_0^{t_{m-1}}(t_{m-1}-t_{m-2})^j t_{m-2}^{m-3}\, dt_{m-2} = t_{m-1}^{m-2+j}\int_0^1 (1-v)^j v^{m-3}\, dv$$

$$= \frac{j!\,(m-3)!\,t_{m-1}^{m-2+j}}{(j+m-2)!}.$$

Therefore,

$$I_j = \frac{a_j j!}{(j+m-2)!}\int_0^w (w-t_{m-1})^{k-m}(1-w-t_{m-1})^{N-k+1-j}t_{m-1}^{m-2+j}\, dt_{m-1}$$

$$= \frac{a_j j!}{(j+m-2)!}w^{k-1+j}(1-w)^{N-m+1-j}$$

$$\times \int_0^1 (1-u)^{k-m}u^{m-2+j}\left(1-\frac{uw}{1-w}\right)^{N-k+1-j}\, du,$$

where $t_{m-1} = uw$. Expanding the terms

$$\left(1-\frac{uw}{1-w}\right)^{N-k+1-j} = \sum_{s=0}^{N-k+1-j}\binom{N-k+1-j}{s}(-1)^s\left(\frac{uw}{1-w}\right)^s,$$

evaluating the integral

$$\int_0^1 (1-u)^{k-m}u^{m-2+j+s}\, du = \frac{(m-2+j+s)!\,(k-m)!}{(k+s+j-1)!},$$

and simplfying the products of the binomial coefficients with the factorial terms yield

$$I_j = \sum_{s=0}^{N-k+1-j}\frac{(-1)^s}{(m-2+j)!}\left[\frac{(m-2+j+s)!}{s!}\right]b(k+s+j-1; N, w).$$

To complete the proof of Lemma 9.1, set $h = s + j$.

Lemma 9.2 (Lemma A.2 in Glaz (1992)). *Let $0 \leq j \leq m - 2$ and $3 \leq m \leq k$ be integers. Define $T(a) = \sum_{n=1}^{a} j_n$, where j_n and a are nonnegative integers and $T(0) = 0$. Then the number of solutions to the equation $T(m - 2) = j$, subject to the constraints $0 \leq j_s \leq s - T(s - 1)$ for $1 \leq s \leq m - 2$, is equal to*

$$c_{j,m-2} = \binom{m-3+j}{j} - \binom{m-3+j}{j-2},$$

where $\binom{j}{i} = 0$ for $i < 0$.

Proof. First, note that the specified constraints for the equation $T(m - 2) = j$ are equivalent to $0 \leq T(s) \leq s$, $0 \leq s \leq j - 1$. It is well known that the number of solutions to the above equation, ignoring the constraints, is given by $\binom{m-3+j}{j}$ (Feller (1968, Chap. II.5)). Therefore, it suffices to show that the number of solutions to $T(m - 2) = j$, that do not satisfy the constraints $0 \leq T(s) \leq s$, $0 \leq s \leq j - 1$, is equal to

$$b_{j,m-2} = \binom{m-3+j}{j-2}.$$

The proof of this fact proceeds by induction on $m^* = m - 2$. For $m^* = 1$ and $0 \leq j \leq 1$, $b_{j,1} = 0$ ($c_{j,1} = 1$). Assume that the formula for b_{j,m^*} is valid for $m^* \geq 1$ and $0 \leq j \leq m^*$. One has to show that the number of solutions to the equation $T(m^* + 1) = j$, that do not satisfy the constraints $0 \leq T(s) \leq s$, $0 \leq s \leq j - 1$, is equal to $b_{j,m^*+1} = \binom{m^*+1}{j-2}$. Fix the value of $j_{m^*+1} = v$ where $0 \leq v \leq j$. For a given value of $j_{m^*+1} = v$, the equation $T(m^* + 1) = j$ simplifies to $T(m^*) = j - v$, with the relevant constraints being $0 \leq T(s) \leq s$, $0 \leq s \leq j - v - 1$, as the specified conditions for $j - v \leq s \leq j - v - 1$ cannot be violated. From the induction hypothesis it follows that, for a specified value of $j_{m^*+1} = v$, the number of solutions to $T(m^* + 1) = j$, that violate the specified constraints is equal to $b_{j-v,m^*} = \binom{m^*-1-v+j}{j-2-v}$. Therefore,

$$b_{j,m^*+1} = \sum_{v=0}^{j-2} b_{j-v,m^*} = \sum_{v=0}^{j-2} \binom{m^* - 1 - v + j}{j - 2 - v}$$

$$= \sum_{v=0}^{j-2} \binom{m^* + 1 + j - 2 - v}{m^* + 1} = \sum_{v=0}^{j-2} \binom{m^* + 1 + v}{m^* + 1} = \binom{m^* + j}{j - 2}.$$

This completes the proof of Lemma 9.2.

Theorem 9.1 (Theorem 1 in Glaz (1992)). *Let $X_{(1)} < \cdots < X_N$ be the order statistics of i.i.d. observations from a uniform distribution on the interval $[0, 1)$. Then for $3 \leq m \leq k \leq N/2$ and $0 < w < .5$:*

$$\alpha_m^* = b(k - 1; N, w) - b(k; N, w)$$

$$+ \sum_{j=m}^{N-k+1} (-1)^j \prod_{i=1}^{m-2} \left[1 - \frac{j(j-1)}{i(i+1)} \right] b(k + j - 1; N, w). \quad (9.36)$$

Proof. From the definition of α_m^* it follows that

$$\alpha_m^* = P\left\{(X_{(k-1)} \le w) \cap \left[\bigcap_{j=1}^{m-1}(X_{(k+j-1)} - X_{(j)} \ge w)\right]\right\}. \tag{9.37}$$

Conditional on $(X_{(1)}, \ldots, X_{(L-1)}) = (t_1, \ldots, t_{L-1})$, $X_{(L)}, \ldots, X_{(n)}$ are distributed as order statistics from a uniform distribution on the interval $[t_{L-1}, 1)$. Therefore,

$$\alpha_m^* = \sum_{s=0}^{m-3} \sum_{j_{s+1}=0}^{s+1-T(s)} I_{j_1, \ldots, j_{m-2}}, \tag{9.38}$$

where

$$I_{j_1, \ldots, j_{m-2}} = \frac{n!}{(n-m+1)!}\binom{n-m+1}{k-m}\prod_{v=1}^{m-2}\binom{n-k+1-T(v-1)}{j_v}$$

$$\times \int_0^w \int_0^{t_{m-1}} \cdots \int_0^{t_2} (w - t_{m-1})^{k-m}(1 - w - t_{m-1})^{n-m+1-T(m-2)}$$

$$\times \prod_{r=2}^{m-1}(t_r - t_{r-1})^{j_r-1}\, dt_{r-1} \cdots dm_{m-1},$$

$0 \le j_s \le s - T(s)$ for $1 \le s \le m - 2$, $T(a) = \sum_{n=1}^{a} j_a$, and $T(0) = 0$. It is elaborate but routine to verify that

$$I_{j_1, \ldots, j_{m-2}} = I_{0, \ldots, 0, T(m-2)}.$$

Therefore, it follows from (9.37) that

$$\alpha_m^* = \sum_{j=0}^{m-2} c_{j,m-2} I_j, \tag{9.39}$$

where $c_{j,m-2}$ is the number of solutions to the equation $T(m - 2) = j$, subject to constraints $0 \le j \le m - 2$. It follows from Lemmas 9.1 and 9.2 that

$$\alpha_m^* = \sum_{j=0}^{m-2} \frac{\left[\binom{m-3+j}{j} - \binom{m-3+j}{j-2}\right]}{(m-2+j)!}$$

$$\times \sum_{h=j}^{N-k+1}(-1)^{h-j}\left[\prod_{i=1}^{m-2+j}(h+i-j)\right]b(k+h-1; N, w)$$

$$= \sum_{h=0}^{N-k+1}(-1)^h \prod_{i=1}^{m-2}(h+i)b(k+h-1; N, w)$$

$$\times \sum_{j=0}^{\min(h,m-2)}(-1)^j \frac{\left[\binom{m-3+j}{j} - \binom{m-3+j}{j-2}\right]}{(m-2+j)!}\prod_{i=1}^{j}(h+i-j). \tag{9.40}$$

Note that

$$\frac{[\binom{m-3+j}{j} - \binom{m-3+j}{j-2}]}{(m-2+j!)} \prod_{i=1}^{j} (h+i-j)$$

$$= \frac{[(m-1)(m-2)-(j-1)j]}{(m-1)!\,(m-2+j)} \prod_{i=1}^{j} (h+i-j)$$

$$= \frac{(m-1-j)}{(m-1)!} \binom{h}{j}.$$

Use the well-known identity (Feller (1968, Chap. II.12, Eq. (12.7))):

$$\sum_{i=0}^{M} (-1)^i \binom{j}{i} = (-1)^M \binom{j-1}{M},$$

to conclude that for $0 \le h \le N-k+1$ and $3 \le m \le k$:

$$\sum_{j=0}^{\min(h,m-2)} (-1)^j \frac{[\binom{m-3+j}{j} - \binom{m-3+j}{j-2}]}{(m-2+j!)} \prod_{i=1}^{j} (h+i-j)$$

$$= \begin{cases} \frac{1}{(m-2+h)!}, & h = 0, 1, \\ 0, & 2 \le h \le m-1, \\ (-1)^{m-2} \prod_{i=1}^{m-2} \frac{h-i-1}{(m-1)!\,(m-2)!}, & m \le h \le N-k+1. \end{cases} \quad (9.41)$$

Substitute the results from (9.41) in (9.40) to get that

$$\alpha_m^* = b(k-1; N, w) - b(k; N, w) + \sum_{j=m}^{N-k+1} \frac{(-1)^{j+m-2}}{(m-1)!\,(m-2)!}$$

$$\times \prod_{i=1}^{m-2} (j+i)(j-i-1)b(k+j-1; N, w).$$

Routine calculation shows that

$$\frac{(-1)^{j+m-2}}{(m-1)!\,(m-2)!} \prod_{i=1}^{m-2} (j+i)(j-i-1) = \prod_{i=1}^{m-2} \left[1 - \frac{j(j-1)}{i(i+1)}\right].$$

This completes the proof of Theorem 9.1.

9.3 Method of Moments Bounds Using Linear Programming

An interesting and entirely different approach to derive inequalities for $P(k; N, w)$, based on the order statistics representation of the scan statistic, is given in Huffer and Lin (1997a, 1999b). Let

$$\xi = \sum_{j=1}^{N-k+1} I_j, \tag{9.42}$$

where

$$I_j = \begin{cases} 1, & X_{(j+k-1)} - X_{(j)} \leq w, \\ 0, & X_{(j+k-1)} - X_{(j)} > w. \end{cases} \tag{9.43}$$

The random variable ξ counts the number of intervals of length w or less that contain k points. It has been referred to in the statistical literature as the multiple scan statistic (Glaz and Naus, 1983). Note that

$$P(k; N, w) = P(\xi \geq 1). \tag{9.44}$$

Huffer and Lin (1999b) show that

$$\min_{X \in H}\{P(X \geq 1\} \leq P(\xi \geq 1) \leq \max_{X \in H}\{P(X \geq 1\}, \tag{9.45}$$

where H is the set of all random variables taking values in $\{0, 1, \ldots, N - k, N - k + 1\}$ and $E(X^k) = E(\xi^k) = \mu_k$, $1 \leq k \leq 4$. The lower and upper bounds given in (9.45) are reformulated as linear programming problems given below:

$$\max_{X \in H}\{P(X \geq 1\} = \max\left\{\sum_{i=1}^{N-k+1} a_i\right\} \tag{9.46}$$

subject to $\sum_{i=1}^{N-k+1} i^k a_i = \mu_k$, $1 \leq k \leq 4$ and $a_i \geq 0$ for all i, and

$$\min_{X \in H}\{P(X \geq 1\} = \min\left\{\sum_{i=1}^{N-k+1} a_i\right\}, \tag{9.47}$$

subject to the same constraints. For $k \leq 10$ both linear programming programs can be solved using Maple.

A different way that allows a simple systematic approach to compute the bounds in (9.45) is presented in Huffer and Lin (1997a, 1999b). Let $\phi(x)$ and $\psi(x)$ be functions that satisfy for all x:

$$\phi(x) \leq I_{(\xi \geq 1)}(x) \leq \psi(x).$$

Then

$$E\phi(X) \leq P(\xi \geq 1) \leq E\psi(X).$$

If one has a tractable class of these functions then one can evaluate

$$\max_{\phi} E\phi(X) \leq P(\xi \geq 1) \leq \min_{\psi} E\psi(X). \tag{9.48}$$

For the problem at hand a tractable class of functions are polynomials of order 4. This leads to the following bounds:

$$\min_{\psi \in G} E\psi(X) = \min \left\{ b_0 + \sum_{i=1}^{4} b_i \mu_i \right\}, \qquad (9.49)$$

where the min is taken over all polynomials

$$\psi(y) = \sum_{i=0}^{4} b_i y^i$$

satisfying $\psi(0) \geq 0$ and $\psi(i) \geq 1$ for all $1 \leq i \leq N - k + 1$, and

$$\max_{\phi \in G} E\phi(X) = \max \left\{ b_0 + \sum_{i=1}^{4} b_i \mu_i \right\}, \qquad (9.50)$$

satisfying $\psi(0) \leq 0$ and $\psi(i) \leq 1$ for all $1 \leq i \leq N - k + 1$. These bounds also can be computed via linear programming and they yield the same bounds as in (9.46) and (9.47) (Huffer, Lin 1999b). Moreover, Huffer and Lin (1999b) show that these upper ((9.46) or (9.49)) and lower ((9.47) or (9.50)) bounds can be expressed as

$$\max_{1 \leq j \leq m-2 \leq N-k-2} E\phi_{j,m}(\xi) \leq P(\xi \geq 1) \leq \min_{1 < j < N-k} E\psi_j(\xi), \qquad (9.51)$$

where

$$\psi_j(y) = 1 - \frac{(y-1)(y-N+k-1)(y-j-1)}{(N-k+1)j(j+1)}$$

and

$$\phi_{j,m}(y) = 1 - \frac{(y-j)(y-j-1)(y-m)(y-m-1)}{j(j+1)m(m+1)}.$$

Since the bounds are achieved for low values of j and j, m an upper bound of $m = 10$ is used in the algorithms for evaluating these bounds. This method is applicable for $k \leq 10$ only. Therefore it will not be useful for evaluating bounds for $E(S_w)$. Numerical results for the inequalities (9.51) are presented in Table 9.1.

9.4   Bounds for $E(S_w)$

We now turn to discuss inequalities for $E(S_w)$. Since S_w is a discrete random variable with values $0 \leq k \leq N$:

$$E(S_w) = \sum_{k=0}^{N-1} P(S_w > k) = \sum_{k=1}^{N} P(k; N, w). \qquad (9.52)$$

Now, $P(1; N, w) = 1$, $P(2; N, w) = \min\{1, 1-[1-(N-1)w]^N\}$ and for $w \leq .5$ and $j \geq [N/2] + 1$, $P(j; N, w) = 2G(j; N, w) + (j/w - N - 1)b(j; N, w)$,

Table 9.1. Comparison of three lower and four upper inequalities for $P(k; N, w)$ for $N = 100$.

k	L	MMLB	BTLB1	BTLB2	BTUB2	BTUB1	MMUB	BTTUB
4	1000	.014	.014	.014	.014	.014	.014	.014
	750	.031	.031	.031	.031	.032	.031	.032
	650	.046	.046	.046	.046	.047	.046	.047
	600	.058	.057	.058	.058	.059	.058	.059
	500	.094	.073	.094	.095	.098	.095	.098
10	50	.011	.012	.012	.012	.012	.012	.012
	40	.048	.050	.050	.051	.051	.056	.051
	35	.102	.111	.112	.115	.116	.129	.116
	30	.221	.198	.253	.273	.279	.315	.280
	25	.462	.453	.508	.674	.695	.780	.700

MMLB and MMUB are method of moments lower and upper bounds in (9.51); BTLB1 and BTUB1 are Bonferroni-type lower and upper bounds in (9.8) and (9.3), respectively; BTLB2 and BTUB2 are Bonferroni-type lower and upper bounds in (9.16)–(9.18); and BTTUB is the Bonferroni-type upper bound in (9.35).

Table 9.2. Comparison of two lower and three upper inequalities for $P(k; N, w)$.

N	k	L	BTLB1	BTLB2	BTUB2	BTUB1	BTTUB
100	11	20	.548	.565	.797	.869	.880
	12		.279	.346	.386	.397	.399
	13		.154	.155	.160	.162	.162
	14		.059	.059	.059	.060	.060
	15		.020	.020	.020	.020	.020
	18	10	.321	.380	.439	.445	.449
	19		.230	.225	.239	.240	.241
	20		.118	.117	.120	.120	.120
	21		.055	.055	.056	.056	.056
	22		.024	.024	.024	.024	.024
500	40	20	.243	.312	.342	.349	.351
	42		.129	.130	.134	.135	.135
	44		.046	.046	.046	.046	.046
	46		.014	.014	.014	.014	.014
	70	10	.185	.186	.190	.191	.192
	72		.092	.093	.093	.094	.094
	74		.042	.042	.043	.043	.043
	76		.018	.018	.018	.018	.018

BTLB1 and BTUB1 are Bonferroni-type lower and upper bounds in (9.8) and (9.3), respectively; BTLB2 and BTUB2 are Bonferroni-type lower and upper bounds in (9.16)–(9.18); and BTTUB is the Bonferroni-type upper bound in (9.35).

where $b(j; N, w)$ and $G(j; N, w)$ are binomial and cumulative binomial probabilities defined in (9.5) and (9.29), respectively. Therefore, to evaluate bounds for

Table 9.3. Bonferroni-type inequalities for $E(S_w)$.

N	w	LB1	LB2	UB2	UB1
100	.010	4.64	4.89	5.18	5.28
	.020	6.44	6.71	6.98	7.08
	.040	9.36	9.69	10.05	10.11
	.050	10.72	11.05	11.41	11.52
	.100	16.84	17.18	17.60	17.66
500	.001	4.30	4.53	4.68	4.78
	.002	5.60	5.83	6.22	6.25
	.005	8.51	8.84	9.30	9.41
	.010	12.54	12.89	13.46	13.61
	.020	19.40	19.88	20.57	20.69
	.050	37.52	38.12	39.12	39.22

LB1 and UB1 are Bonferroni-type lower and upper bounds for
$E(S_w)$ based on (9.8) and (9.3), respectively; LB2 and LB1 are
Bonferroni-type lower and upper bounds for $E(S_w)$ based on
(9.16)–(9.18).

$E(S_w)$ we need to evaluate bounds for $P(k; N, w)$ for $3 \leq k \leq [N/2]$. Since the bounds (9.3) and (9.8) and the bounds based on (9.13), (9.17), and (9.18) are tight we will use them to evaluate the bound for $E(S_w)$. Numerical results are presented in Table 9.3.

9.5 Bounds for the Distribution of a Scan Statistic on a Circle

Let $X_1, \ldots, X_N$ be a sequence of i.i.d. observations from a uniform distribution on a unit circle. Denote by zero the starting point for scanning the circle in the clockwise direction and arc of length w where $0 < w < 1$. For $0 \leq t < 1$, let $Y_t(w)$ be the number of points in the arc $(t, (t+w) \bmod 1]$. We define the *circular* scan statistic

$$S_w^c = \max_{0 \leq t < 1} Y_t(w).$$

The scan statistic on the circle, its use as a test for randomness, and other related problems have been investigated by many researchers including: Ajne (1968), Cressie (1977b, 1978, 1980, 1984), Hüsler (1982), Kokic (1987), Naus (1982), Rothman (1972), Weinberg (1980), and Takacs (1996). Exact distribution of S_w^c has been derived for $w = 1/2$ (Ajne, 1968), $w = 1/3$ (Takacs, 1966), $w = 1/L$, $L \geq 4$ an integer and $k > (N+1)/2$ (Rothman, 1972), and for $w = r/L$ with r and L relatively prime integers, $r < L$, $L \geq 4$ and $k > N(r+1)/L$ (Weinberg,

1980). Approximations for $P_c(k; N, w) = P(S_w^c \geq k)$ is investigated in Naus (1982) and in Wallenstein and Neff (1987).

Assume that $w = 1/L$, $L \geq 4$ is an integer. We present below Bonferroni-type inequalities for $P_c(k; N, w)$. Based on these inequalities we obtain inequalities for $E(S_w^c)$. Divide the unit circle into L arcs of length $w = 1/L$. For $i = 1, \ldots, L$ define the events E_i as in (9.2). Then

$$P_c(k; N, w) = P\left(\bigcup_{i=1}^{L} E_i^c\right).$$

The second-order Bonferroni-type upper inequalities for $P_c(k; N, w)$ are obtained from the inequalities for $P(k; N, w)$ given in (9.3) and in (9.13) and (9.17) by replacing L with $L + 1$. The lower inequalities for $P_c(k; N, w)$ are obtained from (9.8) with

$$t_1 = L(1 - Q_2)$$

and

$$t_2 = .5L(L - 1)(1 - 2Q_2) + LQ_3 + .5L(L - 3)Q_{2,2}$$

and from (9.13) and (9.18) with

$$t_1^* = LP(B_1)$$

and

$$t_2^* = LP(B_1 \cap B_2) + .5L(L - 3)P(B_1 \cap B_3),$$

where $P(B_1)$, $P(B_1 \cap B_2)$, and $P(B_1 \cap B_3)$ are given in (9.19)–(9.22). Inequalities for $E(S_w^c)$ are obtained from the inequalities for $P_c(k; N, w)$ in

$$E(S_w^c) = \sum_{k=1}^{N} P_c(k; N, w).$$

For selected values of the parameters k, w, L, and N we evaluate the inequalities for $E(S_w^c)$ in Table 9.4.

Table 9.4. Bonferroni-type inequalities for $E(S_w^c)$.

N	w	LB1	UB1
100	.010	4.64	5.28
	.020	6.46	7.10
	.040	9.40	10.16
	.050	10.79	11.59
	.100	16.89	17.84
500	.001	4.30	4.78
	.002	5.60	6.25
	.005	8.52	9.41
	.010	12.56	13.62
	.020	19.43	20.72
	.050	37.59	39.33

LB1 and UB1 are Bonferroni-type lower and upper bounds for $E(S_w^c)$ based on the modified (9.8) and (9.3) for the circle.

10

Approximations for the Conditional Case

There is, by now, a voluminous literature on approximations. We will highlight those approximations that are interesting from a methodological point of view and could be considered optimal relative to the effort involved. There are two basic approaches used. The methods of moments and product limit approximations are based on spacings, and the other methods are based on cell occupancy numbers. The approximations based on spacings are described in Sections 10.1–10.4, and those on cell occupancy numbers in Sections 10.5–10.7. In order of computational effort they might be ordered as:

1. Simple one parameter exponential approximation.

2. Crude approximation based on cell occupancy probabilities.

3. (a) Markov-type approximation based on cell occupancy numbers.

   (b) Product limit approximations.

   (c) Method of moments: two-parameter approximations.

4. Average of upper and lower bounds based on three-way intersections.

Section 10.10 will give a short comparison of the various procedures. Section 10.11 will describe how certain approximations can easily be implemented for the circle.

10.1   Spacings: Notation and Approximations Based on First Moment Only

We first order the N observations into order statistics $X_{(1)}, X_{(2)}, \ldots, X_{(N)}$, and let A_j be the event that the distance between k observations starting from the jth observation is less than w, i.e.,

$$A_j = \{X_{(j+k-1)} - X_{(j)} \leq w\}.$$

Let I_j be the indicator variable for the event A_j, that is:

$$I_j = \begin{cases} 1 & \text{if } X_{(k+j-1)} - X_{(j)} \leq w, \\ 0 & \text{otherwise,} \end{cases}$$

and let ξ be the total number of small *spacings*

$$\xi = \sum_{i=1}^{N-k+1} I_j.$$

Then

$$P(k, N, w) = P(\xi > 0) = 1 - P(\xi = 0).$$

In this chapter, we will use probabilities related to these events. The simplest, given by Berman and Eagelson (1985), is

$$P(A_1) = P(I_1 = 1) = E(I_1) = G_b(k - 1, N, w) = \sum_{j=k-1}^{N} b(j; N, w). \quad (10.1)$$

Although the distribution of ξ is very difficult to obtain, the moments can be computed, though with increasing difficulty for higher moments. The first moment obtained from (10.1) is

$$E(\xi) = (N - k + 1)E(I_1) = (N - k + 1)G_b(k - 1, N, w). \quad (10.2)$$

The variance is given in (10.11).

Methods of moments approximations for $P(\xi = 0)$ described in Section 10.4 require us to select another random variable Y^*, for which both the distribution (or, at least, $P(Y^* = 0)$) and m moments are known, to equate the first m moments of the two distributions, and then employ the approximation

$$P(Y^* = 0) \approx P(\xi = 0).$$

The approximation involves both choosing m and a random variable Y^* that is similar, in some sense, to ξ.

The simplest application of the method of moments lets Y^* have a Poisson distribution, and sets $m = 1$ so that

$$P(\xi = 0) \approx 1 - P(Y^* = 0)$$
$$= 1 - e^{-E(\xi)} = 1 - \exp\{-(N - k + 1)G_b(k - 1, N, w)\}. \quad (10.3)$$

This approximation was discussed in Glaz, Naus, Roos, and Wallenstein (1994, equation (2.10)). Other expressions similar in format to (10.3), but with slightly different expressions in the exponent, have been given by McClure (1976); Cressie (1977a), and Glaz (1978).

Recent years has seen more extensive use of approximations of the form of (10.3), chiefly by Karlin and by coauthors and chiefly applied to problems in molecular biology. The development is not so much to get close approximations per se, but to give a rigorous derivation of a limiting formula, bounds on errors, and to see how widely the asymptotic theory can be applied. In our context, these can be viewed as alternate approximations, in which $E(\xi)$ is replaced by asymptotically equivalent expressions that we generically call μ. Dembo and Karlin (1992) (as cited in Glaz, Naus, Roos, and Wallenstein (1994, equation (2.15))) approximate $P(k, N, w)$ by $1 - \exp(-\mu)$, where

$$\mu = (N - k - 1)\left[1 - \exp\left\{-(N + 1)w\sum_{j=0}^{k-2}[w(N + 1)]^j/j!\right\}\right].$$

Leung, Schactel, and Yu (1994) term this the finite Poisson approximation. Karlin and Macken (1991, Theorem 3), Dembo and Karlin (1992), and equation (2.16) of Glaz, Naus, Roos, and Wallenstein (1994) give

$$\mu = (N - 1)[w(N - 1)]^{k-1}/(k - 1)!.$$

It should be noted that the required condition given for convergence for these asymptotic results is

$$wN^{1+1/k} \to 0. \tag{10.4}$$

Glaz, Naus, Roos, and Wallenstein (1994) found (see Section 10.10 below) that in actual application the approximation is often very poor. However, closer examination suggests that when $wN^{1+1/k} < 1.0$, the approximation may be adequate, but when $wN^{1+1/k} > 1.0$, the approximation will be poor. (Of course, $wN^{1+1/k} < 1.0$ implies $w < N^{-(1+1/k)}$ which implies a very sparse distribution of points relative to the window, and is not usually of practical interest.)

There are several approaches that can be viewed as attempts to get more accurate approximations while using spacings. Methods of moments approximations when $m > 1$ are described in Section 10.4, declumping techniques are discussed in Section 10.3, and methods involving probabilities of the A's are described immediately below.

10.2 Approximations Involving Probabilities Associated with Intersections of Order Statistics

As noted in (9.25), Berman and Eagelson (1985) use the Hunter (1976) extension of the Bonferroni inequality to derive an upper bound

$$P(k; N, w) \leq (N - k + 1)P(A_1) - (N - k)P(A_1 \cap A_2), \qquad (10.5)$$

where $P(A_1)$ is given in (10.1) and $P(A_1 \cap A_2)$ in (9.27). They suggest using this bound as an approximation.

Glaz (1992) proposes the approximation

$$P(k; N, w) = 1 - \alpha_{N-k+1} \approx 1 - \alpha_k [\alpha_k/\alpha_{k-1}]^{N-2k+1}, \qquad (10.6)$$

where as in (9.34):

$$\alpha_i = P\left(\bigcap_{j=1}^{i} A_j^c\right).$$

This approximation can be derived as follows. By definition, $P(k; N, w) = 1 - \alpha_{N-k+1}$. Set $M = N - k + 1$ and note that

$$\alpha_M = P(A_1^c \cap A_2^c \cap \cdots \cap A_M^c)$$

$$= P(A_1^c \cap A_2^c \cap \cdots \cap A_k^c) \prod_{j=k+1}^{M} P(A_j^c \mid A_1^c \cap A_2^c \cap \cdots \cap A_{j-1}^c).$$

Now for $j > k$, apply the approximation that conditioning on the entire past is the same as conditioning on the last k events so that

$$P(A_j^c \mid A_1^c \cap A_2^c \cap \cdots \cap A_{j-1}^c) \approx P(A_j^c \mid A_{j-1}^c \cap A_{j-2}^c \cap \cdots \cap A_{j-k}^c)$$

$$= P(A_k^c \mid A_1 \cap A_2^c \cap \cdots A_{k-1}^c) = \alpha_k/\alpha_{k-1}.$$

(This approximation is the same in spirit as the Q_2/Q_3 (Markov) approximation described in Section 10.6.) Replacing the previous equation into the one above, and setting $M = N - k$, yields (10.6).

Computing the α's has been addressed following equation (9.34) and is again discussed in Section 17.2. Specifically, define the indicator variable for an observation starting a new clump (nonoverlapping cluster) as

$$I_j^* = I_j \prod_{i=1}^{r-1} [1 - I_{j-i}], \qquad 1 \leq j \leq n - r. \qquad (10.7)$$

Abbreviate $\alpha_j^* \equiv P[I_j^* = 1]$.

For the conditional case, $P[I_j^*(w) = 1] = \alpha_1^*$ is given by (10.1), while Berman and Eagelson (1985) have shown that $P[I_2^*(w) = 1]$ is given by

$$\alpha_2^* \equiv P(A_1 \cap A_2^c) \equiv P[I_2^* = 1] = \sum_{j=k-1}^{N} (-1)^{j-k-1} b(j; n, w). \qquad (10.8)$$

Equation (9.36), derived in Glaz (1992), gives $\alpha_j^* \equiv P[I_j^*(w) = 1]$. As indicated in Chapter 9, the α's can be expressed in terms of α_j^* based on $\alpha_1 = \alpha_1^*$, and

$$\alpha_i = \alpha_1 - \sum_{j=2}^{i} \alpha_j^*.$$

10.3 Declumping Techniques

A reason that the simple one-parameter approximation, (10.2), does not appear to agree well with simulated results is that the events $A_1, A_2, \ldots$ are highly correlated. Arratia, Goldstein and Gordon (1990) examine the probability of long head runs in which a failure (tail) ends the clump, and use (global) declumping to get a good approximation. For the scan statistic, global declumping is not feasible (Chen and Glaz, 1996), and instead we employ local declumping.

Under the declumping framework, each observation has the potential to be the start of a new clump. Each clump is associated with a random size U. We can view different ways of local declumping as generating different *declumped variables*, $U_1, U_2, \ldots, U_C$, $C \leq N - k$. All these methods, described in more detail in Chapter 17, focus on finding the distribution of multiple clusters, but can be applied to the problem here. We focus here in applying two results to find approximations to the scan statistic.

Glaz, Naus, Roos, and Wallenstein (1994) start a new clump at position j if $I_j = 1$ and if *all* the previous $k - 1$ events are not part of a cluster, i.e., if in (10.7), $I_j^* = 1$. Define the total number of clumps based on this definition as $C^* = \sum I_j^*$. Assuming that C^* follows a Poisson distribution it follows that

$$P(k; N, w) \equiv 1 - P(C^* = 0) \approx 1 - \exp[-E(C^*)],$$

where

$$E[C^*] = \sum_{j=1}^{k-2} \alpha_j^* - (N - 2k + 1)\alpha_{k-1}^*,$$

and where α_i^* is referred to in (10.7) above. Based on simulations, Glaz et al. conclude that this is not a good approximation, and suggest an alternative method ((10.15)). We will return to this method in the chapter on multiple clusters where we will use the Poisson distribution with $E(C^*)$ to approximate the number of nonoverlapping clusters.

Su and Wallenstein (2000) use a Markovian method of declumping in which a *Markovian clump* starts at position j if $I_j = 1$ and $I_{j-1} = 0$. Thus the number of Markovian clumps is

$$C = I_1 + \sum_{j=2}^{N-k-1} (1 - I_{j-1})I_j.$$

This "Markovian" definition of a clump, could be viewed as an extension of an idea by Arratia, Gordon, and Waterman (1990) who examine the probability of long head runs, in which a failure (tail) ends the clump. Su and Wallenstein suggest the approximation

$$P(k; N, w) = 1 - P(C = 0) \approx 1 - \exp[-E(C)], \qquad (10.9)$$

where it follows from the definition that

$$
\begin{aligned}
E(C) &= P(I_1 = 1) + \sum_{j=2}^{N-k-1} P[\{I_{j-1} = 0, I_j = 1\}] \\
&= P(I_1 = 1) + (N - k - 2)P(I_2^* = 1),
\end{aligned}
$$

where the probabilities on the right-hand side are given by (10.1) and (10.8), respectively.

Alternatively, it is of interest to express this result as a "correction" to the asymptotic expressions given in (10.3). To do this, note that for N large and $P(I_1 = 1)$ small:

$$
\begin{aligned}
P(I_1 = 1) + (N - k - 2)P(I_2^* = 1) &\approx (N - k - 1)P(I_2^* = 1) \\
&= (N - k - 1)P(A_1 \cap A_2^c) \\
&= (N - k - 1)P(A_1)P(A_2^c \mid A_1)
\end{aligned}
$$

so that,

$$1 - P(k; N, w) \approx 1 - \exp[-(N - k - 1)P(A_2^c \mid A_1)G_b(k - 1, N, w)] \qquad (10.10)$$

which is the same as the one-moment approximation, (10.3), adding a "correction" of $P(A_2^c \mid A_1)$.

10.4 The Method of Moments Based on Two Moments

To utilize these methods, we have to calculate the variance of ξ. Glaz and Naus (1983) give an expression for $\mathrm{Var}(\xi)$. Huffer and Lin (1997a) find a simpler expression

$$\text{Var}(\xi) = E(\xi) - [E(\xi)]^2 + (N - k + 1)(N - k)[1 - 2F_b(k - 2, N, w)]$$
$$+ 4 \sum_{i=0}^{k-3} [(k - i - 2)(N - k - 0.5(k - i - 1)(k - i - 3)]F_b(i, N, w)$$
$$- 2 \sum_{i=0}^{k-3} \sum_{j=0}^{k-3} [(N - 2k + 3) - 0.5(k - i - 3)(k - j - 3)$$
$$\times \sum_{a=0}^{i} \sum_{b=0}^{j} P(U_1 = a, U_2 = b)]$$
$$+ (N - 2k + 3)(N - 2k + 2) \sum_{a=0}^{k-2} \sum_{b=0}^{k-2} P(U_1 = a, U_2 = b), \quad (10.11)$$

where $(U_1, U_2, N - U_1 - U_2)$ has a trinomial distribution with expected values $2wN, 2wN, N - 4wN$.

10.4.1 Two-Moment "Markov-Chain" Approximation (MC2)

For the matching distribution, Huffer and Lin (1997a) select a random variable $Y^* = \sum_{i=1}^{N-k-1} Z_i$ where $Z_1, Z_2, \dots$ is a Markov chain with states 0 and 1, based on transition probabilities p_{01} and p_{10} where $P(Z_1 = 1) = p_{01}/(p_{01} + p_{10})$.

Re-expressing Y^* in terms of $P(Z_1 = 1)$ and of $\beta = p_{01} + p_{10}$, they find the moments of Y^* are given by

$$E(Y^*) = (N - k + 1)P(Z_1 = 1),$$
$$\text{Var } Y^* = (N - k + 1)P(Z_1 = 1)P(Z_1 = 0) + 2P(Z_1 = 1)P(Z_1 = 0)(\beta - 1)$$
$$\times [N - k + 1 - \beta[1 - (1 - \beta^{-1})^{N-k+1}].$$

Equating moments would require numerical techniques. For a simplification, they ignore the small term, $(1 - \beta^{-1})^{N-k+1}$, and solve a quadratic equation so that (see Lin (1999, p. 209)):

$$P(Z_1 = 1) = G_b(k - 1; N, w),$$

and

$$2\beta = N - k + 2 - \sqrt{[(N - k)^2 + 2(N - k + 1) - 2\text{Var}(\xi^2)]}/[P(Z_1 = 1)P(Z_1 = 0)].$$

Thus, one of several approximations suggested by Huffer and Lin is

$$P(k; N, w) \approx P(Y^* \geq 1) = 1 - [1 - G_b(k - 1, N, w)]$$
$$\times [1 - G_b(k - 1, N, w)/\beta)]^{N-k}. \quad (10.12)$$

10.4.2 Two-Moment Compound Poisson Approximations

These distributions were first applied to the scan problem by Roos (1993a,b) and subsequently by Glaz, Naus, Roos, and Wallenstein (1994), Huffer and Lin (1997a), and Su and Wallenstein (2000). For a matching distribution, one chooses a family of distribution based on weighted sums of Poisson distributed variables

$$Y^* = \sum_i i V_i,$$

where for $i = 1, 2, \ldots$, V_i is a Poisson distribution with parameter λ_i, where $\sum \lambda_i < \infty$ and the V's are independent.

To apply the method of moments set

$$E(Y^*) = \sum_i i\lambda_i = (N - k + 1)G_b(k - 1, N, w) = E(\xi),$$

and

$$E(Y^*) = \sum_i i^2\lambda_i = E(\xi^2).$$

From the definition of Y^* it follows that

$$P(Y^* = 0) = \prod_{i=1}^{\infty} P(V_i = 0) = \exp\left(-\sum_i \lambda_i\right). \qquad (10.13)$$

In this section, we consider the possibly infinite set of parameters λ_i as generated by two parameters (Section 10.4.3 discusses the case where four parameters are used). Different approximations use different functions of the two parameters to generate the possibly infinite sequence of λ's. The goal is to find a pair of parameters so that Y^* mimics ξ, and so that the computational load is not too great.

To motivate the different definitions of λ_j, note that in the compound Poisson approximation λ_j can be viewed as representing the expected number of consecutive runs of j occurrences of A_g. There will be a consecutive run of j occurrences of A starting at i, if

(a) the "first" event in the run is not preceded by a k-spacing less than w, i.e., $\{A_i \cap A_{i-1}^c\}$;

(b) for the next $j - 1$ points the events $\{A_g\}$ occurs, $g = i + 1, \ldots, i + j - 1$; and

(c) the cluster ends because A_{i+j-1} is not followed by a spacing less than w, i.e., $\{A_{i+j-1} \cap A_{i+j}^c\}$.

10.4.3   Two-Parameter Compound Poisson Geometric (CPG2)

We first focus on a method given by Huffer when $m = 2$ denoted by CPG2, both because of its simplicity and its computability over all values. The infinite sequence $(\lambda_1, \lambda_2, \dots)$ is generated by two parameters λ_1 and r, so that, for $i \geq 2$:

$$\lambda_i = \lambda_1 r^{i-1}.$$

Equating moments of ξ and Y^* yields

$$\lambda_1 = E(\xi)(1 - r)^2,$$
$$r = (\text{Var}(\xi) - E(\xi))/(\text{Var}(\xi) + E(\xi)),$$

so that

$$P(k; N, w) \approx 1 - P(Y^* = 0) = 1 - \exp\{-2[E(\xi)]^2/[\text{Var}(\xi) + E(\xi)]\},$$
$$(10.14)$$

where the moments are given in (10.2) and (10.11).

10.4.4   Glaz's et al. Compound Poisson Approximation

Glaz, Naus, Roos, and Wallenstein (1994) give another procedure in which $m = 2$ and the λ's are generated by two parameters λ_1 and ω. Based on the heuristic above, λ_j is proportional to $(1 - \omega)\omega^{j-1}(1 - \omega)$, where $\omega = P(A_2 \mid A_1)$. Multiplying by the (approximate) number of values for the start position i, the expected number of consecutive occurrences of the event A_i is

$$\lambda_j = (N - k + 1)G_b(k - 1, N, w)(1 - \omega)^2\omega^{j-1}, \qquad j = 2, \dots, k - 1.$$

Lastly, to compute ω, note $\omega = (1 - \alpha_2^*)/\alpha_1$ with the α's given in (10.9) and (10.1). Even though the above expression continues to hold for arbitrary j, for computational reasons, Glaz et al. set $\lambda_j = 0$ for $j > k$.

The approximation is made more precise by constraining the sum of the λ_i's so they satisfy

$$\sum_{j=1}^{k-1} j\lambda_j = E(\xi) = (N - k + 1)G_b(k - 1, N, w),$$

so that

$$\lambda_1 = (N - k + 1)G(k - 1, N, w) - \sum_j j\lambda_j$$
$$= (N - k - 1)G_b(k - 1, N, w)(1 - 2\omega + \omega^2 - (k - 1)\omega^k + k\omega^{k-1}).$$

Thus based on (10.13), Glaz et al. derive the approximation

$$P(k, N, w) \approx 1 - \exp\{-(N - k + 1)G_b(k - 1, N, w)$$
$$\times (1 - \omega + \omega^{k-1}(k - 1 + \omega - (k - 1)\omega\}. \quad (10.15)$$

10.4.5   Other Methods of Moments Approximations

Huffer and Lin (1997a) also describe a four-parameter approximation, CPG4, which assumes that the infinite sequence is generated by four parameters λ_i, $i = 1, 3$, and ρ, where for $i \geq 4$:

$$\lambda_i = \lambda_3 \rho^{i-3}.$$

Deriving an explicit representation for λ_i involves a symbolic algebra program such as MAPLE, and involves four, instead of two, moments of Y. These are nontrivial to compute, as the authors themselves admit difficulty when $k > 10$. Further, solutions do not always exist, and the resulting approximations are not necessarily more accurate than the simple approximation. The reader interested in more detail should consult their article. Huffer and Lin also give approximations termed LP2 and LP4 based on linear programming, which we will not describe here.

All the methods given in this section can be extended without undue difficulty to approximate the distribution of the number of clusters, which leads to identification of the mth largest clusters, or smallest spacings. These methods, described in Chapter 17, are useful in molecular biology applications.

10.5   Cell Occupancy Approximations: Introduction

In this section, we compute the probabilities that will be required in the remaining sections of this chapter. The approximations are simplest when T/w is an integer. (We can apply approximations in this section to any w simply by finding approximations for windows of size T/L and $T/(L+1)$ where $L = [T/w]$, and then linearly interpolate between the approximations.) Although approximations could be derived directly for the general case, we shall not in general do so, since this makes the "simple" approximations much more complicated.

Many of the results can be extended to the case of the circle, or to the unconditional case discussed in Chapter 11. We will give some, but not all, of these extensions explicitly.

Let $L = [T/w]$ where $[x]$ is the greatest integer in x. As in Naus (1965a), for $i = 1, \ldots, L$, let n_i be the number of points in each of the disjoint equally spaced cells, $[(i-1)w, iw)$, and let

$$\mathcal{A} = \bigcup_{i=1}^{L} \{n_i \geq k\}.$$

Let E_i^c be the event that a cluster of k events begins in the ith cell

$$E_i^c = \left\{ \sup_{(i-1)w \leq t \leq iw} Y_t(w) \geq k \right\},$$

so that E_i is the complementary event introduced in (9.2):

$$E_i = \left\{ \sup_{(i-1)w \leq t \leq iw} Y_t(w) < k \right\}.$$

We next define two other events whose conditional distribution given $\{n_i\}$ is either zero or is the same as E_i^c. Let $\mathcal{D}_i$ be the event that a cluster of k events begins in the ith cell, even though the *adjoining* cell number occupancy numbers are less than k, and let B_i be the same event except that *all* cell occupancy numbers are less than k. Formally, for $i \leq L - 1$, let

$$\mathcal{D}_i = E_i^c \cap \{n_i < k\} \cap \{n_{i+1} < k\} \qquad (10.16)$$

and let

$$B_i = \mathcal{D}_i \cap \mathcal{A}^c.$$

Then

$$P(k; N, w) = P(\mathcal{A}) + P\left(\bigcup_{i=1}^{L-1} B_i \right). \qquad (10.17)$$

10.5.1 Conditional Probabilities

By the reflection principle (see (8.14)):

$$P(B_1 \mid \{n_i\}) = \frac{n_1! \, n_2!}{k! \, (n_1 + n_2 - k)!}, \qquad n_j < k, \quad j = 1, \ldots, L,$$
$$= 0, \qquad\qquad\qquad \text{otherwise.} \qquad (10.18)$$

Similarly,

$$P(\mathcal{D}_1 \mid n_1, n_2) = \frac{n_1! \, n_2!}{k! \, (n_1 + n_2 - k)!}, \qquad n_1 < k, \quad n_2 < k,$$
$$= 0, \qquad\qquad\qquad \text{otherwise,}$$

and

$$P(E_i^c \mid n_1, n_2) = \frac{n_1! \, n_2!}{k! \, (n_1 + n_2 - k)!}, \qquad n_1 < k, \quad n_2 < k,$$
$$= 0, \qquad\qquad\qquad \text{otherwise.}$$

10.5.2 Unconditional Probabilities

To simplify notation, we assume in this subsection that $T = 1$. The results are in fact correct in general except that each time w is referred to, it denotes the ratio of the window to the total time frame or should be replaced by $W = w/T$. (Where the results can be stated simply allowing the generalization to arbitrary T, we do so, and in all cases, $L = T/w$.)

The unconditional probabilities can be calculated by multiplying the conditional probabilities in the previous section by either $P(n_1, n_2)$ or $P(\{n_i\})$ and then summing. For B or $\mathcal{D}$, we can avoid a summation by noting that for $k \le j \le 2(k-1)$:

$$P(\mathcal{D}_1 \mid n_1 + n_2 = j) = P(B_1 \mid n_1 + n_2 = j, n_j < k, j = 3, \dots, L)$$

$$= \frac{2k - 1 - j}{2^j}\binom{j}{k}.$$

The unconditional probabilities will be different since they are summed over different sets. Specifically,

$$P(\mathcal{D}_1) = \sum_{j=k}^{\min(N,2k-2)} P[\mathcal{D}_1 \mid n_1 + n_2 = j]P[n_1 + n_2 = j],$$

and

$$P(B_1) = \sum_{j=k}^{\min(N,2k-2)} P[\mathcal{D}_1 \mid n_1 + n_2 = j]$$

$$\times P\left[n_i < k, i = 3, \dots, L \mid \sum_{i=3}^{L} n_i = N - j\right] P(n_1 + n_2 = j)$$

$$= \sum_{j=k}^{\min(N,2k-2)} P[\mathcal{D}_1 \mid n_1 + n_2 = j]$$

$$\times H_k(N - j, L - 2)P[N_1 + n_2 = j], \qquad (10.19)$$

where $H_k(M, g)$ is defined following (9.15). Similarly,

$$P(E_1) = \sum_{a=1}^{k-1} \sum_{b=1}^{k-1} P(E_1 \mid a, b)P(n_1 = a, n_2 = b).$$

These equations can each be simplified somewhat. Straightforward substitution yields

$$P(\mathcal{D}_1) = \sum_{j=k}^{\min(N,2k-2)} \frac{2k - 1 - j}{2^j}\binom{j}{k}\binom{N}{j}(2w)^j(1 - 2w)^{N-j}$$

$$= b(k; N, w) \sum_{j=k}^{\min(N,2k-2)} (2k - 1 - j)b[j - k; N - k, w/(1 - w)].$$

A simple expression for $P(B_1)$ is given in (9.19).

To compute $P(E_1)$, set $P(n_1 = a, n_2 = b)$ to be a multinomial, so that

$$P(E_1) = \sum_{a=1}^{k-1} \sum_{b=1}^{k-1} P(E_1 \mid a, b) \binom{N}{a, b} w^{a+b} (1 - 2w)^{N-a-b}.$$

Wallenstein, Naus, and Glaz (1993) give an alternative expression

$$P(E_1) = \sum_{j=0}^{k-1} b(j; N, w) F_b \left(k - 1, N - j, \frac{w}{1 - w} \right)$$

$$- b(k; N, w) \sum_{i=1}^{k-1} F_b \left(k - i - 1, N - k, \frac{w}{1 - w} \right). \quad (10.20)$$

10.5.3 Joint Unconditional Probabilities

The joint conditional probability, as previously derived, is implicit in (9.21):

$$P(\mathcal{D}_1 \cap \mathcal{D}_2 \mid n_1 + n_2 + n_3 = j)$$

$$= 3^{-j} \sum_{x=1}^{k-1} \sum_{y=1}^{\min(k-1, j-1-x)} \left[\frac{j!}{k! \, k! \, (j - 2k)!} \right. \qquad (10.21)$$

$$\left. + \frac{j!}{(2k - y)! \, (x + y - k)! \, (j - x - k)!} - \frac{j!}{(2k - y)! \, y! \, (j - 2k)!} \right],$$

using the convention that $a!/b! = 0$ if $a \geq 0$ and $b < 0$, so that when $j < 2k$ only the middle term is summed. Unconditioning yields that

$$P(\mathcal{D}_1 \cap \mathcal{D}_2) = \sum_j P(\mathcal{D}_1 \cap \mathcal{D}_2 \mid Y_0(3w) = j) b(j; N, 3w).$$

To find $P(B_1 \cap B_2)$ insert in the above summand the probability that $n_i < k$, $i = 4, \ldots, L$, to find that $P(B_1 \cap B_2)$ is given as in (9.20):

$$P(B_1 \cap B_2) = \sum_{j=k+1}^{\min(N, 3k-3)} P(\mathcal{D}_1 \cap \mathcal{D}_2 \mid Y_0(3w) = j)$$

$$\times b(j; N, 3w) H_k(N - j, L - 3). \quad (10.22)$$

To derive $P(E_1 \cap E_2)$ use the relationship

$$P(E_1 \cap E_2) = P(E_1) + P(E_2) + P(E_1^c \cap E_2^c) - 1.$$

Further manipulation, as in Wallenstein, Naus, and Glaz (1993), yields

$$
P(E_1 \cap E_2) = \sum_{j=0}^{k-1} b(j; N, w) \sum_{i=0}^{k-1} b\left(i; N - j, \frac{w}{1-w}\right)
$$

$$
\times F_b\left(k - 1, N - i - j, \frac{w}{1-2w}\right)
$$

$$
- 2\left\{ \sum_{j=0}^{k-1} b(j; N, w) b\left(k; N - j, \frac{w}{1-w}\right) \right.
$$

$$
\times \sum_{i=1}^{k-1} F_b\left(k - i - 1, N - k - j, \frac{w}{1-2w}\right) \biggr\}
$$

$$
+ \sum_{j=1}^{k-1} b(k + j; N, w) \sum_{i=0}^{k-1-j} b\left(i; N - j - k, \frac{w}{1-w}\right)
$$

$$
\times F_b\left(k - 1 - j, N - j - i - k, \frac{w}{1-2w}\right)
$$

$$
+ \sum_{j=1}^{k-2} \left\{ b(k; N, w) b\left(k, N - k, \frac{w}{1-w}\right) \right.
$$

$$
- b(k + j; N, w) b\left(k - j; N - k - j, \frac{w}{1-w}\right) \biggr\}
$$

$$
\times \sum_{i=0}^{k-j-2} F_b\left(i; N - 2k, \frac{w}{1-2w}\right).
$$

(Naus (1982) finds $P(E_1)$ and $P(E_1 \cap E_2)$ indirectly after finding the comparable quantities for the unconditional problem and then summing.)

10.6   Markov-Type Approximation (Naus, 1982)

We begin by assuming that $L = T/w$ is an integer, $L \geq 4$. By construction, see (7.15):

$$
P\left\{ \sup_{0 \leq t \leq 1-w} Y_t(w) < k \right\} = P(E_1 \cap E_2 \cap \cdots \cap E_{L-1})
$$

$$
= P(E_1)P(E_2 \mid E_1)P(E_3 \mid E_1, E_2)
$$

$$
\ldots P(E_{L-1} \mid E_1, E_2, \ldots, E_{L-2}).
$$

As described in Section 7.3, a key assumption is that the probability of an event conditional on the entire past is approximately equal to the probability conditional only on the *recent past*, i.e.,

$$P(E_i \mid E_1, E_2, \dots, E_{i-1}) \approx P(E_i \mid E_{i-1}). \qquad (10.23)$$

Applying (10.23) yields

$$P\left\{ \sup_{0 \le t \le T-w} Y_t(w) < k \right\} \approx P(E_1)P(E_2 \mid E_1)P(E_3 \mid E_2) \dots P(E_{L-1} \mid E_{L-2}),$$
$$(10.24)$$

so that

$$1 - P(k; N, w/T) \approx \prod_{i=1}^{L-2} P(E_i \cap E_{i+1}) / \prod_{i=2}^{L-2} P(E_i).$$

It is useful to note this approximation does not require a uniform density and will be exploited in calculating power. For the probability of interest in this section, apply symmetry to find

$$P\left\{ \sup_{0 \le t \le T-w} Y_t(w) < k \right\} \approx P(E_1) \left[\frac{P(E_1 \cap E_2)}{P(E_1)} \right]^{L-2}. \qquad (10.25)$$

Generalize to the case where L is not an integer to find

$$P(k; N, w/T) \approx 1 - P(E_1) \left[\frac{P(E_1 \cap E_2)}{P(E_1)} \right]^{T/w-2}.$$

Naus (1982) identified $P(E_1)$ by the symbol Q_2, and labeled $P(E_1 \cap E_2)$ as Q_3, so that we often refer to this approximation as the Q_2/Q_3 approximation.

A similar assumption can be used in developing the product-limit approximation in (10.6). The application to the circle is described below.

10.7   Very Simple Approximations based on Multiples of $b(k, N, w)$

In Chapter 2, we used the simple approximation of Wallenstein and Neff (1987):

$$P(k; N, w/T) \approx (Tk/w - N + 1)b(k; N, w/T) + 2G_b(k+1, N, w/T).$$

This approximation is one of many similar approximations that have been derived or could be derived. We first indicate how this approximation is derived and then indicate similar approximations.

10.7.1 Derivation of Wallenstein–Neff Approximations

The notation is simplified if $T = 1$; otherwise, as before, replace w by $W = w/T$ throughout. The derivation by Wallenstein and Neff assumes that $w = T/L$, L an integer, and is based on approximating $P(\mathcal{A})$ by the simple Bonferroni bound, and $P(\bigcup B)$ by the Hunter upper bound in (9.17), so that

$$P(k; N, w) \le LG_b(k, N, w) + (L - 1)P(B_1) - (L - 2)P(B_1 \cap B_2). \quad (10.26)$$

To calculate $P(B_1)$, as given in (10.19) or (9.19), requires calculating $H_k(M, j)$, the probability that if M balls are placed randomly in j urns, each will contain fewer than k balls. To simplify the expression, we would like to avoid calculating this term and further avoid even a one-way summation. To do this, we postulate that when $P(k; N, w)$ is small:

(i) $H_k(N, L)$ will be fairly close to 1.0 and, in general, $H_k(N - j, L - 2)$ will be even closer to 1.0 or, equivalently, $P(B_1) \approx P(D_1)$;

(ii) $b(2k + j; N, 2w)$ will be extraordinarily small and thus the upper bound in the summation in (9.19) can be approximated by N. Thus

$$P(B_1) \approx \sum_{j=k}^{N} \frac{2k - 1 - j}{2^j} \binom{j}{k} b(j; N, 2w)$$
$$= [k - 1 - (N - k)/(L - 1)]b(k; N, w)$$
$$= [(k - wN)/(1 - w) - 1]b(k; N, w), \quad (10.27)$$

the last equality requiring somewhat extensive manipulation of binomials.

Experience with computing the two-way summation in (10.21) suggested that the second term usually predominates. (This is possibly because the other terms involve $1/(j - 2k)!$ and are not even included unless $j > 2k$.) Wallenstein and Neff (1987) choose to approximate the three-term sum in (10.21) by only the second term, so that $P(B_1 \cap B_2)$ is approximated by summing

$$\frac{j!}{(2k - y)! \, (x + y - k)! \, (j - x - k)!} . \quad (10.28)$$

We again, in (9.20), set $H_k(N - j, L - 3) = 1$, ignoring some terms like $b(2k; N, w)$, and apply somewhat extensive manipulation of binomial coefficients to find

$$P(B_1 \cap B_2) \approx G_b(k + 1, N, w) - G_b(2k - 1, N, w) \approx G_b(k + 1, N, w). \quad (10.29)$$

Substituting (10.27) and (10.29) into (10.26) and generalizing to arbitrary w yields

$$P(k; N, w) \approx (k/w - N + 1)b(k; N, w) + 2G_b(k + 1, N, w). \quad (10.30)$$

One could anticipate that since (10.26) is an upper bound, this approximation will tend to exceed the true value.

10.7.2   Related Approximations

Neff (1978) (and possibly Wolf (1968)), independent of these results, had proposed using the approximation just derived (or a computationally equivalent and possibly more complicated variant) since it was the exact result for $N \le 2k$.

Using methods similar to those used to derive (13) and (14) in Wallenstein, Naus, and Glaz (1993) it can be shown that

$$Q_2 \approx 2F_b(k - 1, N, w) - b(k; N, w)[(k - 1) - (N - k)w/(1 - w)] - 1,$$
$$Q_3 \approx 2F_b(k - 1, N, w) - b(k; N, w)[2(k - 1) - 2(N - k)w/(1 - w) - 1] - 1.$$

Substituting these terms in (10.25), and performing some more approximations yields

$$P(k; N, w) \approx (k/w - N)b(k; N, w) + G_b(k, N, w). \tag{10.31}$$

This differs from (10.30) by the usually small term $G_b(k + 1, N, w)$.

Results similar to (10.30) have also been derived based on formal asymptotic theory. Cressie (1980) makes a similar argument to Neff, phrasing it as analogous to methods used by Watson (1967) and Kuiper (1960), in a related context. He then took the argument a step further and invoked a normal approximation

$$P(k; N, w) \approx z\phi(z)/w + 2[1 - \Phi(z)],$$

where $z = (k - Nw)/\sqrt{[w(1 - w)]}$, $\phi(z)$ is the density function, and $\Phi(z)$ is the cumulative probability for the standard normal distribution. He found the approximation "not good enough." However, had he "backed-up" a step and used binomials instead of normal approximation, he would have an expression similar to (10.30), with $k/w - N + 1$ replaced by $k/w - N = (k - Nw)/w$.

Loader (1991), based on a large deviation approximation, finds that $(k/w - N)b(k, N, w)$ is a crude approximation to $P(k; N, w)$. He used endpoint correction(s) and proposes the approximation

$$P(k; N, w) \approx (k/w - N)b(k; N, w) + G_b(k, N, w)$$
$$+ \sum_{j=0}^{k-1} \left[\frac{k(N - k)}{N^2 w(1 - w)} \right]^{2(k-j)} b(j; N, w). \tag{10.32}$$

Judging among (10.30), (10.31), (10.32) and related expressions is difficult. On theoretical grounds, the derivation by Loader is more elegant than the somewhat ad hoc derivations used to derive (10.30), and the extra term does improve precision when $w = 1/2$. However, on practical terms, since (10.30) can exceed 1.0 and tends to result in an overestimation of the probabilities, the additional positive contributions will generally be counterproductive, and further detracts from the simplicity of the approximations.

10.8   Approximations Based on Bounds

The concept of bounds and approximations is heavily intertwined. Any pair of an
upper and lower bound can be used to construct an approximation, by taking any
value between them. In a fortunate case, the bounds may be identical to, say, three
decimal places and that may be all the precision needed. Otherwise, the question
of how to take a weighted average appears to be an open question (see below).

The bounds we will study are based on expressing $P(k; N, w)$ as

$$P(k; N, w) = P(\mathcal{A}) + P\left(\bigcup_{i=1,\dots,L-1} B_i\right),$$

where $P(\mathcal{A}) = 1 - H_k(N, L)$. For these bounds, $P(\mathcal{A})$ is computed exactly
based on the recursion relationship in (9.15) and $P(\bigcup B_i)$ is approximated based
on Bonferroni-type bounds. (Of course, it is also possible to approximate $P(\mathcal{A})$.)

10.8.1   Approximation Based on Two-Way Intersections

Letting s_j denote the sums of all j-way intersections of events B_j (see (9.18)),
upper and lower bounds on $P(\bigcup B_i)$ are given by s_1 and $s_1 - s_2$, respectively.
Wallenstein (1980) proposed averaging the upper and lower bounds to find

$$P\left(\bigcup B_i\right) \approx s_1 - s_2/2.$$

The bounds for $P(\bigcup B_i)$ are sufficiently tight to provide, when combined with
the extra value for $P(\mathcal{A})$, a table of critical values for $N < 100$, for values of w
commonly used by epidemiologists to detect clustering in time (i.e., $w/T = 1/L$,
$L = 3, 4, 6, 8, 12, 24$). Specifically, the resulting bounds were within .001 of each
other for tail probabilities less than .04, and within .0025 of each other for tail
probabilities less than .10. Wallenstein does not dwell on these bounds per se, but
rather takes an average of the upper and lower bounds as an approximation.

However, it would be silly to use this approximation (or these bounds) since
sharper bounds and thus presumably more accurate approximations can be obtained without additional computational effort, using the Kwerel (1975) lower
bound and the Hunter (1976) upper bound. The procedure merely involves averaging the bounds in (9.17) and (9.18) which we symbolically term Hunter and
Kwerel to obtain the approximation

$$P(k; N, w) \approx P(\mathcal{A}) + 0.5(\text{Hunter} + \text{Kwerel})$$
$$= P(\mathcal{A}) + (L-1)(0.5 + a^{-1})P(B_1)$$
$$- 0.5(L-2)P(B_1 \cap B_2) - s_2/(a(a-1)), \quad (10.33)$$

where $a = [2s_2/s_1 + 2]$. In particular, if $a = 2$ (if the Kwerel lower bound were
equal to the Bonferroni), the approximation would be

$$P(\mathcal{A}) + (L-1)P(B_1) - (L-2)P(B_1 \cap B_2) - 0.25(L-2)(L-3)P(B_1 \cap B_3).$$

10.8.2   Approximation Based on Three-Way Intersections

Alternatively, with much extra computational effort, we could compute s_3, the sum of all three-way intersections of the events B_i, yielding a revised upper bound $s_2 - s_2 + s_3$ which could be averaged with $s_1 - s_2$ to yield an approximation $s_1 - s_2 + s_3/2$. Again, we will not consider such an approximation since, as indicated in Chapter 7, sharper bounds are available without any extra computational effort. In particular, we denote the upper bound in (7.11) as HIGH, and that in (7.13) as LOW. Based on these bounds, it is natural to form the approximation

$$\text{Approx} = wt\ \text{LOW} + (1 - wt)\text{HIGH}, \qquad (10.34)$$

where $0 < wt < 1$. For small probabilities the bounds are very tight and any weight, wt, will essentially give the same answer.

Bonferroni-type bounds will usually, but not always, have the property that the absolute error, based on terms including I-way intersections ($I = 2, 3$), is lower than for terms involving ($I - 1$)-way intersections. This might suggest having $wt < 1/2$. However, we posit that we could improve on a fixed weight by letting the decision be data-based, by assigning a larger weight to the bound based on three-way intersections if it shows a large improvement over the simpler Hunter bound (see (9.17)), than if it shows a small improvement over the simple bound. We thus suggest a weight of

$$wt = \frac{\text{Hunter} - \text{High}}{\text{Hunter} - \text{Low}}, \qquad (10.35)$$

where Hunter is given in (9.17), Low in (9.18). Thus a presumably accurate, but computationally intensive, approximation can be obtained by substituting (10.35) into (10.34).

10.9   Other Methods

Gates and Westcott (1984) develop an approximation based on a recursion formula, best for the case when $Nw/(k - 1) \ll 1$ and $N - 2k - 1$ is not too large. The approximation has some use for small values of w and for N not too large.

Berman and Eagelson (1985) give a simplification of the Gates–Westcott result, although they find the Gates–Westcott approximation to be unacceptable when the sample size is large.

Knox and Lancashire (1982) propose two simple approximations. It is somewhat unclear if they have the conditional or unconditional version in mind. Since these approximations are neither more accurate nor more theoretically justified than the Wallenstein–Neff approximation, it would appear to be of historical rather than practical interest.

Anderson and Titterington (1995) review several of the procedures already mentioned and appear to favor the Wallenstein–Neff procedure for calculating critical values near $\alpha = .05$. They also present what they term a direct approximation of critical values. Letting $k_{.05}(N, w)$ denote the critical value for the scan statistic for fixed w and N, they first, for fixed N, fit the polynomial in w/T:

$$k_{.05}(N, w/T)/N = \alpha(N) + \beta(N)w/T + \gamma(N)(w/T)^2.$$

They then assume that the functions $\ln \alpha(N)$, $\ln[\beta(N) - 1]$, and $\ln[-\gamma(N)]$ are linear in $\ln N$ and thus get the very simple approximation

$$k_{.05}(N, w)/N \approx 1.392N^{-.629} + (1 + 3.328N^{-.469})w - 4.835N^{-0.505}w^2.$$

This is in a sense simpler than the other approximations considered in that no probability distribution need be evaluated, although one "price" paid is the limitation to the .05 critical value.

In Chapter 2, a similar approach, based on postulating linear and quadratic relationships and fitting values, was used to estimate the means and variances of S_w as a function of w and N.

Anderson and Titterington (1995), in their equation (5), also consider applying a normal approximation to binomial probabilities. This may give some insight, but probably has the defect noted by Cressie (1980) (see discussion following (10.31)), who utilized a similar normal approximation, of needlessly detracting from the accuracy of the approximation.

10.10   Comparisons

We will summarize and place in context the approximately 10 approximations that are most useful or have been used frequently. Almost all published approximations have included some comparison to simulated values and other approximations, and the reader is referred to these publications in addition to the material here. In general, given that we have done some choosing among approximations, more complicated expressions will give more accurate values, and the decision should be made in that context.

Table 10.1 compares approximations for 15 cases, which are a subset of those presented in Tables 1 and 2 of Huffer and Lin (1997a). (The selection of these 15 cases was haphazard, but was intended to mostly, but not exclusively, focus on the case when $w = 1/L$, L an integer.) The fit of these comparisons to simulated values is summarized by the index

$$\sqrt{\sum (\text{approx} - \text{sim})^2/15}.$$

Although the conclusions we reach below are consistent with Table 10.1, and reflect the ordering of this index, they often reflect additional examination of the results.

We first describe applications that could conceptually be done on a hand-held calculator that would be sophisticated enough to calculate binomial coefficients. The one-parameter approximation ((10.3) and its variants) should not in general be used for numerical work, unless one perhaps checks first the condition in (10.4). The Wallenstein–Neff approximation ((10.30) or its variants), is the next simplest, is adequate for use in hypothesis testing, i.e., to find p-values less than .10, but will fail miserably in the upper tail.

Table 10.1. Comparison of various approximations to simulated values for N = 100.

k	w	Simulation	Three-way bounds 10.34	Huffer MC2 10.12	Lin CPG2 10.14	Glaz Prod 10.6	Naus Q2/Q3 10.25	Wallen. Neff 10.30	Berman Eagels. 10.5	Poisson 10.3	Su 10.10	Glaz Com.P 10.15	Two-way bounds 10.33
4	0.002	0.0942	0.0944	0.0944	0.0944	0.094	0.0943	0.0992	0.0986	0.1029	0.0938	0.094	0.094
4	0.004	0.4738	0.4736	0.4749	0.4739	0.4676	0.4643	0.6247	0.6204	0.5287	0.4615	0.4671	0.4676
4	0.005	0.6804	0.6777	0.6828	0.6809	0.667	0.6571	>1	>1	0.7454	0.6576	0.6693	0.6697
7	0.02	0.5865	0.5864	0.5907	0.5827	0.5674	0.553	0.7875	0.8435	0.7667	0.567	0.5811	0.5685
7	0.025	0.8862	0.8858	0.8933	*	0.8583	0.8339	>1	>1	0.9765	0.8451	0.8746	0.8616
10	0.025	0.0503	0.0503	0.0498	0.0506	0.05	0.0498	0.051	0.0536	0.0818	0.0518	0.0519	0.05
10	0.03	0.1487	0.1487	0.1471	0.1503	0.1458	0.1523	0.1665	0.1668	0.2537	0.1524	0.1532	0.1461
10	0.04	0.5597	0.5588	0.5616	*	0.5331	0.5171	0.7	0.8052	0.8224	0.5483	0.5624	0.5452
10	0.045	0.7806	0.7764	0.7884	*	0.7415	0.7305	0.1	0.1	0.9641	0.7471	0.7753	0.7461
10	0.05	0.9244	0.9276	0.933	0.8837	0.8881	0.8582	>1	>1	0.9968	0.8803	0.9162	0.8954
16	0.1	0.8615	0.8607	0.8707	0.116	0.808	0.77	>1	>1	0.9979	0.8225	0.8574	0.8213
20	0.1	0.1189	0.1185	0.142	0.116	0.116	0.1148	0.1199	0.1473	0.31	0.1345	0.1348	0.116
26	0.2	0.897	0.9095	0.9239	0.901	0.8437	0.79	>1	>1	0.9999	0.8496	0.8847	0.8669
30	0.2	0.2738	0.2739	0.2678	0.2678	0.2648	0.2588	0.2768	0.4033	0.7586	0.3228	0.3228	0.2661
34	0.2	0.0291	0.0291	0.0247	0.029	0.029	0.0289	0.0291	0.0373	0.0987	0.0357	0.0357	0.029
			0.004	0.009		0.027	0.047			0.177	0.029	0.015	0.019

* Failed to converge.

$s = \sqrt{\sum (\text{Approx.} - \text{Sim.})^2 / 15}.$

If one were programming from scratch, it would be hard to do better than the Glaz et al. approximation (10.15). The work required to get an alternating sum is essentially the same as an ordinary sum. Any other approximation will require considerably more computational effort. The similar approximation (10.10) is a bit simpler and perhaps more intuitive, but apparently not as accurate.

We next review approximations that require a "short, easy-to-write" computer program that "runs quickly," in addition to the ones just noted. The Markov-like approximation (Q_2/Q_3) of Naus (10.25) is widely applicable, relatively easy to compute, and fairly accurate over the entire range. It makes use only of exact and cumulative binomial probabilities. The Glaz (1992) product limit approximation (10.6) is conceptually similar, and unlike the Naus approximation, has a simple-to-state formula but may involve numerical problems. Another procedure based on cell occupancy methods, (10.33), is competitive, and apparently more accurate than the Q_2/Q_3 approximation, but requires first using a recursive relationship to find the probability of placing N balls in J urns subject to restrictions.

Getting even more accurate results requires more programming, but much less computer time than would be required by the exact methods. Huffer and Lin's (1997a) higher-order approximations require MAPLE, and may not result in tighter approximations. Huffer and Lin recommend different procedures depending on the relative size of k, but it is not clear if this suggestion is based on some theoretical consideration or perhaps just a small number of results. The approximations based on bounds involving three-way intersections of events (10.34) requires fairly extensive calculation and would be best done over the net. The web site address that computes these bounds, at least for $N < 100$, and $w > .01$, is http://c3.biomath.mssm.edu/scan.html. These approximations will not be so good for very high p-values (perhaps $> .95$), but appear better than other approximations otherwise.

Except for the approximation such as (10.34), which is complicated to program (although not necessarily so computationally intensive), the most accurate approximations appear to be those by Huffer and Lin. Equation (10.12) (MC2) converges for all cases and, based on these examples, gives the best approximation among all procedures not requiring extensive coding.

This chapter has dealt somewhat extensively with approximations for the conditional case, focusing on the line. In the remaining chapters of the book, we will discuss approximations for other cases. Often it might be possible to modify some of the techniques presented here for these other scenarios.

10.11   Circular Case

The cell occupancy methods lend themselves to extensions on the circle. We use the same notation as in Section 10.5, based on cutting the circle of unit circumference at an arbitrary point. We copy the points on $[0, w)$ to $(1, 1 + w)$ so that for $t = (i - 1)L + s$, $(s \leq w)$, $Y_t(w)$ includes the events in the last interval of length $1 - s$ as well as the points in the first interval of length s. This allows us to define the event E_L and its complement exactly as on the line, and also to define the event

$$\mathcal{D}_L = E_L^c \cap \{n_L < k\} \cap \{n_1 < k\}.$$

We then note that

$$P_c(k; N, w) = P\left\{\bigcup_{i=1}^{L}(\mathcal{A}_i \cup \mathcal{D}_i)\right\},$$

where $\mathcal{A}_i = \{n_i \geq k\}$ and $\mathcal{A} = \bigcup \mathcal{A}_i$. We then can define bounds based on the extension of the Bonferroni procedure as we did in Section 10.8. Wallenstein, Weinberg, and Gould (1989) manipulate these bounds using various combinatorial identities, generalized to the case where L need not be an integer, and suggest the approximation

$$P_c(k; N, w) \approx \frac{k - wN}{w(1 - w)}b(k; N, w).$$

As noted in Section 10.7, there are several variants of this approximation. Nevertheless, a comparison of a small number of exact values with this approximation indicated much better agreement than one usually expects from these Bonferroni bounds, and the authors conjecture that this may be the case because the terms that are ignored cancel out with one another.

Lastly, the Q_2/Q_3 approximation can be extended by noting

$$1 - P_c(k; N, w) = \Pr\left\{\sup_{0 \leq t \leq T} Y_t(w) < k\right\} = P(E_1 \cap E_2 \cap \cdots \cap E_{L-1} \cap E_L)$$

$$= P(E_1)P(E_2 \mid E_1)P(E_3 \mid E_1, E_2)$$

$$\ldots P(E_{L-1} \mid E_1, E_2, \ldots, E_{L-2})$$

$$\times P(E_L \mid E_1, E_2, \ldots, E_{L-2}E_{L-1}).$$

As described in Section 7.5, a key assumption is that the conditional probability of an event conditional on the entire past is approximately equal to the probability conditional only on the *recent past*, i.e.,

$$P(E_i \mid E_1, E_2, \ldots, E_{i-1}) \approx P(E_i \mid E_{i-1}).$$

Applying the previous assumption yields

$$P\left\{\sup_{0 \leq t \leq T} Y_t(w) < k\right\} \approx P(E_1)P(E_2 \mid E_1)P(E_3 \mid E_2)$$

$$\ldots P(E_{L-1} \mid E_{L-2})P(E_L \mid E_{L-1}),$$

so that

$$1 - P(k; N, w/T) \approx \prod_{i=1}^{L-1} P(E_i \cap E_{i+1})/\prod_{i=2}^{L-1} P(E_i)$$

so that

$$P(k; N, w/T) \approx 1 - Q_2 \left(\frac{Q_3}{Q_2} \right)^{T/w-1}, \qquad (10.36)$$

where Q_2 and Q_3 are given at the end of Sections 10.5.2 and 10.5.3, respectively.

11
Scanning Points in a Poisson Process

11.1   Poisson Distribution of Events

Let $Y_t(w)$ denote the number of points (X's) in the interval $\{t, t + w)$. The scan statistic $S_w = \max\limits_{0 \le t \le T-w} \{Y_t(w)\}$, denotes the largest number of points to be found in any subinterval of $[0, T)$ of length w. Let $X_{(1)} \le X_{(2)} \le \ldots$, denote the ordered values of the X's. The statistic W_k, the size of the smallest subinterval of $[0, T)$ that contains k points, equals $\min\limits_{0 \le w \le T} \{w : S_w \ge k\} = \min\limits_{1 \le i}\{X_{(i+k-1)} - X_{(i)}\}$. For the case where the N points are uniformly distributed on $[0, T)$, the common probabilities $P(S_w \ge k) = P(W_k \le w)$ are denoted $P(k; N, w/T)$. The maximum cluster S_w is called the *scan statistic*, and the smallest interval W_{r+1} is called the *r-scan statistic*.

11.1.1   The Poisson Process

Let λ denote the (expected) average number of events in any unit interval. The number of events Z_t in any interval of length t is Poisson distributed with mean λt. That is, $P(Z_t = k) = p(k; \lambda t) = \exp\{-\lambda t\}(\lambda t)^k/k!$ for $k = 0, 1, 2, \ldots$. The numbers of events in any disjoint (nonoverlapping) intervals are independently distributed. There are various other ways to characterize the Poisson process. For the Poisson process the arrival times between points are independent exponential random variates. Conditional on there being a total of N points from the Poisson process in $[0, T)$, these N points are uniformly distributed over $[0, T)$.

Given a point process on $[0, \infty)$, let $T_{k,w}$ denote the waiting time until we first observe at least k points in an interval of length w. Formally, $T_{k,w} = X_{(i+k-1)}$ for the smallest i, such that $X_{(i+k-1)} - X_{(i)} \leq w$. The three scan statistics, S_w, W_k, and $T_{k,w}$, are related by

$$P(S_w \geq k) = P(W_k \leq w) = P(T_{k,w} \leq T).$$

For the Poisson process, with mean λ *per unit time*, we denote these common probabilities by $P^*(k; \lambda T, w/T) = 1 - Q^*(k; \lambda T, w/T)$.

For some applications the researcher may need exact results, or at least bounds on the probability as a supplement to the approximation. Section 11.2 gives exact formulas for $P^*(k; \lambda T, w/T)$. In cases where one needs accurate but not necessarily exact results, the approximations of Section 11.4 can be supplemented by bounds on the probability. Section 11.3 gives tight bounds for the probability.

11.2   Exact Results for $P^*(k; \lambda T, w/T)$

Chapter 8 gives exact formulas for $P(k; N, w)$, for various combinations of k, N, and w, given N uniformly distributed points over $[0, 1)$. For N points distributed uniformly over $[0, T)$, $P(S_w \geq k) = P(k; N, w/T)$, and in the formula in Chapter 8 we can simply rewrite w by w/T. For the case where the events occur according to a Poisson process on $[0, \infty)$, with average number of points λ per unit interval, $P(S_w \geq k) = P^*(k; \lambda T, w/T)$. For the Poisson process, the total number of points in $[0, T)$ is a random variable $\tilde{N}$ with expectation λT. Further, given that the points are generated by a Poisson process, then conditional on $\tilde{N} = N$, the N points are uniformly distributed on $[0, T)$ and $P(S_w \geq k \mid \tilde{N} = N) = P(k; N, w/T)$. Thus, we can find $P^*(k; \lambda T, w/T)$ by averaging $P(k; N, w/T)$ over the Poisson distribution of $\tilde{N}$. This proves:

Theorem 11.1. *For* $1 < k$, $0 < w < T$, $0 < \lambda$, *and* $V = [T/w](k - 1) + k$:

$$P^*(k; \lambda T, w/T) = \sum_{N=k}^{\infty} P(k; N, w/T) p(N; \lambda T) \tag{11.1}$$

and

$$Q^*(k; \lambda T, w/T) = \sum_{N=0}^{V} Q(k; N, w/T) p(N; \lambda T). \tag{11.2}$$

The form of (11.2) makes clear that only a finite number of values of $Q(k; N, w/T)$ are needed to evaluate $Q^*(k; N, w/T)$. We can use Theorem 11.1 together with exact results for $P(k; N, w/T)$ to find either specific numbers or general expressions for $P^*(k; \lambda T, w/T)$. For example, Chapter 8 gives exact expressions for $P(k; N, 1/2)$ and $P(k; N, 1/3)$. Averaging these over the Poisson distribution of N and simplifying, gives the following results for $P^*(k; 2\psi, 1/2) = 1 - Q^*(k; 2\psi, 1/2)$ and $P^*(k; 3\psi, 1/3) = Q^*(k; 3\psi, 1/3)$ where $\psi = \lambda w$.

Theorem 11.2. *For $k > 2, 0 < \psi$:*

$$Q^*(k; 2\psi, 1/2) = (F_p(k - 1; \psi))^2 - (k - 1)p(k; \psi)p(k - 2; \psi)$$
$$- (k - 1 - \psi)p(k; \psi)F_p(k - 3; \psi) \tag{11.3}$$

and

$$Q^*(k; 3\psi, 1/3) = (F_p(k - 1; \psi))^3 - A_1 + A_2 + A_3 - A_4, \tag{11.4}$$

where $F_p(i; \psi) = 0$ for $i < 0$, and

$$A_1 = 2p(k; \psi)F_p(k - 1; \psi)\{(k - 1)F_p(k - 2; \psi) - \psi F_p(k - 3; \psi)\},$$
$$A_2 = .5(p(k; \psi))^2\{(k - 1)(k - 2)F_p(k - 3; \psi)$$
$$- 2(k - 2)\psi F_p(k - 4; \psi) + \psi^2 F_p(k - 5; \psi)\},$$
$$A_3 = \sum_{r=1}^{k-1} p(2k - r; \psi)(F_p(r - 1; \psi))^2,$$
$$A_4 = \sum_{r=2}^{k-1} p(2k - r; \psi)p(r; \psi)\{(r - 1)F_p(r - 2; \psi) - \psi F_p(r - 3; \psi)\}.$$

Theorem 11.2, in addition to giving exact results for the Poisson case for $w/T = 1/2, 1/3$, also provides the basis for the highly accurate approximation for $Q^*(k; \lambda T, w/T)$ given in Section 11.4. We can similarly apply (11.1) to other results from Chapter 8 to derive general results for the unconditional (Poisson) case

$$1 - P^*(k; \psi L, 1/L) = \Pr\left\{\sup_{i,t}[n_i - v_i(t) + v_{i+1}(t)] < k\right\}$$

$$= \sum_{\sigma^*} \Pr\left\{\sup_{i,t}[n_i - v_i(t) + v_{i+1}(t)] < k \mid \{n_i\}\right\}$$

$$\times \left(\exp\{-\psi L\}(\psi L)^{\sum n_i} / \prod n_i!\right), \tag{11.5}$$

where the sum is over the set σ^* of all sets of integers $n_1, n_2, \ldots, n_L$ each less than k. We can write the sum over σ^* as a double sum where the first summation is over $N = \sum n_i$, and the following summation is over the set s of all partitions of N into L integers $n_1, n_2, \ldots, n_L$ each less than k. Equation (8.21) gives an expression for

$$\Pr\left\{\sup_{i,t}[n_i - v_i(t) + v_{i+1}(t)] < k \mid \{n_i\}\right\},$$

and substituting this into (11.5) gives Theorem 11.3.

Theorem 11.3. *Let k and L be integers, $2 \leq k$, L and let $0 < \psi$. Then*

$$P^*(k; \psi L, 1/L) = 1 - \exp\{-\psi L\} \sum_{N=0}^{\infty} (\psi L)^N \sum_{\sigma} \det |1/c_{ij}!|, \qquad (11.6)$$

where

$$c_{ij} = (j-i)k - \left(\sum_{r=i}^{j-1} n_r\right) + n_i, \qquad i < j,$$

$$= (j-i)k + \sum_{r=j}^{i} n_r, \qquad i \geq j,$$

and where the sum is over the set σ of all partitions of N into L positive integers $n_i < k$ for $i = 1, 2, \dots, L$ for all N.

Theorem 11.4. *Given k an integer, $2 \leq k$ and $0 < w < T$; let H denote the largest integer in T/w and let $d = 1 - wH/T$. Let*

$$M = \sum_{j=0}^{H} m_{2j+1},$$

and

$$R^* = N! \, d^M \{(w/T) - d\}^{N-M} p(N; \lambda T).$$

Then,

$$Q^*(k; \lambda T, w/T) = \sum_{V^*} R^* \det |1/h_{ij}!| \det |1/v_{ij}!|, \qquad (11.7)$$

where the summation is over the set V^* of all partitions of N into $(2H + 1)$ nonnegative integers m_i satisfying $m_i + m_{i+1} < k$ for $i = 1, 2, \dots, 2H$, and where

$$h_{ij} = \sum_{s=2j-1}^{2i-1} m_s - (i-j)k, \qquad 1 \leq j \leq i \leq H+1,$$

$$= -\sum_{s=2i}^{2j-2} m_s + (j-i)k, \qquad 1 \leq i < j \leq H+1,$$

$$v_{ij} = \sum_{s=2j}^{2i} m_s - (i-j)k, \qquad 1 \leq j \leq i \leq H,$$

$$= -\sum_{s=2i+1}^{2j-1} m_s - (j-i)k, \qquad 1 \leq i < j \leq H.$$

Hwang (1977) derives an alternative general formula for $P(k; N, w)$ that extended somewhat the range of direct computation. Hwang's result is based on a generalized version of the Karlin–McGregor theorem that led (through the Barton and Mallows' corollary) to the proof of Theorem 8.4 of Chapter 8. Average the result for $Q(k; N, w)$ over the Poisson distribution of $\tilde{N}$; note that $Q(k; N, w) = 1$, $0 \le N \le k - 1$, and $Q(k; N, w) = 0$, $(k - 1)w < N$, to find:

Theorem 11.5. *Define the units so that $T = 1$. Given k an integer, $2 \le k$ and $0 < w < 1$, let $L = [1/w]$, $v = 1 - wL$. Then,*

$$Q^*(k; \lambda, w) = F_p(k - 1; \lambda) + \sum_{N=k}^{w(k-1)} e^{-\lambda} \lambda^N \sum_{\Phi} \det |g_{ij}/(\beta_j - \alpha_i)!|, \quad (11.8)$$

where,

$$g_{ij} = w^{(\beta_j - \alpha_i)} \sum_{S=\zeta}^{\beta_j - \alpha_i} b(s; \beta_j - \alpha_i, v/w), \quad j \le L, \quad \beta_j - \alpha_i \ge 0,$$

$$= v^{(\beta_j - \alpha_i)}, \qquad\qquad j = L + 1, \quad (\beta_j - \alpha_i) \ge 0,$$

$$= 0, \qquad\qquad\qquad (\beta_j - \alpha_i) < 0, \qquad (11.9)$$

where the second sum is over the set Φ of all partitions of N into $L + 1$ integers each less than k and $\zeta = \max\{0, (\beta_{L+1} + 1 - \alpha_i)\}$.

11.3 Bounds for the Distribution of the Scan Statistic

Let $\Xi(T)$ be the number of events that have occurred in the interval $[0, T)$, $T \ge 0$. Assume that $\{\Xi(T)\}_{T \ge 0}$ is a Poisson process with a constant intensity $\lambda > 0$. $\Xi(T)$ has a Poisson distribution with mean λT. Let $Y_t(w)$, $t > 0$, be its scanning process, i.e.,

$$Y_t(w) = \Xi(t + w) - \Xi(t) \qquad (11.10)$$

is the number of events that have occurred in the interval $[t, t + w)$ for some fixed constant $w > 0$. In this section we present the bounds for

$$P^*(k; \lambda T, w/T) = P(S_w \ge k), \qquad (11.11)$$

where S_w is defined in Section 11.1. The material presented in this section is based on Janson (1984).

For $0 < w \le t \le u$ and $k \ge 2$ an integer, define

$$N_{t,u} = \max_{t \le s \le u} Y_{s-w}(w) \qquad (11.12)$$

and abbreviate $N_{w,t}$ to N_t. Let

$$\tau = \inf_{t \geq w} \{Y_{t-w}(w) \geq k\} \qquad (11.13)$$

and for $t \geq w$:

$$G(t) = P(\tau > t) = P(N_t \leq k - 1). \qquad (11.14)$$

For $0 < t < w$, define $G(t) = P(\Xi(t) \leq k - 1)$. Then

$$P^*(k; \lambda T, w/T) = 1 - G(T). \qquad (11.15)$$

The following results in Janson (1984) play a key role in deriving the bounds for $P^*(k; \lambda T, w/T)$.

Lemma 11.1. *Let f and g be two nonnegative increasing (or decreasing) functions of a Poisson process Ξ. Then*

$$E[f(\Xi)g(\Xi)] \geq E[f(\Xi)]E[g(\Xi)].$$

The proof of Lemma 11.1, given in Janson (1984), is based on a correlation inequality for nonnegative increasing (or decreasing) functions of a finite sequence of independent random variables in Esary, Proschan, and Walkup (1967). We will not present this proof here.

Lemma 11.2. *The distribution of τ has a mass point at w and a density function $f(t)$ on (w, ∞), where*

$$P(\tau = w) = P(Y_0 \geq k) \qquad (11.16)$$

and for $t > w$:

$$f(t) = \lambda P\{(Y_{t-w} = k - 1) \cap (N_t \leq k - 1)\}. \qquad (11.17)$$

Proof. Equation (11.16) follows from the fact that $P(\tau = w) = P(Y_0 \geq k) > 0$. For $t > w$, $\tau = t$ if and only if $N_t \leq k - 1$ and $\lim_{0 < h \to 0} Y_{t-w+h} \geq k$. Since the interarrival times between events in a Poisson process have an exponential distribution, the probability that two events are separated by exactly w is equal to 0, and therefore $\tau = t$ if and only if $\Xi(t) = k$ and the event $(Y_{t-w} = k - 1) \cap (N_t \leq k - 1)$ occurs. From the properties of a Poisson process we get that for any $u > w$:

$$P(w < \tau \leq u) = \int_w^u P\{(Y_{t-w} = k - 1) \cap (N_t \leq k - 1)\} \lambda \, dt. \qquad (11.18)$$

Equation (11.17) follows.

Lemma 11.3. *Let $f(t)$ be the density in (11.17). Then*

$$f(t) \leq f(2w)G(t - 2w), \qquad t \geq 3w, \qquad (11.19)$$

and

$$f(t) \geq f(2w)G(t - w), \qquad t \geq 2w. \qquad (11.20)$$

Proof. For $t \geq 3w$ let $E_1 = (Y_{t-w} = k - 1) \cap (N_{t-w,t} \leq k - 1)$ and let $E_2 = (N_{t-2w} \leq k - 1)$. Then $f(t) = \lambda P(E_1 \cap (N_{t-2w,t-w} \leq k - 1) \cap E_2)$. It follows that $f(t) \leq \lambda P(E_1 \cap E_2)$. Since the events E_1 and E_2 are independent we get

$$f(t) \leq \lambda P(E_1 \cap E_2) = \lambda P(E_1)P(E_2). \qquad (11.21)$$

From homogeneity of the Poisson process we get $f(2w) = \lambda P(E_1)$. Since $P(E_2) = G(t - 2w)$, inequality (11.19) follows.

Let E_1 be defined as above and let $E_3 = (N_{t-w} \leq k - 1)$. Then $f(t) = \lambda P(E_1 \cap E_3)$. For $t \geq 2w$, define Ξ_1 to be the restriction of Ξ to the interval $[t - w, t)$ (i.e., the events that occur in $[t - w, t)$ generated by the Poisson process Ξ), and let $\Xi_2 = \Xi - \Xi_1$, i.e., the restriction of Ξ to the complement of $[t - w, t)$. Then Ξ_2 is a Poisson process and conditional on Ξ_1, the indicator functions of E_1 and E_3 are decreasing functions of Ξ_2. Lemma 11.1 implies that

$$P(E_1 \cap E_3 \mid \Xi_1) \geq P(E_1 \mid \Xi_1)P(E_3 \mid \Xi_1). \qquad (11.22)$$

Since E_3 is independent of Ξ_1, $P(E_3 \mid \Xi_1) = P(E_3) = G(t - w)$. We have seen that $f(2w) = \lambda P(E_1)$. Therefore,

$$f(t) = \lambda P(E_1 \cap E_3) \geq \lambda P(E_1)P(E_3) = f(2w)G(t - w).$$

This concludes the proof of Lemma 11.3.

Lemma 11.4. *If $t \geq w$ and $u \geq 0$, then*

$$G(t + u) \geq G(t)G(u + w) \qquad (11.23)$$

and

$$G(t + u + w) \leq G(t)G(u + w). \qquad (11.24)$$

Proof. For $t \geq w$ and $u \geq 0$ we have

$$G(t + u) = P(N_{t+u} \leq k - 1) = P\{(N_t \leq k - 1) \cap (N_{t,t+u} \leq k - 1)\}$$
$$\geq P(N_t \leq k - 1)P(N_{t,t+u} \leq k - 1) = G(t)G(u + w). \qquad (11.25)$$

As the indicator functions of the events $(N_t \leq k - 1)$ and $(N_{t,t+u} \leq k - 1)$ are decreasing functions of Ξ, inequality (11.25) follows from the correlation inequality in Lemma 11.1. This establishes the inequality given in (11.23).

Now,

$$
\begin{aligned}
G(t + u + w) &= P(N_{t+u+w} \leq k - 1) \\
&= P\{(N_t \leq k - 1) \cap (N_{t,t+w} \leq k - 1) \\
&\quad \cap (N_{t+w,t+u+w} \leq k - 1)\} \\
&\leq P\{(N_t \leq k - 1) \cap (N_{t+w,t+u+w} \leq k - 1)\} \\
&= P(N_t \leq k - 1)P(N_{t+w,t+u+w} \leq k - 1) \\
&= G(t)G(u + w). \quad\quad\quad (11.26)
\end{aligned}
$$

Equation (11.26) follows from the fact that the events $(N_t \leq k-1)$ and $(N_{t+w,t+u+w} \leq k - 1)$ are independent. This completes the proof of Lemma 11.4.

To evaluate the bounds for $G(T)$ we have to evaluate $f(2w)$.

Lemma 11.5. *Let Y be a Poisson random variable with mean λw. Then*

$$
f(2w) = \lambda P(Y = k - 1)[P(Y \leq k - 1) - \frac{\lambda w}{k} P(Y \leq k - 2)]. \quad (11.27)
$$

Proof. It follows from Lemma 11.2 that

$$
f(2w) = \lambda P(Y_w = k - 1)P(N_{2w} \leq k - 1 \mid Y_w = k - 1).
$$

We first evaluate $P(N_{2w} \leq k - 1 \mid Y_w = k - 1, Y_0 = m)$ for $0 \leq m \leq k - 1$. Denote by $\xi_1, \ldots, \xi_{k-1}$ and $\eta_1, \ldots, \eta_m$ the realizations of the Poisson process Ξ in the intervals $[w, 2w)$ and $[0, w)$, respectively. Then, for $0 \leq s \leq w$:

$$
\begin{aligned}
Y_s &= \#\{i; \xi_i < s + w\} + \#\{j; \eta_j \geq s\} \\
&= k - 1 - \#\{i; \xi_i \geq s + w\} + \#\{j; \eta_j \geq s\},
\end{aligned}
$$

Therefore,

$$
\begin{aligned}
N_{2k} \leq k - 1 &\Leftrightarrow \quad Y_s \leq k - 1 \\
&\Leftrightarrow \quad \#\{i; \xi_i \geq s + w\} \geq \#\{j; \eta_j \geq s\},
\end{aligned}
$$

for every $0 \leq s \leq w$. Since, $\#\{j; \eta_j \geq s\} = \#\{j; \eta_j + w \geq s + w\}$, we get that $N_{2w} \leq k - 1$ if and only if we count $\{\xi_i\}$ and $\{\eta_j + w\}$ in decreasing order then at any instance we observe at least as many ξ_i's as $(\eta_j + w)$'s. It follows from the properties of the Poisson process that $\{\xi_i\}$ and $\{\eta_j + w\}$ are uniformly distributed on $[w, 2w)$. From the classical ballot problem (Feller 1968, p. 69) it follows that

$$
P(N_{2w} \leq k - 1 \mid Y_w = k - 1, Y_0 = m) = 1 - \frac{m}{k}.
$$

Therefore,

$$P(N_{2w} \leq k - 1, Y_w = k - 1) = \sum_{m=0}^{k-1} P(N_{2w} \leq k - 1, Y_w = k - 1, Y_0 = m)$$

$$= P(Y_w = k - 1) \sum_{m=0}^{k-1} \left(1 - \frac{m}{k}\right) P(Y_0 = m)$$

$$= P(Y_w = k - 1)E\left(1 - \frac{Y_0}{k}\right)_+$$

and

$$f(2w) = \lambda P(Y_w = k - 1)E\left(1 - \frac{Y_0}{k}\right)_+,$$

where $(x)_+ = \max(x, 0)$. Since Y_0 has a Poisson distribution with mean λw:

$$E\left(1 - \frac{Y_0}{k}\right)_+ = \sum_{m=0}^{k-1}\left(1 - \frac{m}{k}\right) P(Y_0 = m) = P(Y_0 \leq k-1) - \frac{\lambda w}{k} P(Y_0 \leq k-2).$$

Equation (11.27) follows. This completes the proof of Lemma 11.5.

We are now ready to present the bounds for $G(t)$. For the lower bounds, (11.23) yields for $t \geq 3w$:

$$G(t) \geq G(3w)G(t - 2w).$$

From Lemma 11.3, (11.19), we get that for $t \geq 3w$:

$$f(t) \leq \frac{f(2w)}{G(3w)}G(t).$$

Since

$$\frac{d}{dt}[e^{tf(2w)/G(3w)}G(t)] = \frac{f(2w)}{G(3w)}e^{tf(2w)/G(3w)}G(t) - e^{tf(2w)/G(3w)}f(t) \geq 0,$$

$e^{tf(2w)/G(3w)}G(t)$ is an increasing function for $t \geq 3w$. Therefore, for any value of $T \geq 3w$:

$$G(T) \geq e^{-f(2w)(T-3w)/G(3w)}G(3w). \tag{11.28}$$

Define $\gamma_1 = f(2w)/G(3w)$ and $\gamma_{k+1} = f(2w)e^{3w\gamma_k}$, $k \geq 1$. By induction, we get

$$f(t) \leq \gamma_k G(t), \qquad t \geq (2k + 1)w,$$

and

$$G(t) \geq A_k e^{-\gamma_k t}, \qquad t \geq (2k + 1)w, \tag{11.29}$$

where $A_k = e^{(2k+1)w\gamma_k} G((2k+1)w)$. It follows from repeated application of (11.24) that

$$G(t)^j \geq G(jt).$$

It follows from (11.29) that

$$G(t) \geq A_k e^{-\gamma_k jt}$$

and as $j \to \infty$ we get

$$G(t) \geq e^{-\gamma_k t}. \tag{11.30}$$

The sequence $\{\gamma_k\}$ is either decreasing or increasing. Let $\alpha(x) = f(2w)e^{2wx} - x$. Then if $2wf(2w) < 1/e$ then the equation $\alpha(x) = 0$ has two roots $x_1 = \beta_1 f(2w)$ and $x_2 > x_1$ and $\alpha'(x_2) = 2wf(2w)e^{2wx_2} - 1 = 2wx_2 - 1$. Therefore, if $2wf(2w)/G(3w) \leq 1$ then $\gamma_1 = f(2w)/G(3w) \leq x_2$. If $\gamma_2 \leq \gamma_1$ or $2wf(2w)/G(3w) \leq 1$ and $2wf(2w) < 1/e$, then $\gamma_k \to \beta_1 f(2w)$. It follows from (11.30) that

$$G(T) \geq e^{-\beta_1 f(2w)T} \tag{11.31}$$

for $T > 3w$ and when $G(3w)e^{2wf(2w)/G(3w)} < 1$ or $2wf(2w) \leq \min(G(3w), 1/e)$. To evaluate the lower bound in (11.31) note that β_1 is the smallest root of the equation $e^{-wf(2w)\beta_1} = \beta_1$.

Now, assume that $(T - w)/2w = n$ an integer. It follows from Lemma 11.4, (11.23) that

$$G(T) = G(n(2w) + w) \geq G((n-1)2w + w)G(3w).$$

Repetitive application of this inequality results in

$$G(T) \geq G(3w)^{(T-w)/2w}, \tag{11.32}$$

if $(T - w)/2w$ is an integer.

Janson (1984) concluded that when T is close to $3w$ the sharpest lower bound is (11.28). When T is large, the sharpest lower bound is (11.32) when $(T-w)/2w$ is an integer and $G(3w)e^{2wf(2w)/G(3w)} > 1$, and (11.31) when $G(3w)e^{2wf(2w)/G(3w)} < 1$.

For the upper bounds, (11.20) implies for $t \geq 2w$:

$$f(t) \geq f(2w)G(t - w) \geq f(2w)G(t).$$

Therefore for $t \geq 2w$:

$$\frac{d}{dt}[e^{tf(2w)}G(t)] = f(2w)e^{tf(2w)}G(t) - e^{tf(2w)}f(t) \leq 0,$$

and $e^{tf(2w)}G(t)$ is a decreasing function of t. For $2w \leq s \leq t$ we have that

$$e^{tf(2w)}G(t) \leq e^{sf(2w)}G(s). \tag{11.33}$$

Let $t = T$ and $s = 2w$ or $3w$. It follows from (11.33) that for $T > 2w$:

$$G(T) \leq e^{-f(2w)(T-2w)} G(2w) \tag{11.34}$$

and for $T > 3w$:

$$G(T) \leq e^{-f(2w)(T-3w)} G(3w). \tag{11.35}$$

For large T it is possible to improve the upper bound for $G(T)$. For $t \geq 3w$, it follows from (11.33) that

$$e^{wf(2w)} G(t) \leq G(t-w)$$

and therefore from (11.20) we get, for $t \geq 3w$:

$$f(t) \geq f(2w) e^{wf(2w)} G(t).$$

Set $\delta_1 = f(2w)$ and $\delta_2 = f(2w) e^{wf(2w)}$. Then applying the same method as above we get that $e^{\delta_2 t} G(t)$ is a decreasing function for $t \geq 3w$ and therefore

$$G(t) \leq e^{-\delta_2 t} e^{3w\delta_2} G(3w).$$

Define for $k \geq 2$, $\delta_{k+1} = f(2w) e^{w\delta_k}$. It follows that $t \geq (k+1)w$, $f(t) \geq \delta_k G(t)$ and, therefore, $e^{\delta_k t} G(t)$ is a decreasing function for $t \geq (k+1)w$. For $k \geq 2$, let $B_k = e^{(k+1)w\delta_k} G((k+1)w)$. Then for $t \geq (k+1)w$:

$$G(t) \leq B_k e^{-\delta_k t}. \tag{11.36}$$

For fixed values of $t > w$ and $k \geq 2$ and large positive integers j, it follows from repeated applications of Lemma 11.4, (11.23), that

$$G(t)^j \leq G(j(t-w)) \leq B_k e^{-\delta_k j(t-w)},$$

and therefore

$$G(t) \leq B_k^{1/j} e^{-\delta_k(t-w)}.$$

As $j \to \infty$ we get for $t > w$:

$$G(t) \leq e^{-\delta_k(t-w)}. \tag{11.37}$$

This implies that $B_k \leq 1$ and therefore the inequality (11.36) is tighter than (11.37).

Note that the $\{\delta_k\}$ is a bounded increasing sequence. Let $\delta = \lim_{k \to \infty} \delta_k$. It follows from the definition of δ_{k+1} that $\delta = f(2w) e^{w\delta}$ and therefore $\delta = f(2w)\beta_2$, where β_2 is the smallest root of $\delta = e^{wf(2w)\delta}$. From (11.37) we get for $T > w$:

$$G(T) \leq e^{-\beta_2 f(2w)(T-w)}. \tag{11.38}$$

Janson (1984) states that the sharpest upper bound for $G(T)$ is (11.35), when T is close to $3w$ and (11.38), when T is large. Numerical results to evaluate the bounds for $G(T)$ are given in Table 11.1.

11.4   Approximations for the Distribution of the Scan Statistics

Theorems 11.3 through 11.5 gave exact results for $P^*(k; \lambda T, w/T)$. For the case where w/T is small, these results are computationally impractical for direct calculation. This has led to work on a variety of approximations and asymptotic results. In this section we describe several approximations to $P^*(k; \lambda T, w/T)$, including one that is higly accurate over the full distribution.

Newell (1963) and Ikeda (1965) derive the asymptotic formula

$$P^*(k; \lambda T, w/T) \approx 1 - \exp\{-\lambda^k w^{k-1} T/(k-1)!\}. \qquad (11.39)$$

This formula gives useful rough approximations for certain purposes when P^* is sufficiently small. The asymptotic convergence of this formula is very slow. Conover, Bement, and Iman (1979) give an alternative approximation where $\psi = \lambda w$:

$$
\begin{aligned}
P^*(k; \psi L, 1/L) \approx{} & 1 - 1.5 F_p(k-1; \psi) \exp\{-\psi(L-1) \\
& \times (1 - (F_p(k-2; \psi)/F_p(k-1; \psi)))\} \\
& + .5 \exp\{-\psi L (1 - F_p(k-2; \psi))\}. \qquad (11.40)
\end{aligned}
$$

This formula is intended for cases where $k \le 7$, and is most accurate for P^* small.

Naus (1982) gives the approximation

$$P^*(k; \psi L, 1/L) \approx 1 - Q_2(Q_3/Q_2)^{L-2}, \qquad (11.41)$$

where $Q_2 = Q^*(k; 2\psi, 1/2)$ and $Q_3 = Q^*(k; 3\psi, 1/3)$ are given in readily computable forms in (11.3) and (11.4). Approximation (11.41) is accurate even when $L = T/w$ is not an integer. Section 7.5 details the reasoning underlying approximations (11.41).

To further reduce computational effort, with a slight loss of accuracy, Wallenstein, Naus, and Glaz (1993) note that

$$Q_2 \approx 2F_p(k-1; \psi) - 1 - (k-1-\psi)p(k; \psi)$$

and

$$Q_3 \approx 2F_p(k-1; \psi) - 1 - (2k-1-2\psi)p(k; \psi).$$

Substituting these into (11.41) leads to a simpler approximation. An even simpler approximation suggested by Wallenstein, Naus, and Glaz (1995) is

$$P^*(k; \lambda L, 1/L) \approx 1 - \{1 - (k-\psi)p(k; \psi)\}^{L-1}. \qquad (11.42)$$

Wallenstein and Neff (1987) suggest, in analogy to their approximation (10.30), that for $P^*(k; \lambda L, 1/L)$ small ($< .1$):

$$P^*(k; \lambda L, 1/L) \approx (L-1)(k-\psi)p(k; \psi) + 2\{1 - F_p(k; \psi)\}. \qquad (11.43)$$

11.4.1   Alm's Approximation

Alm (1983) develops the approximation

$$P^*(k; \lambda T, w/T) \approx 1 - F_p(k-1; \lambda w)$$
$$\cdot \exp\{-[(k-w\lambda)/k]\lambda(T-w)p(k-1; \lambda w)\}. \quad (11.44)$$

Alm gives further simplifications of approximation (11.44) for cases where k is large (relative to λw), and a further simplification if in addition w/T is small. Alm provides some tables and quantiles for the approximation (11.44) for the case $T = 3600$, $\{w = 1, 2, 5$ and $\lambda = 1(1)70\}$, and for $\{w = 1, \lambda = 10(5)50\}$.

Alm (1983, 1997, 1999) develops a method of approximating the probability $P(S_w \geq k) = P^*(k; \lambda T, w/T)$ and its generalization to higher dimensions. In this section we describe Alm's approach and reasoning for the one-dimensional case.

Let $Y_a(b)$ denote the number of points in $[a, b)$. Let $Y_0(t)$ denote the number of points in the time interval $[0, t)$. In this chapter we deal with $Y_0(t)$, a Poisson process for t in $[0, T)$ with mean number of points λ per unit time. $Y_{t-w}(w)$ denotes the number of points in the interval $\{t - w, t)$. The scan statistic $S_w = \max_{w \leq t \leq T}\{Y_{t-w}(w)\}$. The event $S_w \geq k$ occurs if for some t in (w, T), $Y_{t-w}(w) \geq k$. Since the number of points in the sliding window starts at zero, the first occurrence of $Y_{t-w}(w) \geq k$ must occur either if $Y_0(w) \geq k$ or for a t^* such that $Y_{t^*-w}(w)$ passes from $k-1$ to k at t^*. Alm calls the passing of $Y_{t-w}(w)$ from state $k-1$ to k an *upcrossing of level k*.

Given that $M_k(T)$ is the number of upcrossings of level k, Alm finds the expectation of $M_k(t)$:

$$E\{M_k(T)\} = (T - w)\lambda p(k-1; \lambda w). \quad (11.45)$$

For cases where $P(S_w \geq k)$ is small, the chance of an upcrossing of level k is small, and since it is a rare event, we might approximate the distribution of the number of upcrossings by a Poisson distribution with mean given by (11.45). We could then approximate

$$P(S_w < k) = P\{(M_k(T) = 0) \cap (Y_0(w) < k)\} \approx \exp\{-E\{M_k(T)\}\}. \quad (11.46)$$

Alm notes that approximation (11.46) is not good, because upcrossings are highly dependent, and the number of upcrossings is not fit well by the Poisson. Alm adjusts the approximation to take into account the dependence of upcrossings. Specifically given that one upcrossing has just occurred, and thus the process is at a high level, it is easier for another upcrossing to take place. To handle this dependence, Alm distinguishes between primary and secondary upcrossings. The first upcrossing is primary, and until the process drops to a level k_0, any other upcrossing is secondary. Once the process drops to k_0, the next upcrossing is primary, and so on. The primary upcrossings are less dependent on each other and $U_k(T)$, the number of primary upcrossings, is approximately Poisson with mean

μ_k:

$$P(S_w < k) = P\{(U_k(T) = 0) \cap (Y_0(w) < k)\}$$
$$= P(Y_0(w) < k) P(U_k(T) = 0 \mid Y_0(w) < k)$$
$$\approx P(Y_0(w) < k) \exp\{-\mu_k\}, \tag{11.47}$$

where $P(Y_0(w) < k) = F_p(k - 1; \lambda w)$.

Alm now proceeds to estimate $E(U_k(T)) = \mu_k$. The total number of upcrossings equals the sum of the primary upcrossings and the secondary upcrossings following them. Let Z_i denote the number of secondary upcrossings following the ith primary upcrossing:

$$M_k(T) = U_k(T) + \sum_{i=1}^{U_k(T)} Z_i = \sum_{i=1}^{U_k(T)} (1 + Z_i). \tag{11.48}$$

$M_k(T)$ is the sum of a random number of independent and identically distributed (i.i.d.) random variables, and its expectation satisfies, by Wald's lemma,

$$E(M_k(T)) = E(U_k(T))(1 + E(Z_1)). \tag{11.49}$$

The rest of the argument approximates

$$E(Z_1) \approx w\lambda/(k - w\lambda). \tag{11.50}$$

Substituting the right-hand side of (11.45) and (11.50) into (11.49) gives

$$E(U_k(T)) \approx \{(k - w\lambda)/k\}\lambda(T - w)p(k - 1; \lambda w). \tag{11.51}$$

Substitute the right-hand side of (11.51) into (11.47) to find

$$P(S_w < k) \approx F_p(k - 1; \lambda w) \exp\{-\{(k - w\lambda)/k\}\lambda(T - w)p(k - 1; \lambda w)\}\}. \tag{11.52}$$

Alm gives further simplifications of approximation (11.52) for cases where n is large, and a further simplification if, in addition, w/T is small.

The approximation (11.50) for $E(Z_1)$ is as follows. Consider the case where the number of points in the sliding window, $Y_t(w)$, starts at a value $k \geq k_0$. Z_1 denotes the number of upcrossings of level k, before dropping to level k_0. Alm notes that close to k, the number of points in the sliding window, $Y_t(w)$, behaves somewhat like a random walk, where the probability of an up move is $p = w\lambda/(w\lambda + k)$ and of a down move is $q = 1 - p$. It follows that $E(Z_1)$ is approximately $p/(q - p)$ = right-hand side of (11.50).

Alm provides some tables and quantiles for the approximation (11.51) for the case $T = 3600$, $\{w = 1, 2, 5$, and $\lambda = 1(1)70\}$, and for $\{w = 1, \lambda = 10(5)50\}$. A comparison of approximation (11.51) with the Janson (1984) bounds, discussed in the previous section, is given for $T = 3600$, $w = 1$, and $\lambda = 40$ in Alm's

Table 11.1. Comparison of Alm's Approximation (11.51) with Janson bounds and approximation (11.41), for $P^*(k \mid \lambda T, w/T)$, $T = 3600$, $w = 1$, $\lambda = 40$.

k	LB	Alm's (11.51)	Approx (11.41)	UB
66	.9812	.9812	.9813	.9814
67	.9150	.9150	.9152	.9153
68	.7777	.7777	.7779	.7780
69	.5946	.5946	.5947	.5948
70	.413594	.413590	.41365	.413692
71	.267083	.267081	.267103	.267125
72	.1632	.1632	.1632	.1632
73	.0958	.0958	.0958	.0958
74	.0545	.0545	.0545	.0545

Table 3, and we compare a few values below with approximation (11.41). (Alm's Table 3 tabulates $P(S_w \le n) = Q^*(n + 1 \mid \lambda T, w/T)$.) For the comparison in Table 11.1, we give the corresponding figures for $P^*(k \mid \lambda T, w/T)$. For this example, Alm's approximation (11.51) and Naus' approximation (11.41) are both highly accurate, and Janson's bounds are very tight. Alm's approximation agrees to four decimal places to Janson's lower bound, and approximation (11.41) falls between the bounds. Alm notes that the approximation for $P^*(k; \psi L, 1/L)$ can drop slightly below the lower bound (this is illustrated for $k = 70, 71$ in Table 11.1). This effect is not of practical concern for the present example. Alm notes that the errors tend to be small for k large (relative to λw) and for w/T small (or even for moderate to large w/T for small tail probabilities). For further comparisons, see Chapter 3.

11.4.2 Moments of Scan Statistics

Recall that S_w denotes the largest number of points to be found in any subinterval of $[0, T)$ of length w; W_k denotes the size of the smallest subinterval of $[0, T)$ that contains k points; $T_{k,w}$ denotes the waiting time until we first observe at least k points in an interval of length w. The distribution of all three variables are directly related to $P^*(k; \lambda T, w/T)$. Chapter 2 described results for the first two moments for S_w and W_k for the conditional-on-N case. Chapter 3 discusses moments for the unconditional case.

12

The Generalized Birthday Problem

12.1 Binomial Distribution of Events: Discrete Time, Unconditional Case

Many researchers deal with data that can be viewed as a series of trials, each with two possible outcomes. We will arbitrarily label the two alternative possible outcomes of a trial as *success* and *failure*. The maximum number within any m contiguous trials within the N trials, denoted S'_m, is called the *scan statistic*. For the special case where $S'_m = m$, a *success run* of length m has occurred within the N trials. For the general case where $S'_m = k$, a *quota* of at least k successes within m consecutive trials has occurred.

In some applications, the researcher conditions on a known observed value of the total number of successes in the N trials. The present chapter deals with this *conditional* or *retrospective* case. In other applications the total number of successes in N trials is treated as a random variable. Chapter 13 deals with this *unconditional* or *prospective* case. Chapter 4 gives applications for both the conditional and unconditional cases.

12.2 The Conditional Case: Exact Results

Consider a sequence of N trials, where each trial results in either a success or a failure. Let S'_m denote the maximum number of successes within any m contiguous trials within the N trials. S'_m is called the *discrete scan statistic*. For the general case where $S'_m \geq k$, a *quota* of at least k successes within m consecutive trials has occurred.

This section gives formulas and applications for the distribution of S'_m given that there are exactly a successes in N trials. The distribution of S'_m is computed for the simple probability model where all $N!/a! \, (N-a)!$ sequences of a successes and $N-a$ failures are equally likely. For this case denote $P(S'_m \geq k)$ by $P(k \mid m; N, a)$.

Saperstein (1972) derives the exact distribution of $P(k \mid m; N, a)$ for the case $k > a/2$. Naus (1974) derives the exact distribution for all a and k for $m/N = 1/L$, L an integer, and more generally for $m = cR$, $N = cL$ where c, R, and L are integers and $c > 1$.

Theorem 12.1. *For $N/m = L \geq 2$ and L, a, m, N, k integers, $2 \leq k \leq$ a. Let $(n_1, n_2, \ldots, n_L)$, denote a partition of a into L nonnegative integers. Let Θ_k denote the set of all partitions of a into L nonnegative integers each less than k:*

$$1 - P(k \mid m; N, a) = \left\{ (m!)^L \Big/ \binom{N}{a} \right\} \sum \det |d_{rs}|, \qquad (12.1)$$

where the sum is over Θ_k and $d_{rs} = 1/c_{rs}! \, (m - c_{rs})!$, where

$$c_{rs} = (s-r)k + n_r + \sum_{i=1}^{s-1} n_i, \qquad r < s,$$

$$= (s-r)k + \sum_{i=s}^{r} n_i, \qquad r \geq s, \qquad (12.2)$$

$d_{rs} = 0$ if $c_{rs} < 0$ or $m - c_{rs} < 0$.

Proof. Divide the N trials into L nonoverlapping sets each of m contiguous trials. The ith set consists of trials $(i-1)m + 1$, $(i-1)m + 2, \ldots, im$. Let n_i denote the number of successes in the ith set of trials. Given that all $\binom{N}{a}$ sequences of a successes and $N-a$ failures are equally likely, the joint distribution of $(n_1, n_2, \ldots, n_L)$ is

$$P(n_1, n_2, \ldots, N_L \mid a) = \binom{m}{n_1}\binom{m}{n_2} \cdots \binom{m}{n_L} \Big/ \binom{N}{a}. \qquad (12.3)$$

We find $1 - P(k \mid m; N, a) = P(S'_m < k)$ by conditioning on $(n_1, n_2, \ldots, n_L)$, finding $P(S'_m < k \mid (n_1, n_2, \ldots, n_L))$, and averaging this conditional probability over the distribution (12.3). We find the conditional probability $P(S'_m < k \mid (n_1, n_2, \ldots, n_L))$.

Let $V_i(t)$ denote the number of successes in trials $(i-1)m+1, \ldots, (i-1)m+t$. Let

$$\alpha_r = (L-r)k - \sum_{i=r}^{L-1} n_i, \qquad r = 1, \ldots, L-1. \qquad (12.4)$$

$n_i - V_i(t) + V_{i+1}(t)$ describes the number of successes in a particular position of the scanning interval. The event $\{S'_m < k\}$ is equivalent to the event that, for every position of the scanning interval, the number of successes is less than k. That is, for all $t = 1, 2, \ldots, m$ and for all $i = 1, 2, \ldots, L - 1, n_i - V_i(t) + V_{i+1}(t) < k$ or, equivalently, that $V_i(t) + \alpha_i > V_{i+1}(t) + \alpha_{i+1}$.

The $V_i(t) + \alpha_i$ are L nondecreasing functions of t for $t = 1, 2, \ldots, m$, and each can be viewed as describing a path of a particle. The path corresponding to $V_i(t) + \alpha_i$ starts at α_i and ends at $\alpha_i + n_i$. We only need to find the conditional probability for the case where $n_i < k$ for all i. This implies that $\alpha_1 > \alpha_2 > \cdots > \alpha_L$ and that $\alpha_1 + n_1 > \alpha_2 + n_2 > \cdots > \alpha_L + n_L$. The ith path starts and ends above the $(i + 1)$st path. The event $V_i(t) + \alpha_i > V_{i+1}(t) + \alpha_{i+1}$ for $t = 1, 2, \ldots, m$ describes the ith path always being above the $(i + 1)$st path.

The event $S'_m < k$ is equivalent to none of the L paths crossing. Apply the Karlin and McGregor (1959) theorem (see Chapter 7) to L independent Bernoulli processes with identical transition probabilities $P_{u,v}(m) = \binom{m}{v-u}(.5)^m$. Given L labeled particles independently follows this process and start, respectively, at $\alpha_1 > \alpha_2 > \cdots > \alpha_L$ and end at $\alpha_1 + n_1 > \alpha_2 + n_2 > \cdots > \alpha_L + n_L$, the probability that none of the paths coincide is

$$\det |m!\,(.5)^m/(\alpha_r + n_r - \alpha_s)!\,(m - \alpha_r - n_r + \alpha_s)!|. \tag{12.5}$$

Note that the Karlin and McGregor result gives the probability joint with $(n_1, n_2, \ldots, n_L)$. To find the probability conditional on $(n_1, n_2, \ldots, n_L)$, it is necessary to divide the term (12.5) by

$$P(n_1, n_2, \ldots, n_L) = \prod_r m!\,(.5)^m/(n_r)!\,(m - n_r)!.$$

This gives

$$P(S'_m < k \mid (n_1, n_2, \ldots, n_L)) = \det |h_{rs}|, \tag{12.6}$$

where

$$h_{rs} = (n_r)!\,(m - n_r)!/(\alpha_r + n_r - \alpha_s)!\,(m - \alpha_r - n_r + \alpha_s)!. \tag{12.7}$$

Substitute (12.4) into (12.6) and average the result over the distribution in (12.3) to find (12.1).

Corollary 12.1. For $k > a/2$ and $N/m = L$ an integer, let $H(s, a, m, N)$ denote the hypergeometric probability

$$H(s, a, m, N) = \binom{m}{s}\binom{N - m}{a - s} \Big/ \binom{N}{a}, \tag{12.8}$$

then

$$P(k \mid m; N, a) = 2 \sum_{s=k}^{a} H(s, a, m, N) + (Lk - a - 1)H(k, a, m, N). \tag{12.9}$$

Proof. Define the events

$$A_i = (n_i \geq k),$$ (12.10)

$$B_i = A^c \cap \left\{ \bigcup_{t=1}^{m} (n_i - V_i(t) + V_{i+1}(t) \geq k) \right\}.$$ (12.11)

Note that for $k > a/2$, the A_i's are mutually exclusive events, and that while $B_i \cap B_{i+1}$ can occur, $B_i \cap B_{i+2}$ cannot.

$$P(k \mid m; N, a) = P\left(\bigcup A_i\right) + P\left(\bigcup B_i\right)$$
$$= \sum P(A_i) + \sum P(B_i) - \sum P(B_i \cap B_{i+1}).$$ (12.12)

By symmetry,

$$P(k \mid m; N, a) = L P(A_1) + (L - 1) P(B_1) - (L - 2) P(B_1 \cap B_2),$$ (12.13)

where

$$P(A_1) = \sum_{s=k}^{a} H(s, a, m, N).$$ (12.14)

To find $P(B_1)$ and $P(B_1 \cap B_2)$, condition on $(n_1, n_2, \ldots, n_L)$. $P(B_1 \mid (n_1, n_2))$ and $P(B_1 \cap B_2 \mid (n_1, n_2, n_3))$ can be found from formula (12.6). Average over the distribution in (12.3), substitute the resulting expressions and (12.14) into (12.13), and simplify to find (12.9).

Theorem 12.1 deals with the case $N/m = L$ an integer. Theorem 12.2 generalizes the result to the case where $m = cR$, $N = cL$ for c, R, L integers, $c > 1$. The theorem is most useful for c large. The approach is to divide the N trials into L disjoint groups of $c = N/L$ each. Let n_i denote the number of successes in the ith group. Let $J(u, v) = n_u + n_{u+1} + \cdots + n_v$ for $u \leq v$ (and zero otherwise).

Theorem 12.2. *Let $m = cR$, $N = cL$, and let c, R, L, k, a be positive integers where $c > 1$, R, and L have greatest common denominator of one, $1 \leq R \leq L$ and $2 \leq k \leq$ a:*

$$1 - P(k \mid m; N, a) = \left[(c!)^L \Big/ \binom{N}{a} \right] \sum_{U(k)} \prod_{i=1}^{R} \det |d_{rs}(i)|,$$ (12.15)

where $U(k)$ is the set of all partitions of a into L nonnegative numbers $(n_1, n_2, \ldots, n_L)$, satisfying $J(i, i + R - 1) < k$ for $i \leq L - R + 1$, and

$$d_{rs}(i) = 1/c_{rs}(i)! \, (c - c_{rs}(i))!$$ (12.16)

and

$$c_{rs}(i) = (s - r)k - J(i + 1 + (r - 1)R, i - 1 + (s - 1)R), \quad r < s,$$
$$= (s - r)k + J(i + (s - 1)R, i + (r - 1)R), \quad r \geq s.$$ (12.17)

The proof follows Wallenstein and Naus (1973), and the approach is described in Section 8.7 of Chapter 8 for the conditional continuous case. Many of the other results of Chapter 8 can be modified to handle the conditional discrete case of this chapter.

12.3   Bounds for the Conditional Scan Statistic for 0–1 Bernoulli Trials

Let $X_1, \ldots, X_N$ be independent and identically distributed (i.i.d.) 0–1 Bernoulli trials. Suppose that a successes (ones) and $N - a$ failures (zeros) have been observed. Then

$$P\left(X_1 = x_1, \ldots, X_N = x_N \mid \sum_{i=1}^{N} X_i = a\right) = \frac{1}{\binom{N}{a}}. \tag{12.18}$$

In this case the joint distribution of the observed 0–1 trials assigns equal probabilities to all the $\binom{N}{a}$ arrangements of a ones and $N - a$ zeros. We are interested in deriving tight bounds for the upper tail probabilities for a conditional scan statistic denoted by

$$P(k; m, N, a) = P\left(S'_m \geq k \mid \sum_{i=1}^{N} X_i = a\right), \tag{12.19}$$

where S'_m is defined in Section 12.2.

Let $U_1, \ldots, U_N$ be the random variables denoting one of the $\binom{N}{a}$ sequences of 0–1 trials that contain a ones and $N - a$ zeros. For $N = Lm$, $L \geq 4$, and $1 \leq i \leq L - 1$ define the events

$$D_i = \bigcap_{j=1}^{m+1} (U_{(i-1)m+j} + \cdots + U_{im+j-1} \leq k - 1). \tag{12.20}$$

It follows that

$$P(k; m, N, a) = P\left(\bigcup_{i=1}^{L-1} D_i^c\right). \tag{12.21}$$

Employing the second-order Bonferroni-type inequality in Hunter (1976) and Worsley (1982) given in (7.4), and the fact that D_i are stationary events, we get

$$P(k; m, N, a) \leq \sum_{i=1}^{L-1} P(D_i^c) - \sum_{i=2}^{L-1} P(D_i^c \cap D_{i-1}^c)$$
$$= 1 + (L - 3)q_{2m}(a) - (L - 2)q_{3m}(a), \tag{12.22}$$

where for $1 \leq i \leq L-1$, $q_{2m}(a) = P(D_i)$, $q_{3m}(a) = P(D_i \cap D_{i-1})$ and $r = 2, 3$:

$$q_{rm}(a) = \sum_{j=0}^{\min(rk-r,a)} q(rm \mid j) \frac{\binom{rm}{j}\binom{n-rm}{a-j}}{\binom{n}{a}}, \tag{12.23}$$

where $q(rm \mid j) = 1 - P(k; m, rm, j)$ are evaluated via Theorem 12.1.

To derive a Bonferroni-type lower bound for $P(k; m, N, a)$ an inequality in Kwerel (1975) presented in (7.12) gives

$$P\left(\bigcup_{i=1}^{L-1} D_i^c\right) \geq \frac{2s_1}{b} - \frac{2s_2}{b(b-1)} \tag{12.24}$$

where $b = [2s_2/s_1 + 2]$:

$$s_1 = \sum_{i=1}^{L-1} P(D_i^c) = (L-1)(1 - q_{2m}(a)) \tag{12.25}$$

and

$$\begin{aligned}
s_2 &= \sum_{1 \leq i < j \leq L-1} P\left(D_i^c \cap D_j^c\right) \\
&= \sum_{i=1}^{L-2} P\left(D_i^c \cap D_{i+1}^c\right) + \sum_{1 \leq i < j-1 \leq L-2} P\left(D_i^c \cap D_j^c\right) \\
&= (L-2)[1 - 2q_{2m}(a) + q_{3m}(a)] \\
&\quad + .5(L-2)(L-3)[1 - 2q_{2m}(a) + q_{2m,2m}(a)] \\
&= (L-2)q_{3m}(a) + .5(L-2)(L-3)q_{2m,2m}(a) \\
&\quad + .5(L-1)(1 - 2q_{2m}(a)),
\end{aligned} \tag{12.26}$$

where

$$\begin{aligned}
q_{2m,2m}(a) &= \sum_{j_1=0}^{\min(2k-2,a)} \sum_{j_2=0}^{\min(2k-2,a-j_1)} q(2m \mid j_1)q(2m \mid j_2) \\
&\quad \times \frac{\binom{2m}{j_1}\binom{2m}{j_2}\binom{N-4m}{a-j_1-j_2}}{\binom{N}{a}}
\end{aligned} \tag{12.27}$$

and $q(rm \mid j)$, $r = 2, 3$, are defined above in (12.23).

Different bounds are obtained based on an alternate representation for $P(k; m, N, a)$. For $1 \leq i \leq L$, denote the events that the total number of ones in trials $(i-1)m + 1, \ldots, im$ is at least k by

$$A_i^* = \left(U_{(i-1)m+1} + \cdots + U_{im} \geq k\right), \tag{12.28}$$

and let $A^* = \bigcup_{i=1}^{L} A_i^*$. Set

$$G_i = D_i^c \cap A^{*c} \tag{12.29}$$

and let $G = \bigcup_{i=1}^{L-1} G_i$ where the event D_i is defined in (12.20). It follows that

$$P(k; m, N, a) = P(A^*) + P(G). \tag{12.30}$$

To obtain bounds for $P(k; m, N, a)$ we evaluate $P(A^*)$ exactly using a recursive formula presented below, and bound $P(G)$ by second-order Bonferroni-type inequalities.

Let $h^*(a, l, m, k)$ be the number of ways to arrange a ones among $N = lm$ trials so that the l groups, consisting of m trials each, will have at most $k - 1$ ones. Abbreviate $h^*(a, l, m, k)$ to $h^*(a, l)$ and define

$$H^*(a, l) = \frac{h^*(a, l)}{\binom{N}{a}}. \tag{12.31}$$

$H^*(a, l)$ is the cumulative distribution function (c.d.f.) of the largest-order statistic of an l-dimensional multivariate hypergeometric random vector with parameter a and cell size m, evaluated at $k - 1$. Condition on the number of ones in the first group of m trials being equal to j. The following recursion in a and l for $H^*(a, l)$ holds:

$$H^*(a, l) = \sum_{j=0}^{\min(m, k-1)} \frac{\binom{N}{j}\binom{N-m}{a-j}}{\binom{N}{a}} H^*(a - j, l - 1), \tag{12.32}$$

with initial conditions $H^*(a, 1) = 1$ for $a < k$ and $H^*(a, 1) = 0$ for $a \geq k$. It follows that

$$P(A^*) = 1 - H^*(a, L). \tag{12.33}$$

Second-order Bonferroni-type inequalities given in (7.4) and (7.12) yield

$$P(G) \leq \sum_{i=1}^{L-1} P(G_i) - \sum_{i=2}^{L-1} P(G_i \cap G_{i-1})$$
$$= (L - 1)P(G_1) - (L - 2)P(G_1 \cap G_2) \tag{12.34}$$

and

$$P(G) \geq \frac{2s_1^*}{b^*} - \frac{2s_2^*}{b^*(b^* - 1)} \tag{12.35}$$

where $b^* = [2s_2^*/s_1^* + 2]$,

$$s_1^* = \sum_{i=1}^{L-1} P(G_i) \tag{12.36}$$

and

$$s_2^* = \sum_{1 \le i < j \le L-1} P(G_i \cap G_j) = \sum_{i=1}^{L-2} P(G_i \cap G_{i+1}) + \sum_{1 \le i < j-1 \le L-2} P(G_i \cap G_j)$$
$$= (L-2)P(G_1 \cap G_2) + .5(L-2)(L-3)P(G_1 \cap G_3). \qquad (12.37)$$

Equation (12.37) follows from the fact that the events G_i are stationary.

To evaluate $P(G_1)$, $P(G_1 \cap G_2)$, and $P(G_1 \cap G_3)$ let $n_i = U_{(i-1)m+1} + \cdots + U_{im}$ be the number of ones in trials $(i-1)m+1, \ldots, im$, $1 \le i \le L$. To evaluate $P(G_1)$, recall that the event G_1 says that, in the first $2m$ trials, there is a sequence of m consecutive trials has at least k ones and any sequence of m consecutive trials starting at trial $(i-1)m+1$ for $1 \le i \le L$, has at most $k-1$ ones. Condition on n_1 and n_2 to get that

$$P(G_1) = \sum_{n_1=0}^{\min(a,k-1)} \sum_{n_2=\max(0,k-n_1)}^{\min(a-n_1,k-1)} P(D_1^c \mid n_1, n_2) H^*(a - n_1 - n_2, L - 2)$$
$$\times \frac{\binom{m}{n_1}\binom{m}{n_2}\binom{N-2m}{a-n_1-n_2}}{\binom{N}{a}}, \qquad (12.38)$$

where the event D_1^c and the function H^* are defined above in (12.20) and (12.31), respectively. Note that the range for the indexes in both sums was chosen to satisfy the requirement that there are only a ones and that the event $A_1^{*c} \cap A_2^{*c}$ occurs. Also, conditional on n_1 and n_2, the events $D_1^c \cap A_1^{*c} \cap A_2^{*c}$ and $\cap_{i=1}^{L-2} A_i^{*c}$ are independent and therefore

$$P\left(D_1^c \cap \left[\bigcap_{i=1}^{L-2} A_i^{*c}\right] \Big| n_2, n_2\right) = P(D_1^c \mid n_1, n_2) H^*(a - n_1 - n_2, L - 2),$$
$$(12.39)$$

which leads to the expression for $P(G_1)$ given above. Using a similar approach, by conditioning on n_1, n_2, n_3 and n_1, n_2, n_3, n_4, respectively, we get

$$P(G_1 \cap G_2) = \sum_{n_1=0}^{\min(a,k-1)} \sum_{n_2=\max(0,k-n_1)}^{\min(a-n_1,k-1)} \sum_{n_3=\max(0,k-n_2)}^{\min(a-n_1-n_2,k-1)} P(D_1^c \cap D_2^c \mid n_1, n_2, n_3)$$
$$\times H^*(a - n_1 - n_2 - n_3, L - 3) \frac{\binom{m}{n_1}\binom{m}{n_2}\binom{m}{n_3}\binom{N-3m}{a-n_1-n_2-n_3}}{\binom{N}{a}} (12.40)$$

Table 12.1. Inequalities for $P(k; m, N, a)$.

N	m	a	k	BTLB	BTUB
100	10	5	3	.166	.166
			4	.009	.009
		10	3	.830	.907
			4	.231	.233
			5	.026	.026
	20	10	5	.350	.351
			6	.075	.075
			7	.010	.010
500	10	50	4	.766	1.000
			5	.238	.250
			6	.027	.027
	20	25	4	.659	.759
			5	.168	.171
			6	.027	.027
			7	.002	.002
	20	75	8	.419	.465
			9	.124	.127
			10	.026	.026

BTLB and BTUB are Bonferroni-type lower and up-per bounds based on (12.30)–(12.37).

and

$$P(G_1 \cap G_3) = \sum_{n_1=0}^{\min(a,k-1)} \sum_{n_2=\max(0,k-n_1)}^{\min(a-n_1,k-1)} \sum_{n_3=0}^{\min(a-n_1-n_2,k-1)}$$
$$\times \sum_{n_3=\max(0,k-n_2)}^{\min(a-n_1-n_2-n_3,k-1)} P\left(D_1^c \cap D_3^c \mid \{n_i\}_{i=1}^4\right)$$
$$\times H^*(a - n_1 - n_2 - n_3 - n_4, L - 4)$$
$$\times \frac{\binom{m}{n_1}\binom{m}{n_2}\binom{m}{n_3}\binom{m}{n_4}\binom{N-4m}{a-n_1-n_2-n_3-n_4}}{\binom{N}{a}}. \tag{12.41}$$

To evaluate these probabilities we use the fact that

$$P(D_1^c \cap D_2^c \mid n_1, n_2, n_3) = 1 - P(D_1 \mid n_1, n_2) - P(D_2 \mid n_2, n_3)$$
$$+ P(D_1 \cap D_2 \mid n_1, n_2, n_3) \tag{12.42}$$

and

$$P(D_1^c \cap D_3^c \mid n_1, n_2, n_3, n_4) = P(D_1^c \mid n_1, n_2, n_3, n_4)$$
$$\times P(D_3^c \mid n_1, n_2, n_3, n_4)$$
$$= [1 - P(D_1 \mid n_1, n_2)][1 - P(D_3 \mid n_3, n_4)], \tag{12.43}$$

Table 12.2. Inequalities for $E(S'_m)$.

N	m	a	LB	UB
100	10	5	2.05	2.10
		10	3.09	3.17
	20	10	4.28	4.33
		20	7.06	7.14
500	10	25	2.89	3.04
		50	4.02	4.28
	20	50	5.56	5.93
		75	7.19	7.62

LB and UB are Bonferroni-type lower and upper bounds based on (12.30)–(12.37).

where $P(D_1 \mid n_1, n_2)$ and $P(D_1 \cap D_2 \mid n_1, n_2, n_3)$ are evaluated using Naus (1974, Equations (2.7) and (2.5), respectively) and are discussed in Section 12.2.

Remark. Since $E\left(S'_m \mid \sum_{i=1}^{N} X_i = a\right) = \sum_{k=1}^{m} P(k; m, N, a)$, tight inequalities for $P(k; m, N, a)$ will yield useful inequalities for the expected size of this conditional scan statistic.

We now turn to discuss the extension on the inequalities derived above to a circular scan statistic. Let $X_1, \ldots, X_N$ be i.i.d. 0–1 Bernoulli trials arranged in a circular fashion. Assume that there are a successes (ones) and $N - a$ failures (zeros) among N observed trials. For $1 \leq i \leq L$, define the events D_i as in (12.20). Denote by

$$P_c(k; m, N, a) = P\left(S'^c_m \geq k \,\Big|\, \sum_{i=1}^{N} X_i = a\right) = P\left(\bigcup_{i=1}^{L} D_i^c\right) \quad (12.44)$$

the upper tail probabilities of a discrete circular scan statistic.

The upper bounds for $P_c(k; m, N, a)$ are obtained from the respective upper bounds for $P(k; m, N, a)$ given in (12.22) and (12.30)–(12.34) by replacing L with $L + 1$. The lower bounds for $P_c(k; m, N, a)$ are obtained from (12.24) with

$$s_1 = \sum_{i=1}^{L} P(D_i^c) = L(1 - q_{2m}(a)) \quad (12.45)$$

and

$$s_2 = \sum_{1 \leq i < j \leq L} P(D_i^c \cap D_j^c) = LP(D_1^c \cap D_2^c) + .5L(L-3)P(D_1^c \cap D_3^c)$$
$$= Lq_{3m}(a) + .5L(L-3)q_{2m,2m}(a) + .5L(L-1)(1 - 2q_{2m}(a)), \quad (12.46)$$

and from (12.35):

$$s_1^* = \sum_{i=1}^{L} P(G_i) = LP(G_1) \quad (12.47)$$

Table 12.3. Comparison of Bonferroni-type inequalities for $P_c(k; m, n, a)$.

n	m	a	k	$\hat{P}_c(k; n, m, a)$	BTLB1	BTLB2	BTUB2	BTUB1
100	10	10	4	.2492	.2448	.2469	.2497	.2593
			5	.0289	.0284	.0284	.0285	.0291
	20	15	7	.2211	.2212	.2213	.2233	.2339
			8	.0491	.0494	.0494	.0496	.0514
			9	.0073	.0075	.0075	.0075	.0077
500	10	25	4	.1368	.1330	.1364	.1392	.1426
			5	.0101	.0098	.0098	.0098	.0098
	20	50	7	.1947	.1881	.1933	.2002	.2049
			8	.0380	.0387	.0388	.0390	.0390
			9	.0058	.0058	.0058	.0058	.0058

BTLB1 and BTUB1 are Bonferroni-type lower and upper bounds based on the extension of (12.24) and (12.22) to the circle, respectively. BTLB2 and BTUB2 are Bonferroni-type lower and upper bounds based on the extension of (12.30)–(12.37) to the circle.

Table 12.4. Bonferroni-type inequalities for $E(S_m^c)$.

n	m	a	$\hat{E}(S_m^c)$	LB1	LB2	UB2	UB1
100	10	5	2.1095	1.9902	2.0758	2.1380	2.1944
		10	3.1444	3.0094	3.1215	3.2282	3.2903
	20	10	4.4152	4.2958	4.3814	4.4866	4.5373
		20	7.2330	7.0772	7.1593	7.3101	7.3737
500	10	25	2.9361	2.7233	2.8900	3.0547	3.1529
		50	4.1449	3.8839	4.0253	4.2837	4.2946
	20	50	5.8493	5.5365	5.5525	5.9595	6.0478
		75	7.4734	7.1111	7.1952	7.6418	7.6720

LB1 and UB1 are Bonferroni-type lower and upper bounds based on the extension of (12.24) and (12.22) to the circle, respectively. LB2 and UB2 are Bonferroni-type lower and upper bounds based on the extension of (12.30)–(12.37) to the circle.

and

$$s_2^* = \sum_{1 \le i < j \le L} P(G_i \cap G_j) = LP(G_1 \cap G_2) + .5L(L - 3)P(G_1 \cap G_3).$$

$$(12.48)$$

Remark. The inequalities for $E(S_m^{\prime c} \mid \sum_{i=1}^{N} X_i = a) = \sum_{k=1}^{m} P_c(k; m, N, a)$ are obtained from the inequalities of $P_c(k; m, N, a)$.

Table 12.5. Comparison of six approximations to $P(k; m, N, a)$ for the Bernoulli model for the conditional case for $N = 100$.

m	a	k	$\hat{P}(k; n, m, a)$	(12.59)	(12.62)	(12.63)	(12.79)	(12.80)
20	5	2	.8941	.7885	.8355	.6703	.7207	.6945
		3	.1678	.1598	.1988	.1534	.1573	.1546
		4	.0098	.0090	.0110	.0090	.0090	.0090
	10	3	.8563	.7665	.8080	.6583	.7321	.6779
		4	.2287	.2210	.2641	.2095	.2266	.2115
		5	.0247	.0261	.0314	.0260	.0271	.0260
		6	.0016	.0016	.0018	.0016	.0016	.0016
	15	3	.9997	.9835	.9786	.8570	.9566	.8948
		4	.7316	.6753	.7237	.5890	.6690	.6031
		5	.2031	.1946	.2302	.1859	.2057	.1873
		6	.0261	.0268	.0318	.0266	.0284	.0267
		7	.0018	.0021	.0024	.0021	.0021	.0021
	20	4	.9864	.9445	.9448	.8141	.9209	.8426
		5	.5964	.5441	.5977	.4857	.5584	.4946
		6	.1431	.1402	.1652	.1356	.1507	.1363
		7	.0196	.0187	.0219	.0186	.0199	.0186
		8	.0021	.0014	.0016	.0014	.0014	.0014
20	5	3	.5350	.5167	.5097	.4155	.4351	.4278
		4	.0835	.0824	.0947	.0795	.0791	.0798
		5	.0042	.0043	.0049	.0043	.0042	.0043
	10	4	.8714	.8254	.7487	.6107	.7183	.6342
		5	.3465	.3433	.3563	.2967	.3358	.3022
		6	.0752	.0748	.0844	.0724	.0785	.0727
		7	.0121	.0096	.0108	.0096	.0100	.0096
	15	5	.9585	.9218	.8313	.6744	.8335	.7037
		6	.5654	.5496	.5321	.4417	.5350	.4532
		7	.0192	.1875	.2033	.1729	.2026	.1746
		8	.0423	.0414	.0464	.0407	.0456	.0407
		9	.0062	.0062	.0069	.0062	.0067	.0062
	20	6	.9820	.9581	.8694	.7014	.8885	.7351
		7	.7079	.6809	.6360	.5265	.6614	.5421
		8	.2948	.2973	.3101	.2625	.3229	.2664
		9	.0882	.0862	.0955	.0830	.0981	.0834
		10	.0163	.0177	.0197	.0176	.0199	.0176
		11	.0037	.0026	.0029	.0026	.0029	.0026

12.4   Approximations for the Conditional Scan Statistic

12.4.1   Approximations for i.i.d. 0–1 Bernoulli Trials

12.4.1.1   Product-Type Approximations

Let $X_1, \ldots, X_N$ be a sequence of N i.i.d. 0–1 Bernoulli trials. Suppose we know that a successes (ones) and $N - a$ failures (zeros) have been observed. Then all

$\binom{N}{a}$ arrangements of a ones and $N - a$ zeros are equally likely, i.e.,

$$P\left(X_1 = x_1, \ldots, X_N = x_N \,\Big|\, \sum_{i=1}^{N} X_i = a\right) = \frac{1}{\binom{N}{a}}.$$

We seek to approximate

$$P(k; m, N, a) = P\left(S'_m \geq k \,\Big|\, \sum_{i=1}^{N} X_i = a\right), \tag{12.49}$$

where S'_m is defined in Section 12.1.

For integers $k, m, L \geq 2$ and $N = mL$ an exact formula for $P(k; m, N, a)$ has been derived in Naus (1974, Theorem 1) and is presented in Section 12.2. If N, m, L are large and $k < a/2$, computing $P(k; m, N, a)$ using Naus (1974, Theorem 1) becomes impractical. In this section we derive product-type approximations for $P(k; m, N, a)$ that are valid for any values of the parameters.

Record the total number of ones in m consecutive trials along the entire sequence. For $N = Lm$, $L \geq 4$, and $1 \leq i \leq L - 1$ define the events

$$D_i = \bigcap_{j=1}^{m+1} (U_{(i-1)m+j} + \cdots + U_{im+j-1} \leq k - 1), \tag{12.50}$$

where $U_1, \ldots, U_N$ is a sequence of 0–1 trials that contains a ones and $N - a$ zeros. Then

$$P\left(S'_m \leq k - 1 \,\Big|\, \sum_{i=1}^{N} X_i = a\right) = P\left(\bigcap_{i=1}^{L-1} D_i\right)$$

$$= P\left(\bigcap_{i=1}^{v} D_i\right) \prod_{i=v+1}^{L-1} P\left(D_i \,\Big|\, \bigcap_{j=1}^{i-1} D_j\right). \tag{12.51}$$

The following *Markov-like* approximations will be examined for $v = 1$ and $v = 2$, respectively,

$$P\left(S'_m \leq k - 1 \,\Big|\, \sum_{i=1}^{N} X_i = a\right) \approx P(D_1 \cap D_2) \prod_{i=3}^{L-1} P(D_i \mid D_{i-1}) \tag{12.52}$$

and

$$P\left(S'_m \leq k - 1 \,\Big|\, \sum_{i=1}^{N} X_i = a\right)$$

$$\approx P(D_1 \cap D_2 \cap D_3) \prod_{i=4}^{L-1} P(D_i \mid D_{i-1} \cap D_{i-2}). \tag{12.53}$$

Equations (12.52) and (12.53) yield the following approximations, respectively,

$$P(k; m, N, a) \approx 1 - P(D_1 \cap D_2) \prod_{i=2}^{L-2} \frac{P(D_i \cap D_{i+1})}{P(D_i)} \qquad (12.54)$$

and

$$P(k; m, N, a) \approx 1 - P(D_1 \cap D_2 \cap D_3) \prod_{i=2}^{L-3} \frac{P(D_i \cap D_{i+1} \cap D_{i+2})}{P(D_i \cap D_{i+1})}. \qquad (12.55)$$

For $1 \leq i \leq L - 3$, $P(D_i) = q_{2m}(a)$, $P(D_i \cap D_{i+1}) = q_{3m}(a)$, and $P(D_i \cap D_{i+1} \cap D_{i+2}) = q_{4m}(a)$, where for $r = 2, 3, 4$:

$$q_{rm}(a) = \sum_{j=0}^{\min(rk-r,a)} q(rm \mid j) \frac{\binom{rm}{j}\binom{N-rm}{a-j}}{\binom{N}{a}} \qquad (12.56)$$

and

$$q(rm \mid j) = P(k; m, rm, j) \qquad (12.57)$$

can be evaluated via Theorem 12.1. Substituting (12.56) into (12.54) and (12.55), respectively, yields the following *product-type approximations*:

$$P(k; m, N, a) \approx 1 - q_{3m}(a) \left[\frac{q_{3m}(a)}{q_{2m}(a)} \right]^{L-3}, \qquad L \geq 4, \qquad (12.58)$$

and

$$P(k; m, N, a) \approx 1 - q_{4m}(a) \left[\frac{q_{4m}(a)}{q_{3m}(a)} \right]^{L-4}, \qquad L \geq 5. \qquad (12.59)$$

In Table 12.5 for values of L, k, m, N, and a we present numerical results for approximation (12.59). This approximation is the most accurate one.

12.4.1.2 Poisson Approximations

Let $D_1, \ldots, D_{l-1}$ be the events defined in (12.51) above. For $1 \leq j \leq l - 1$ set

$$H_j = \begin{cases} 1 & \text{if } D_j^c \text{ occur,} \\ 0 & \text{otherwise.} \end{cases} \qquad (12.60)$$

Then a Poisson approximation for $P(k; m, N, a)$ is given by

$$P(k; m, N, a) \approx 1 - \exp(-\gamma_D), \qquad (12.61)$$

where

$$\gamma_D = E\left(\sum_{j}^{L-1} H_j \right) = (L - 1)(1 - q_{2m}(a)). \qquad (12.62)$$

Since events D_j often occur in clumps the following declumping approach is useful. For $1 \le j \le L - 1$ let

$$H'_j = \begin{cases} 1 & \text{if } D^c_j \cap D_{j-1} \text{ occur,} \\ 0 & \text{otherwise,} \end{cases}$$

where D_0 is defined to be the entire space. Since

$$\sum_{j=1}^{L-1} H_j = 0 \quad \Leftrightarrow \quad \sum_{j=1}^{L-1} H'_j = 0,$$

the following Poisson approximation for $P(k; m, N, a)$ is recommended:

$$P(k; m, N, a) \approx 1 - \exp(-\lambda'_D), \tag{12.63}$$

where

$$\lambda^*_D = E\left(\sum_{j=1}^{L-1} H'_j\right) = 1 - q_{2m}(a) + (L-2)(q_{2m}(a) - q_{3m}(a)). \tag{12.64}$$

Numerical results for these Poisson approximations are presented in Table 12.5.

12.4.1.3   Compound Poisson Approximations

In this section we examine five compound Poisson approximations for $P(k; m, N, a)$. A brief introduction to compound Poisson approximations is given in Chapter 7. The first approximation is based on the clump heuristic of Aldous (1989) as it was applied in Glaz, Naus, Roos, and Wallenstein (1994). A set of m γ_j's is used with the following approximations

$$\gamma_1 \approx \gamma^*_1 = (N - m + 1)\pi(a)[1 - 2p(a) + p^2(a)$$
$$- mp^{m+1}(a) + (m+1)p^m(a)], \tag{12.65}$$
$$\gamma_j \approx \gamma^*_j = (N - m + 1)\pi(a)(1 - p(a))^2 p^{j-1}(a), \quad j = 2, \ldots, m, \tag{12.66}$$

where

$$\pi(a) = P(H_1 = 1) = 1 - q_m(a), \tag{12.67}$$
$$p(a) = P(H_1 = 1, H_2 = 1)/P(H_1 = 1)$$
$$= (1 - 2q_m(a) + q_{m+1}(a))/(1 - q_m(a)), \tag{12.68}$$

where $q_m(a)$ is defined in (12.56), H_j is defined in (12.60), and

$$q_{m+1}(a) = \sum_{k_1=0}^{1} \sum_{k_3=0}^{1} \sum_{k_2=0}^{\min(k-1-k_1, k-1-k_3)} \frac{\binom{1}{k_1}\binom{m-1}{k_2}\binom{1}{k_3}\binom{N-m-1}{a-(k_1+k_2+k_3)}}{\binom{N}{a}}. \tag{12.69}$$

This yields the following approximation:

$$P(k; m, N, a) \approx 1 - \exp\left(-\sum_{i=1}^{m} \gamma_i^*\right), \tag{12.70}$$

where γ_j^*'s are given in (12.65) and (12.66).

The second compound Poisson approximation uses

$$\gamma_j \approx \gamma_j^* = (N - m + 1)\pi(a)(1 - p(a))^2 p^{j-1}(a), \quad j = 1, \ldots, 2m - 1. \tag{12.71}$$

This yields the following approximation:

$$\begin{aligned} P(k; m, N, a) &\approx 1 - \exp\left(-\sum_{i=1}^{2m-1} \gamma_i^*\right) \\ &= 1 - \exp\{(N - m + 1)\pi(a) \\ &\quad \times (1 - p(a))(1 - p^{2m-1}(a))\}. \end{aligned} \tag{12.72}$$

In the third compound Poisson approximation we have

$$\begin{aligned} \gamma_1 \approx \gamma_1^* &= \sum_{i=2}^{\infty} \gamma_i - \sum_{i=2}^{2m-1} \gamma_i \\ &= (N - m + 1)\pi(a)\{(1 - p(a))^2 + p^{2m-1}(a) \\ &\quad \times [2m - (2m + 1)p(a)]\} \end{aligned} \tag{12.73}$$

and

$$\gamma_j \approx \gamma_j^* = (N - m + 1)\pi(a)(1 - p(a))^2 p^{j-1}(a), \quad j = 2, \ldots, 2m - 1. \tag{12.74}$$

This yields the following approximation:

$$P(k; m, N, a) \approx 1 - \exp\left(-\sum_{i=1}^{2m-1} \gamma_i^*\right). \tag{12.75}$$

The fourth compound Poisson approximation is based on Roos (1993a, Lemma 3.3.4), where

$$\gamma_i = (N - m + 1)\pi(a)(1 - p(a))^2 p^{i-1}(a), \quad i = 1, \ldots, m - 1, \tag{12.76}$$

$$\begin{aligned} \gamma_i &= \frac{(N - m + 1)\pi(a)}{i}[2(1 - p(a))p^{i-1}(a) + (2m - i - 2) \\ &\quad \times (1 - p(a))^2 p^{i-1}(a)], \quad i = m, \ldots, 2m - 2, \end{aligned} \tag{12.77}$$

and

$$\gamma_{2m-1} = \frac{(N - m + 1)(1 - q_m(a))p^{2m-2}(a)}{2m - 1}. \tag{12.78}$$

This yields the following approximation:

$$P(k; m, N, a) \approx 1 - \exp\left(-\sum_{i=1}^{2m-1} \gamma_i\right). \tag{12.79}$$

The fifth compound Poisson approximation based on Roos (1993a, 1994) is given by

$$P(k; m, N, a) \approx 1 - \exp\left(-\sum_{i=1}^{3} \gamma_i\right), \tag{12.80}$$

where for $i = 1, 2, 3$:

$$\gamma_i = \frac{1}{i} P(E_1^c)\{2\pi_{1,i}^* + (l - 3)\pi_{2,i}^*\}, \tag{12.81}$$

$$P(E_1^c) = 1 - q_{2m}(a), \tag{12.82}$$

$$\pi_{1,i}^* = P(H_2 = i - 1 \mid H_1 = 1),$$

and

$$\pi_{2,i}^* = P(H_1 + H_3 = i - 1 \mid H_2 = 1).$$

The formulas for $\pi_{1,i}^*$ and $\pi_{2,i}^*$ have the same general form as the ones for $\pi_{1,i}$ and $\pi_{2,i}$ in Chen and Glaz (1999, Equations (2.41)–(2.48)). The only difference is that we have to replace q_{rm} by $q_{rm}(a)$, $2 \le r \le 4$, and q_{2m}^2 by $q_{2m,2m}(a)$. In Table 12.5 we present numerical results for approximations (12.79) and (12.80), for selected values of the parameters k, m, N, and a.

12.4.1.4 Approximations for the Expected Size and Standard Derivation of the Scan Statistic

Approximations for $E(S_m' \mid \sum_{i=1}^{N} X_i = a)$ and $SD(S_m' \mid \sum_{i=1}^{N} X_i = a)$ can be obtained by approximating $P(k; m, N, a)$ in

$$E\left(S_m' \mid \sum_{i=1}^{N} X_i = a\right) = \sum_{k=1}^{m} P(k; m, N, a) \tag{12.83}$$

and

$$\mathrm{Var}\left(S_m' \mid \sum_{i=1}^{N} X_i = a\right) = 2\sum_{k=1}^{m} k P(k; m, N, a)$$

$$- E\left(S_m' \mid \sum_{i=1}^{N} X_i = a\right)\left[1 + E\left(S_m' \mid \sum_{i=1}^{N} X_i = a\right)\right]. \tag{12.84}$$

In Table 12.6 we present approximations for $E(S_m' \mid \sum_{i=1}^{N} X_i = a)$ and $SD(S_m' \mid \sum_{i=1}^{N} X_i = a)$, based on the product-type approximation (12.59), improved Poisson approximation (12.63), and the best compound Poisson approximation (12.79), for selected values of the parameters for 0–1 i.i.d. Bernoulli trials model. To evaluate the performance of these approximations we present simulated values for $\hat{E}(S_m' \mid \sum_{i=1}^{N} X_i = a)$ and $\widehat{SD}(S_m' \mid \sum_{i=1}^{N} X_i = a)$ based on 10,000 trials.

Table 12.6. Approximations for the expected value and standard deviation for the conditional Bernoulli model, $N = 100$.

a	$\hat{E}(S'_m \mid a)$	(12.59)	(12.63)	(12.79)	$\widehat{SD}(S'_m \mid a)$	(12.59)	(12.63)	(12.79)
10	4.30	4.25	3.72	3.99	.82	.86	1.30	1.22
20	7.10	7.04	6.32	6.92	1.01	1.05	1.70	1.35

12.4.2   Scan Statistics for Binomial and Poisson Distributions Conditional on the Total Number of Events

12.4.2.1   Poisson Model

Let $X_1, \ldots, X_N$ be i.i.d. Poisson random variables. Suppose we know that the total number of events $\sum_{i=1}^{N} X_i = a$. In this case, the sequence of i.i.d. Poisson random variables, conditional on $\sum_{i=1}^{N} X_i = a$, has a multinomial distribution given by

$$P\left(X_1 = x_1, \ldots, X_N = x_N \,\middle|\, \sum_{i=1}^{N} X_i = a\right) = \binom{a}{x_1, x_2, \ldots, x_N}\left(\frac{1}{N}\right)^a.$$

(12.85)

We are interested to approximate the tail probability of the conditional scan statistic

$$P_p(k; m, N, a) = P\left(S'_m \geq k \,\middle|\, \sum_{i=1}^{N} X_i = a\right).$$

(12.86)

Since there are no exact results available for $q^p_{rm}(a) = P_p(k; m, rm, a)$, their simulated values denoted by $\hat{q}^p_{rm}(a)$, $r = m, m+1, \ldots, 4m$, based on 100,000, will be used to approximate $q^p_{rm}(a)$ in product-type approximation (12.59), Possion approximations (12.61) and (12.63), and compound Poisson approximations (12.80). The performance of these approximations is exhibited in Table 12.7.

12.4.2.2   Binomial Model

Let $X_1, \ldots, X_N$ be a sequence of N i.i.d. binomial (n, p) random variables. Suppose we know that the total number of successes $\sum_{i=1}^{N} X_i = a$ has been observed. In this case, the joint distribution of $X_1, \ldots, X_N$, conditional on $\sum_{i=1}^{N} X_i = a$, has the following multivariate hypergeometric distribution:

$$P\left(X_1 = x_1, \ldots, X_N = x_N \,\middle|\, \sum_{i=1}^{N} X_i = a\right)$$
$$= \frac{\binom{n}{x_1}\binom{n}{x_2} \cdots \binom{n}{a - \sum_{i=1}^{N-1} x_i}}{\binom{nN}{a}}.$$

(12.87)

We seek to approximate the tail probability of the conditional scan statistic

$$P_b(k; m, N, a) = P\left(S'_m \geq k \,\middle|\, \sum_{i=1}^{N} X_i = a\right).$$

(12.88)

Table 12.7. Comparison of six approximations to $P_p(k; m, N, a)$ for the Poisson model for the conditional case for $N = 100$.

m	a	k	$\hat{P}_p(k; n, m, a)$	(12.59)	(12.62)	(12.63)	(12.79)	(12.80)
10	5	2	.9075	.7956	.8454	.6716	.8418	.7204
		3	.1943	.1819	.2413	.1731	.1962	.1728
		4	.0137	.0132	.0177	.0134	.0172	.0172
	10	4	.3060	.2879	.3496	.2706	.2929	.2805
		5	.0514	.0496	.0662	.0498	.0503	.0498
		6	.0055	.0049	.0063	.0048	.0055	.0055
20	5	3	.5578	.5352	.5287	.4273	.5096	.4346
		4	.0970	.0967	.1115	.0919	.0894	.0862
		5	.0058	.0058	.0061	.0063	.0049	.0018
	10	4	.8876	.8459	.7667	.6217	.7732	.7096
		5	.4082	.3980	.4095	.3363	.3881	.3820
		6	.1070	.1061	.1212	.1019	.0891	.0862
		7	.0176	.0177	.0205	.0179	.0232	.0232
		8	.0019	.0019	.0020	.0017	.0024	.0024

Since there are no exact results available for $q_{rm}^b(a) = P_b(k; m, rm, a)$, we use the Patefield (1981) algorithm to simulate the values for $q_{rm}^b(a)$ denoted by $\hat{q}_{rm}^b(a)$, $r = 1, 2, 3, 4$, based on 100,000. Product-type approximation (12.59), Poisson approximations (12.61) and (12.63), and the compound Poisson approximation (12.80) are evaluated by using $\hat{q}_{rm}^b(a)$, $r = 1, 2, 3, 4$, instead of $q_{rm}^b(a)$. Numerical results for these approximations are presented in Table 12.8. For both models the product-type approximation is the most accurate one.

Table 12.8. Comparison of six approximations to $P_b(k; m, N, a)$ for the binomial model for the conditional cases.

N	m	n	a	k	$\hat{P}_b(k; n, m, a)$	(12.59)	(12.62)	(12.63)	(12.79)	(12.80)
100	10	5	50	10	.4882	.4490	.5122	.4117	.4991	.4989
				11	.2096	.1973	.2319	.1913	.2043	.2043
				12	.0727	.0739	.0819	.0688	.0778	.0778
				13	.0216	.0212	.0278	.0209	.0313	.0313
				14	.0059	.0054	.0060	.0055	.0027	.0027
			25	5	.9672	.9096	.9185	.7777	.8953	.8809
				6	.6247	.5701	.6308	.5004	.5780	.5736
				7	.2331	.2192	.2585	.2094	.2276	.2272
				8	.0625	.0617	.0748	.0582	.0778	.0778
				9	.0126	.0131	.0158	.0125	.0154	.0154
	20	5	50	14	.8751	.8455	.7629	.6287	.8175	.8169
				15	.6426	.6232	.5890	.4874	.6302	.6299
				16	.3928	.3849	.3898	.3280	.4240	.4240
				17	.2017	.1964	.2130	.1814	.2302	.2302
				18	.0918	.0902	.0995	.0872	.1187	.1187
				19	.0379	.0376	.0417	.0378	.0436	.0436
				20	.0137	.0132	.0140	.0133	.0161	.0161
		10	50	14	.8921	.8591	.7769	.6366	.8342	.8335
				15	.6750	.6516	.6139	.5066	.6654	.6653
				16	.4230	.4111	.4080	.3487	.4433	.4433
				17	.2334	.2293	.2379	.2097	.2738	.2738
				18	.1117	.1108	.1205	.1041	.1237	.1237
				19	.0474	.0475	.0529	.0467	.0567	.0567
				20	.0187	.0185	.0206	.0177	.0240	.0240
				21	.0069	.0073	.0071	.0072	.0073	.0073
500	20	5	100	9	.8159	.7418	.8153	.7064	.8370	.8369
				10	.4583	.4172	.4854	.4032	.4598	.4598
				11	.1829	.1646	.1921	.1682	.1790	.1790
				12	.0608	.0513	.0594	.0537	.0829	.0829
				13	.0170	.0146	.0209	.0143	.0107	.0096
				14	.0041	.0031	.0034	.0029	.0048	.0048
	10	10	100	10	.4682	.3929	.5027	.4084	.4755	.4752
				11	.1945	.1618	.2261	.1641	.1949	.1947
				12	.0651	.0498	.0666	.0607	.0741	.0741
				13	.0183	.0122	.0181	.0176	.0284	.0284
				14	.0052	.0041	.0048	.0036	.0039	.0039

13

Scan Statistics for a Sequence of Discrete I.I.D. Variates

13.1 Binomial Distribution of Events. Discrete Time, Unconditional Case. The Bernoulli Process

Let $X_1, X_2, \ldots, X_N$ be a sequence of independently and identically distributed (i.i.d.) discrete random variables, where $P(X_i = 1) = p = 1 - P(X_i = 0)$. We refer to the X's as a sequence of Bernoulli trials, and to the process as a Bernoulli process. For m an integer, and $i = 1, 2, \ldots, N - m + 1$, define the random variables

$$Y_i(m) = \sum_{j=1}^{i+m-1} X_j.$$

The $Y_i(m)$'s define a moving sum of the X's. The scan statistic, S'_m is defined as the maximum of the moving sums, that is, the maximum number of ones in any m consecutive trials:

$$S'_m = \max_{1 \leq i \leq N-m+1} \{Y_i(m)\}.$$

A related statistic is W_k, the smallest number of consecutive trials that contain k ones. That is, $W_k = \min_{k \leq m \leq N} \{m: \text{such that, } S'_m = k\}$. Given a Bernoulli process on $(1, \infty)$, let $T_{k,m}$ denote the waiting time until we first observe at least k ones in an interval of length m. Formally, $T_{k,m}$ is the smallest i (greater than or equal to m) such that $Y_{i-m+1}(m) \geq k$. The three statistics, S'_m, W_k, and $T_{k,m}$, are related by

$$P(S'_m \geq k) = P(W_k \leq m) = P(T_{k,m} \leq N). \tag{13.1}$$

We denote these common probabilities for the Bernoulli process by $P'(k \mid m; N, p)$. These three statistics have similar counterparts in the continuous-time Poisson process considered in Chapter 3.

A fourth statistic defined for the discrete-time Poisson process considered in the present chapter is the length of the longest number of consecutive trials, V_r, that have at most r zeros. For the special case, $r = 0$, V_r is the length of the longest run of ones. For a sequence of N trials, the statistic V_r is probabilistically related to the scan statistic S'_m, by the relation

$$P(V_r \geq k + r) = P(S'_{k+r} \geq k) = P'(k \mid k + r; N, p). \qquad (13.2)$$

Note: In the matching in aligned DNA sequence examples of Chapter 6, researchers sometimes focus on the length of the longest, almost perfectly matching, sequence, and this is directly measured by V_r. For the special case $r = 0$, the researcher is looking at the length of the longest, perfectly matching, sequence, and this is directly related to the length of the longest run of ones.

13.2   Exact Results for the Distribution of the Scan Statistics

13.2.1   The Distribution of the Length of the Longest Success Run: $P'(k \mid k; N, p)$

The random variable V_0 denotes the length of the longest run of ones (*successes*), and $P(V_0 \geq m) = P'(m \mid m; N, p)$. The distribution of the length of the longest run of ones in a sequence of N Bernoulli trials is a classical problem in probability theory. A recursion relation going back to Abraham de Moivre (1738) is

$$P(V_0 \geq m \mid N + 1\} = P(V_0 \geq m \mid N) + (1 - p)p^m (1 - P(V_0 \geq m \mid N - m\}). \qquad (13.3)$$

Various exact and approximate expressions are given for $P(V_0 \geq m \mid N\}$ in Uspensky (1937, p. 79), Bradley (1968, p. 267), Bateman (1948, p. 112), and elsewhere. Bateman's exact formula is relatively simple and is

$$P(V_0 \geq m \mid N\} = \sum_{j=1}^{[N/m]} (-1)^{j+1} \{p + ((N - jm + 1)q/j)\} \binom{N - jm}{i - 1} p^{jm} q^{j-1},$$

$$(13.4)$$

where $q = 1 - p$ and $[y]$ denotes the largest integer in y. Work on the distribution of the longest run and its variations continue through to today. Results are derived for both exact and limiting distributions. The book by Godbole and Papastavridis (1994) contains several papers focusing on the length of the longest success run for various models.

13.2.2   Exact Results for $P'(k \mid m; N, p)$

Chapter 12 gives results for the conditional probability $P(S'_m \geq k \mid \mathbf{a})$ where the total number of successes in N trials is a constant $\mathbf{a}$. We can find the unconditional probability $P'(k \mid m; N, p) = P(S'_m \geq k)$, by averaging the conditional probability $P(S'_m \geq k \mid \mathbf{a})$. We describe the approach in Chapter 7 and illustrate it in the proof of Theorem 13.1 below.

Let $Q'(k \mid m; N, p) = 1 - P'(k \mid m; N, p)$, and abbreviate $Q'(k \mid m; Lm, p)$ by Q'_L. The following theorem, in the spirit of Theorem 11.2, gives exact results for Q'_2 and Q'_3. These results are of interest in themselves, but even more importantly, we use them in Section 13.3 to provide a highly accurate approximation for Q'_L.

Theorem 13.1 (Theorem 2 in Naus (1982)). *For* $2 < k < N$, $0 < p < 1$, *let*

$$b(k; m, p) = \binom{m}{k} p^k (1 - p)^{m-k} \qquad and \qquad F_b(r; s, p) = \sum_{i=0}^{r} b(i; s, p).$$

Then

$$Q'_2 = (F_b(k - 1; m, p))^2 - (k - 1)b(k; m, p) F_b(k - 2; m, p)$$
$$+ mpb(k; m, p) F_b(k - 3; m - 1, p) \qquad (13.5)$$

and

$$Q'_3 = (F_b(k - 1; m, p))^3 - A_1 + A_2 + A_3 - A_4, \qquad (13.6)$$

where

$$A_1 = 2b(k; m, p) F_b(k - 1; m, p)\{(k - 1) F_b(k - 2; m, p)$$
$$- mp F_b(k - 3; m - 1, p)\},$$

$$A_2 = .5(b(k; m, p))^2\{(k - 1)(k - 2) F_b(k - 3; m, p)$$
$$- 2(k - 2)mp F_b(k - 4; m - 1, p) + m(m - 1)p^2 F_b(k - 5; m - 2, p)\},$$

$$A_3 = \sum_{r=1}^{k-1} b(2k - r; m, p)(F_b(r - 1; m, p))^2,$$

$$A_4 = \sum_{r=2}^{k-1} b(2k - r; m, p)b(r; m, p)\{(r - 1) F_b(r - 2; m, p)$$
$$- mp F_b(r - 3; m - 1, p)\},$$

where $F_b(i, n, p) = 0$ *for* $i < 0$.

Proof. To find Q'_2, we average over the conditional probability in Corollary 12.1 (Corollary 1 from Naus (1974)). To find Q'_3, divide the $3m$ trials into three disjoint sets each of m trials; condition on the numbers n_i, $i = 1, 2, 3$, of successes in the three sets and apply Theorem 12.1 (Theorem I from Naus (1974)) and expand terms; finally, average the resulting probability over the joint distribution of n_i, $i = 1, 2, 3$.

Recently, Fu (2000) employed a *finite Markov chain embedding* method to derive an exact formula for $P(S'_m < k)$, that can be easily computed for all values of N, m, and k. This method has been developed in a series of articles by Fu (1986), Fu and Hu (1987), Fu and Koutras (1994b), Koutras and Alexandrou (1995), Koutras (1996), and Boutsikas and Koutras (2000). Until now, $P(S'_m < k)$ could be evaluated for limited values of N, m, and k, since the dimension of the state space of the embedded Markov chain could be as high as $2^{m-1} + 1$. With that approach it is impossible to evaluate $P(S'_m < k)$ for $m = 50$. For the problem at hand, Fu (2000) constructed an embedded Markov chain with a state space that contains at most $2m$ elements. We present below a brief outline of his approach.

For $m \leq j \leq N$ let an *ending block* U_j be defined as

$$U_j = \left(\sum_{i=j-m+1}^{j} X_i, X_j - m + 1 \right).$$

Given k, define for $m \leq j \leq N$ a sequence of *index functions*

$$I_j(k) = \begin{cases} 0 & \text{if } S'_m(i) < k \quad \text{for all } i, \quad m \leq i \leq j, \\ 1 & \text{if } S'_m(i) \geq k \quad \text{some } i, \quad m \leq i \leq j, \end{cases}$$

where $S'_m(i)$ is the scan statistic for a sequence of i Bernoulli trials. It follows that

$$P(S'_m < k) = P(I_N(k) = 0).$$

To evaluate $P(S'_m < k)$, the random variable $I_j(k)$, $m \leq j \leq N$, is embedded as a component of a homogeneous Markov chain given by

$$O_j = \begin{cases} (I_j(k), U_j), & S'_m(j) < k \quad \text{and} \quad I_j(k) = 0, \\ \delta, & I_k(k) = 1, \end{cases}$$

with state space

$$\left\{ (0, (0, 0)), (0, (1, 0)), (0, (1, 1)), \ldots, (0, (k - 1, 0)), (0, (k - 1, 1)), \delta \right\}.$$

This state space has $2k$ elements. We now present, without proof, the main result in Fu (2000).

Theorem 13.2. *For $0 < k \leq m < N$:*

$$P(S'_m < k) = \tau \mathbf{M}^{N-1} \mathbf{J}',$$

where τ is a $1 \times 2k$ vector of initial probabilities with the ith component, $2 \le i = 2j \le 2k - 1$, $1 \le j \le k - 1$, given by

$$\tau_i = \begin{cases} \binom{m-1}{j} p^j q^{m-j}, & i = 2j, \\ \binom{m-1}{j-1} p^j q^{m-j}, & i = 2j + 1, \end{cases}$$

$$\tau_1 = \binom{m-1}{0} q^m \quad and \quad \tau_{2k} = 1 - \sum_{n=0}^{k-1} \binom{m}{n} p^n q^{m-n};$$

J' *is the transpose of* $\mathbf{J} = (1, 1, \ldots, 1, 0)_{1 \times 2k}$ *and* $\mathbf{M} = [M_{(u,v),(x,y)}]$ *is the transition probability matrix for the embedding Markov chain of dimension $2k \times 2k$, where, for $1 \le u \le k - 1$:*

$$M_{(u,1),(x,y)} = \begin{cases} \frac{u-1}{m-1} p, & x = u, \ y = 1, \\ \frac{m-u}{m-1} p, & x = u, \ y = 0, \\ \frac{u-1}{m-1} q, & x = u - 1, \ y = 1, \\ \frac{m-u}{m-1} q, & x = u - 1, \ y = 0, \end{cases}$$

and for $0 \le u \le k - 1$:

$$M_{(u,0),(x,y)} = \begin{cases} \frac{u}{m-1} p, & x = u + 1, \ y = 1, \\ \frac{m-u-1}{m-1} p, & x = u + 1, \ y = 0, \\ \frac{u}{m-1} q, & x = u, \ y = 1, \\ \frac{m-u-1}{m-1} q, & x = u, \ y = 0, \end{cases}$$

$M_{(k-1,0),r} = p$, $M_{\tau,\tau} = 1$, *and* $M_{(u,v),(x,y)} = 0$ *elsewhere.*

Fu (2000) presents numerical results for $P(S_m' < k)$ using the S-Plus software.

13.3 Bounds for S_m' for i.i.d. Integer Valued Random Variables

Let $X_1, \ldots, X_N$ be i.i.d. integer valued random variables that are bounded from below. We will assume without loss of generality that $X_i \ge 0$. If $X_i \ge -n_0$, where n_0 is a positive integer, we will consider $X_i + n_0$. The following model will be assumed throughout this section: $P(X_i = j) = p_j$, $p_j \ge 0$, $j = 0, 1, 2, \ldots$, $c, \ldots$, $P(X_i = j) = 0$ elsewhere, where $\sum_{j=0}^{\infty} p_j = 1$. If the X_i's are bounded by an integer c, one replaces the ∞ in the sum with the integer c.

For integers $2 \le m < N$ and $-m + 2 \le t \le N - m + 1$ let $Y_t = \sum_{i=t \vee 1}^{t+m-1} X_i$, and for $t < -m + 2$ set $Y_t = 0$. For $1 \le N_0 < N$ define

$$S_m'(N_0, N) = \max\{Y_t; N_0 \le t \le N - m + 1\},$$

$$\tau_{k,m} = \inf\{t \ge 1; Y_{t-m+3} \ge k\}, \tag{13.7}$$

where $a \vee b = \max\{a, b\}$. We abbreviate $S'_m(1, N)$ to $S'_m(N)$ and abbreviate it to S'_m when the value of N is apparent. The random variable $\tau_{k,m}$ is the waiting time for the moving sums of m X_i's to exceed the value $k - 1$. Let

$$G_{k,m}(N) = P(\tau_{k,m} > N) = P(S'_m < k), \qquad f_{k,m}(t) = P(\tau_{k,m} = t). \quad (13.8)$$

When the value of k and m is understood we delete the subscripts k, m from the above terms.

We are interested in deriving accurate inequalities for $G(N)$ that will yield inequalities for $P(S'_m \geq k)$. Based on these inequalities we get inequalities for the expected value and variance of $\tau_{k,m}$ and S'_m. Two methods for deriving lower and upper bounds are given below. The first method is based on utilizing the dependence structure inherent in the moving sums. These inequalities will be called *product-type inequalities*. The second method is the method of *Bonferroni-type inequalities* for probabilities of union of dependent events.

The following is the main result for obtaining product-type inequalities for $G(N)$.

Theorem 13.3. *For integers* $i, j, n \geq 1$ *and* $m \geq 2$, *let*

$$A_{1,n} = f((n + 1)m), \qquad A_{j,n} = A_{1,n}(1 - A_{j-1,n})^{-nm+1}, \qquad (13.9)$$

and

$$B_{1,n} = f(nm)/G((n + 1)m - 1), \qquad B_{j,n} = f(nm)(1 + B_{j-1,n})^{nm}. \quad (13.10)$$

Then,

$$G(N) \leq G(im)(1 - A_{j,n})^{N-im} \qquad for \quad N \geq (i \vee (n + 1))m \qquad (13.11)$$

and

$$G(N) \geq G(im)/(1 + B_{j,n})^{N-im} \qquad for \quad N \geq (i \vee n)m. \qquad (13.12)$$

To prove Theorem 13.3 we need the following three preliminary lemmas. The first one is a known result (Esary, Proschan, and Walkup, 1967) and will be stated without proof.

Lemma 13.1. *If* $X_1, \dots, X_n$ *are independent random variables, then for any two* n-*variable real-valued functions* g *and* h, *that are both coordinatewise increasing (decreasing),*

$$E[g(X_1, \dots, X_n)h(X_1, \dots, X_n)] \geq E[g(X_1, \dots, X_n)]E[h(X_1, \dots, X_n)]. \qquad (13.13)$$

Lemma 13.2. *For integers* $t \geq nm$ *and* $n \geq 1$:

$$f(t) \leq G(t - nm)f(nm). \qquad (13.14)$$

Proof. For $t \geq (n+1)m$:

$$f(t) = P\left([S_m'(t-1) \leq k-1] \cap \left[\bigcup_{i=1}^{c \wedge k} D_i\right]\right) = \sum_{i=1}^{c \wedge k} f_i(t), \qquad (13.15)$$

where

$$D_i = (Y_{t-m} = k - i) \cap (X_t \geq i), \qquad (13.16)$$

$a \wedge b = \min\{a, b\}$ and

$$f_i(t) = P\big([S_m'(t-1) \leq k-1] \cap D_i\big). \qquad (13.17)$$

Write

$$
\begin{aligned}
f_i(t) &= P\big([S_m'(t-nm) \leq k-1] \cap [S_m'(t-(n+1)m+2, t-1) \leq k-1] \cap D_i\big) \\
&\leq P\big([S_m'(t-nm) \leq k-1] \cap [S_m'(t-nm+1, t-1) \leq k-1] \cap D_i\big) \\
&= G(t-nm) f_i(nm), \qquad (13.18)
\end{aligned}
$$

where

$$f_i(nm) = P\big([S_m'(nm-1) \leq k-1] \cap [Y_{(n-1)m} = k-i] \cap [X_{nm} \geq i]\big). \qquad (13.19)$$

It follows from (13.15) and (13.18) that

$$f(t) \leq G(t-nm) \sum_{i=1}^{c \wedge k} f_i(nm) = G(t-nm) f(nm), \qquad (13.20)$$

proving Lemma 13.2 for $t \geq (n+1)m$. To verify that the result holds for $nm \leq t \leq (n+1)m - 1$, set $G(0) = 1$, $G(t) = P(X_1 + \cdots + X_t \leq k-1)$ for $1 \leq t \leq m$, and replace $S_m'(t-nm)$ by $\sum_{i=1}^{t-nm} X_i$ and drop the event $[S_m'(t-nm+1, t-1) \leq k-1]$ for $n = 1$ in (13.18).

Lemma 13.3. *For integers $n \geq 1$ and $t \geq (n+1)m$:*

$$f(t) \geq f((n+1)m)G(t-nm). \qquad (13.21)$$

Proof. For $1 \leq i \leq c \wedge k$, define the events

$$E_1 = (S_m'(t-nm) \leq k-1) \qquad \text{and}$$
$$E_{2,i} = (S_m'(t-(n+1)m+1, t-1) \leq k-1) \cap (Y_{t-m} = k-i).(13.22)$$

Then,

$$f_i(t) = P(E_1 \cap E_{2,i}) P(X_t \geq i), \qquad (13.23)$$

where $f_i(t)$ was defined above in (13.17). Note that E_1 depends on $X_1, \ldots,$ X_{t-nm} and $E_{2,i}$ depends on $X_{t-(n+1)m+1}, \ldots, X_{t-1}$. Let $V = (X_{t-nm+1}, \ldots,$ $X_{t-1})$ be the random vector that includes the random variables that $E_{2,i}$ depends on and excludes the random variables that both E_1 and $E_{2,i}$ depend on. Conditional on V, the indicator functions of the events E_1 and $E_{2,i}$, denoted by $I(E_1)$ and $I(E_{2,i})$, respectively, are both coordinatewise decreasing functions of $X_1, \ldots, X_{t-nm}$. It follows from Lemma 13.1 that

$$P(E_1 \cap E_{2,i} \mid V) \geq P(E_1 \mid V)P(E_{2,i} \mid V) = P(E_1)P(E_{2,i} \mid V). \quad (13.24)$$

Averaging both sides of (13.24) over the distribution of the random vector V we get

$$P(E_1 \cap E_{2,i}) \geq P(E_1)P(E_{2,i}) = G(t - nm)P(E_{2,i})$$
$$= G(t - nm)f_i((n + 1)m)/P(X_t \geq i). \quad (13.25)$$

Substitute (13.25) into (13.23) and sum over $i = 1, \ldots, c \wedge k$ to complete the proof of Lemma 13.3.

Proof of Theorem 13.3. Lemmas 13.3 and 13.2 are used to find upper and lower bounds that were given in (13.11) and (13.12), respectively. For $t \geq (n+1)m$, it follows from Lemma 13.3 that

$$f(t) = G(t - 1) - G(t) \geq f(n + 1)(G(t - nm))$$
$$\geq f((n + 1)m)G(t - 1). \quad (13.26)$$

The second inequality in (13.26) follows from the fact that $G(t)$ is a decreasing function of t. For $n \geq 1$, let $A_{1,n} = f((n + 1)m)$. From (13.26) we get

$$G(t - 1)/(1 - A_{1,n})^{t-1} \geq G(t)/(1 - A_{1,n})^t, \quad (13.27)$$

so that $G(t)/(1 - A_{1,n})^t$ is decreasing in t. Therefore, for $N \geq im \vee (n + 1)m$:

$$G(N) \leq G(im)(1 - A_{1,n})^{N-im}. \quad (13.28)$$

This is the upper bound for $G(N)$ given in (13.11) for $j = 1$. Since $G(t)/(1 - A_{1,n})^t$ is decreasing in t for $t \geq (n + 1)m$:

$$G(t - nm) \geq G(t - 1)(1 - A_{1,n})^{t-nm}/(1 - A_{1,n})^{t-1}. \quad (13.29)$$

Substitute (13.29) into (13.26) to get

$$G(t) \leq G(t - 1) - f((n + 1)m)G(t - nm)$$
$$\leq G(t - 1) - A_{1,n}G(t - 1)(1 - A_{1,n})^{-nm+1}$$
$$\leq G(t - 1)(1 - A_{2,n}), \quad (13.30)$$

where $A_{2,n} = A_{1,n}(1 - A_{i,n})^{-nm+1}$. Now proceed through the steps that led to (13.27) and (13.28) to obtain the upper bound for $j = 2$ in (3.11). Iterating in this fashion will give the upper bound for $G(N)$ for any $j \geq 2$.

To derive the lower bounds in (13.12), start with Lemma 13.2 to get, for $t \geq nm$:

$$f(t) = G(t-1) - G(t) \leq G(t-nm)f(nm). \qquad (13.31)$$

Since the indicator functions of the events $(S_m'(u) \leq k-1)$ and $(S_m'(u-m+2, u+v) \leq k-1)$ are decreasing function of the X_i's, it follows from Lemma 13.1 that for $u \geq m$ and $v \geq 0$:

$$G(u+v) = P\big([S_m'(u) \leq k-1] \cap [S_m'(u-m+2, u+v) \leq k-1]\big)$$
$$\geq G(u)G(v+m-1). \qquad (13.32)$$

In particular, for $t \geq nm$, $u = t - nm$, and $v = nm$, inequality (12.32) implies that

$$G(t-nm) \leq G(t)/G((n+1)m-1). \qquad (13.33)$$

Substituting (13.33) into (13.31) yields

$$G(t-1) \leq (1 + B_{1.n})G(t), \qquad (13.34)$$

where $B_{1.n} = f(nm)/G((n+1)m-1)$. The approach used above to derive the upper bounds for $G(N)$ yields the lower bounds given in (13.12). This completes the proof of Theorem 13.3.

Remarks. 1. The proof of Theorem 13.3 is based on the approach of Janson (1984), who derived bounds for the distribution of a scan statistic for a Poisson process.

2. For $j = 1$, the bounds in (13.11) and (13.12) converge as $G(nm) \to 1$ and $f(nm) \to 0$.

3. If we let the total number of trials become large, the bounds will be tight if $(1 - f((n+1)m))^{T-im}$ is close to $1/[1 + f(nm)/G((n+1)m-1)]^{I-im}$.

4. The bounds improve for $j \geq 2$, but in most cases the improvement is of limited value and therefore we recommend the bounds with $j = 1$.

To implement the results of Theorem 13.3 for $j = 1$ we have to evaluate $f(nm)$, $G(im)$, and $G((n+1)m-1)$ for integers $i \geq 1$, $m \geq 2$, and $n \geq 1$. The larger i and n are, the better the bounds appear, though the harder it is to evaluate these quantities. For the general case of i.i.d. integer valued random variables, using the algorithms that have been developed so far, we can evaluate the bounds that require $f(3m)$, $G(3m)$, and $G(3m-1)$. For some special models, such as the i.i.d. 0–1 trials and the i.i.d. trinomial $-1, 0, +1$ trials, we are able to evaluate $G(4m)$ and $G(4m-1)$, and so, higher-order, more accurate, bounds can be obtained. We now present these bounds for $j = 1$ only.

The upper bounds are

$$G(N) \leq G(2m)[1 - f(2m)]^{n-2m} \qquad \text{for} \quad N \geq 2m \qquad (13.35)$$

and

$$G(N) \le G(3m)[1 - f(2m)]^{N-3m} \qquad \text{for} \quad N \ge 3m. \qquad (13.36)$$

The lower bounds are

$$G(N) \ge G(2m)/[1 + f(2m)/(G(2m)G(2m - 1))]^{N-2m} \qquad \text{for} \quad N \ge 2m \qquad (13.37)$$

and

$$G(N) \ge G(3m)/[1 + f(2m)/G(3m - 1)]^{N-3m} \qquad \text{for} \quad N \ge 3m. \qquad (13.38)$$

These upper and lower bounds are evaluated using an algorithm developed recently in Karwe and Naus (1997). For more details see, Section 13.5.

We now derive the Bonferroni-type inequalities for $G(N) = P(S'_m \le k - 1)$. Let $N = (l - 1)m + m_1$, where $1 \le m_1 \le m$ and $l \ge 3$. For $1 \le i \le l - 2$, let

$$B_i = \bigcap_{j=1}^{m+1} (X_{(i-1)m+j} + \cdots + X_{im+j-1} \le k - 1) \qquad (13.39)$$

and

$$B_{l-1} = \bigcap_{j=1}^{m_1+1} (X_{(l-2)m+j} + \cdots + X_{(l-1)m+j-1} \le k - 1).$$

Then $(S'_m \le k - 1) = \bigcap_{i=1}^{l-1} B_i$ and

$$P(S'_m \ge k) = P\left(\bigcup_{i=1}^{l-1} B_i^c\right). \qquad (13.40)$$

It follows from (7.4) that a second-order Bonferroni-type upper bound for $P(S'_m \ge k)$ is given by

$$P(S'_m \ge k) \le \sum_{i=1}^{l-1} P(B_i^c) - \sum_{i=2}^{l-1} P(B_{i-1}^c \cap B_i^c).$$

Since $\{B_i^c; 1 \le i \le l - 2\}$ are stationary, for $1 \le i \le l - 1$, $P(B_i^c) = P(B_1^c)$, $P(B_{i-1}^c \cap B_i^c) = P(B_1^c \cap B_2^c)$, and the inequality given above simplifies to

$$P(S'_m \ge k) \le (l - 2)P(B_1^c) + P(B_{l-1}^c) - (l - 3)P(B_1^c \cap B_2^c) - P(B_{l-2}^c - B_{l-1}^c)$$
$$= (l - 2)(1 - P(B_1)) - (l - 3)[1 - P(B_1) - P(B_2) + P(B_1 \cap B_2)]$$
$$\quad + (1 - P(B_{l-1})) - [1 - P(B_{l-2}) - P(B_{l-1}) + P(B_{l-2} \cap B_{l-1})]$$
$$= 1 + (l - 3)[G(2m) - G(3m)] - G(2m + m_1). \qquad (13.41)$$

A second-order Bonferroni-type lower bound for $P(S'_m \geq k)$ follows from (7.12):

$$P(S'_m \geq k) \geq \frac{2}{a} t_1 - \frac{2}{a(a-1)} t_2, \tag{13.42}$$

where

$$t_1 = \sum_{i=1}^{l-1} P(B_i^c) = (l-2)(1 - G(2m)) + (1 - G(m+m_1)),$$

$$t_2 = \sum_{j=2}^{l-1} \sum_{i=1}^{j-1} P(B_i^c \cap B_j^c) = \sum_{j=2}^{l-1} \sum_{i=1}^{j-1} [1 - 2G(2m) + P(B_i \cap B_j)]$$

$$+ \sum_{i=1}^{l-2} P(B_i^c \cap B_{l-1}^c)$$

$$= .5(l-2)(l-3)(1 - 2G(2m)) + (l-3)G(3m) + \sum_{j=3}^{l-2} \sum_{i=1}^{j-2} P(B_i \cap B_j)$$

$$+ \sum_{i=1}^{l-3} P(B_i^c \cap B_{l-1}^c) + P(B_{l-2}^c \cap B_{l-1}^c) \tag{13.43}$$

and a is the integer part of $2 + 2t_2/t_1$. To evaluate $P(B_i \cap B_j)$ note that for $j-i \geq 2$ the events B_i and B_j are independent and therefore $P(B_i \cap B_j) = [G(2m)]^2$. Hence

$$t_2 = .5(l-2)(l-3)(1 - 2G(2m)) + (l-3)G(3m) + .5(l-3)(l-4)[G(2m)]^2$$
$$+ (l-3)G(2m)G(m+m_1) + (l-2)(1 - G(2m) - G(m+m_1))$$
$$+ G(2m+m_1). \tag{13.44}$$

For the special case of $N = lm$, the upper bound (13.41) simplifies to

$$P(S'_m \geq k) \leq 1 + (l-3)G(2m) - (l-2)G(3m). \tag{13.45}$$

The lower bound (13.42) simplifies with

$$t_1 = (l-1)[1 - G(2m)] \tag{13.46}$$

and

$$t_2 = .5(l-1)(l-2)(1 - 2G(2m))$$
$$+ (l-2)G(3m) + .5(l-2)(l-3)[G(2m)]^2. \tag{13.47}$$

13.4   Approximations for $P'(k \mid m; N, p)$

Let $Q'(k \mid m; N, p) = 1 - P'(k \mid m; N, p)$, and abbreviate $Q'\{k \mid m; Lm, p\}$ by Q'_L. Naus (1982) provides the following highly accurate approximation for Q'_L

in terms of Q'_2 and Q'_3:

$$Q'_L \approx Q'_2 \{Q'_3/Q'_2\}^{((N/m)-2)}. \tag{13.48}$$

Equations (13.5) and (13.6) give exact results for Q'_2 and Q'_3.

Approximation (13.48) is highly accurate over the entire range. To further reduce computational effort, with a slight loss of accuracy, Wallenstein, Naus, and Glaz (1995) note that

$$Q'_2 \approx \hat{Q}'_2 = 2F_b(k-1, N, p) - 1 - (k-1-mp)b(k, N, p),$$
$$Q'_3 \approx \hat{Q}'_3 = 2F_b(k-1, N, p) - 1 - (2k-1-2mp)b(k, N, p).$$

Substituting these two into (13.48) yields a simpler approximation

$$Q'_L \approx \hat{Q}'_2 \{\hat{Q}'_3/\hat{Q}'_2\}^{((N/m)-2)}.$$

An even simpler approximation suggested in Wallenstein, Naus, and Glaz (1995) is

$$P(S_m \geq k) \approx 1 - \{1 - (k-1-mp)b(k, N, p)\}^{((N/m)-2)}.$$

A useful related approximation (see Arratia, Gordon, and Waterman (1990)) is

$$P(S_m \geq k) \approx 1 - \exp\{(N-m)(k-mp)b(k, N, p)/m\}.$$

13.4.1   The Special Case $k = m$: The Length of the Longest Run

For many cases of practical interest the number of trials N is large, and the length of the longest run of ones, m, is much smaller. For example, in $N = 200,000$ tosses of a fair coin ($p = P(H) = .5$), it is fairly unusual ($< .003$) to get a run of heads as long as 25. In this case, the exact formula (13.4) involves a sum of $[N/m] = 8000$ terms. For large N, various approximate and asymptotic formula and bounds have been developed.

Feller (1957, p. 310) gives a simple approximation

$$P'(m \mid m; N, p) \approx 1 - \exp\{-N(1-p)p^m\}. \tag{13.49}$$

Approximation (13.5) gives

$$P'(m \mid m; N, p) \approx 1 - Q'_2 \{Q'_3/Q'_2\}^{((N/m)-2)}, \tag{13.50}$$

where we can apply (13.4) directly, for $(N/m) = 2, 3$, to find

$$Q'_2 = 1 - P'(m \mid m; 2m, p) = 1 - p^m(1 + mq)$$

and

$$Q'_3 = 1 - P'(m \mid m; 3m, p) = 1 - p^m(1 + 2mq) + .5p^{2m}(2mq + m(m-1)q^2). \tag{13.51}$$

Comparisons with exact tables of runs (e.g., Grant (1947)) or with tight bounds, such as the generating function bounds of Uspensky, the Chen–Stein bounds, or Glaz–Naus bounds, show that approximation (13.50) is highly accurate over a wide range of the distribution. For example, $P^*(7 \mid 7; 50, .5) = .1653$ from Grant's tables, .1653 from approximation (13.50), as compared to .1774 from approximation (13.49).

13.4.2 Erdös–Rényi Laws

A substantial literature on the asymptotic results appears under the heading of Erdös–Rényi laws or Erdös–Rényi–Shepp theorems. Deheuvels (1985a) reviews some of the important results, gives a powerful and general theorem applied to arrays, and relates it to runs, spacings, and other problems. We will focus on parts of their summary.

Let $X_1, X_2, \ldots, X_N$ be a sequence of i.i.d. discrete random variables, with zero expectation, unit variance, and moment generating function $G_X(t) = G(t) = E(e^{tX})$. Let t_0 denote the largest t for which the moment generating function is finite, and assume $t_0 > 0$. Let $G'(t) = \partial G(t)/\partial t$. For m an integer, and $i = 1, 2, \ldots, N - m + 1$, define the random variables

$$Y_i(m) = \sum_{j=1}^{i+m-1} X_j.$$

The $Y_i(m)$'s define a moving sum of m of the X's. The scan statistic, $S'_m = \max_{1 \le i \le N-m+1} \{Y_i(m)\}$ is the maximum of the moving sums, that is, the maximum number of ones in any m consecutive trials. Deheuvels denotes S'_m by $I(N, m)$.

Erdös and Revesz derive limit results to runs (1975). Erdös and Rényi (1970) give results for quotas of i.i.d. random variables and prove the following limiting theorem for S'_m: Let $c = c(\mu)$ be defined by

$$e^{-1/c} = \inf_t G(t)e^{-t\mu}, \tag{13.52}$$

then for each μ in $\{G'(t)/G(t), 0 < t < t_0\}$:

$$\lim_{N \to \infty} S'_{[c \log N]}/[c \log N] = \mu, \tag{13.53}$$

almost surely, where $[x]$ denotes the largest integer in x.

To find c in (13.52), we need to find the value of t, call it t^*, that minimizes $G(t)e^{-t\mu}$. Note that taking the derivative of the right-hand side of (13.52) and setting equal to zero gives

$$G'(t^*)e^{-t^*\mu} - \mu G(t^*)e^{-t^*\mu} = 0,$$

or

$$\mu = G'(t^*)/G(t^*). \tag{13.54}$$

Thus,

$$e^{-1/c} = \inf_t G(t)e^{-t\mu} = G(t^*)e^{-t^*}\mu$$

and

$$1/c = t^*\mu - \log G(t^*). \tag{13.55}$$

Deheuvels (1985a) notes how Csorgo and Steinbach (1981) improved on the precision of the Erdös–Rényi (1970) theorem, and how the best possible rate of convergence of the Erdös–Rényi theorem is given by the following theorem of Deheuvels and Devroye (1983):

Theorem 13.4. *Given previous notations and assumptions, define c by (13.55) and* $t^* = t^*(\alpha)$ *by solving (13.54). Then*

$$\limsup_{N \to \infty}\left\{(S'_{[c\log N]} - \mu[c\log N])/\log\log N\right\} = 1/2t^* \tag{13.56}$$

and

$$\liminf_{N \to \infty}\left\{(S'_{[c\log N]} - \mu[c\log N])/\log\log N\right\} = 1/2t^*.$$

To use this asymptotic result as an approximation, choose a value for μ, then derive t^* from (13.55), then substitute into (13.55) to find c. Then, roughly speaking, for N sufficiently large, there will be a good chance that

$$\mu[c\log N] - (1/2t^*)\log\log N \le S'_{[c\log N]} \le \mu[c\log N] + (1/2t^*)\log\log N. \tag{13.57}$$

For the special case of Bernoulli trials, Deheuvels (1985a) states in Corollary 1 (page 93, previously derived in Deheuvels and Devroye (1983)) that for any $p < \mu < 1$ or, equivalently, $c > -1/\log p$:

$$t^* = \log\{\mu(1-p)/p(1-\mu)\} \tag{13.58}$$

and $c = c(\mu)$ is given by

$$1/c = \mu\log(\mu/p) + (1-\mu)\log\{(1-\mu)/(1-p)\}. \tag{13.59}$$

Note: It is useful to go through some of the details of the derivation of (13.58) and (13.59) to illustrate how to apply their approach to the charge problem (where X can take the values 0, 1, 2) in Section 4.2 of Chapter 4.

For the Bernoulli case, $P(X = 1) = p$, $P(X = 0) = 1 - p = q$:

$$G(t) = E(e^{tX}) = qe^{t0} + pe^{t1} = q + pe^t$$
$$G'(t) = pe^t.$$

Choose a μ, $p < \mu < 1$. Write

$$G'(t^*)/G(t^*) = pe^{t^*}/\{q + pe^{t^*}\} = \mu.$$

Solving for t^* gives (13.58). To find (13.59), recall that t^* is the value for t for which $G'(t^*)/G(t^*) = \mu$. Then

$$\inf_t G(t)e^{-t\mu} = G(t^*)e^{-t^*\mu},$$

and

$$e^{-1/c} = G(t^*)e^{-t^*\mu}.$$

Taking logs, and using t^* from (13.58), and

$$G(t^*) = G'(t^*)/\mu = pe^{t^*}/\mu$$

gives, upon simplification, (13.59). Note also that letting $V_i = X_i - E(X_i)$, and dealing with V_i's (whose expectation is zero, according to conditions of the theorem), will leave the value of c unchanged, but will lead to a new $\mu_v = \mu_x - E(X_i)$. Equation (13.56) will be unchanged since the $S'_{[c \log N]} - \mu[c \log N]$ in the X's, will become the equivalent $\{S'_{[c \log N]} - E(X_i)[c \log N]\} - (\mu - E(X_i))[c \log N]$, in terms of the V's.

Application 13.1. $N = 10000$, $p = .1$. Choose a $\mu = .3$ (say). Then from (13.59), $c = 6.5077226$ and $m = [c \log N] = [59.9] = 59$. From (13.58), $1/2t^* = .3704$. The asymptotic approximation (13.57), together with (13.58) and (13.59), implies that S'_{59} is likely (assuming N is large enough) to be between 16.9 and 18.5. N is quite large and one would hope that the asymptotic results would give an accurate approximation. Use approximation (13.48) to generate $P(S'_{59} \geq k) = P^*(k \mid 59; 10000; .1)$. Subtracting successive probabilities gives $P(S'_{59} = k)$:

k	12	13	14	15	16	17	18	19	20
$P(S'_{59} \geq k)$	1.00	.980	.799	.449	.183	.060	.017	.0046	.0011
$P(S'_{59} = k)$	.02	.18	.35	.27	.12	.043	.012	.004	.001

There is only a small chance of exceeding the asymptotic results upper limit of 18.5. However, there is a 94% chance of being less than the lower limit of 16.9. Further, based on approximation (13.48) distribution, the expectation of S'_{59} for this example is 14.5, as compared to the centering of 17.7 based on the asymptotic result (13.57) or (13.53).

13.4.3 Approximating the Discrete Problem by the Continuous

Whitworth (1901) derives the distribution of the sample range of points on a line and a circle by taking the limit of the discrete version of the problem. In a converse way one can use the results for the continuous problem to approximate the discrete version of the problem. Karlin and Brendel (1992) apply this approach to a cluster of the location of a particular DNA pattern (DAM sites) in a long sequence. See Application 6.1 in Chapter 6.

13.5   The Charge Problem

Application 6.4 of Chapter 6 deals with scanning a DNA sequence for a region of large positive net charge. The scores for any letter in the sequence can be -1, 0, or 1, and we seek the distribution of the maximum moving sum of such scores.

Let $X_1, X_2, \ldots, X_N$ be a sequence of i.i.d. discrete random variables, where $P(X_i = -1) = p_{-1}$, $P(X_i = 0) = p_0$, $P(X_i = 1) = p_1$. For m an integer, and $i = 1, 2, \ldots, N - m + 1$, define the random variables $Y_t(m)$:

$$Y_t(m) = \sum_{i=t}^{t+m-1} X_i.$$

The $Y_t(m)$'s define a moving sum of m of the X_i's. The scan statistic, S'_m is defined as the maximum of the moving sums as the window of m trials scans the sequence. This section emphasizes the dependence of S'_m on N, by using the expanded notation

$$S'_m = S'_m(N) = \max_{1 \leq t \leq N-m+t} \{Y_t(m)\}.$$

Denote

$$G_{k,m}(N) = P(S'_m(N) < k). \tag{13.60}$$

Glaz and Naus (1991) give bounds and approximations for $G_{k,m}(N)$ for the special case of a sequence of i.i.d. integer values X_i's. These results are given in their general form below. Equation (13.72) gives a highly accurate approximation. To compute these bounds and approximations one needs the simpler component probabilities $G_{k,m}(r)$ for $r = 2m - 1, 2m, 3m - 1$, and $3m$. We now describe the results for computing these (and some other) special case probabilities exactly for the charge problem.

13.5.1   Exact Results

Saperstein (1976) derives useful recursion formulas for computing $G_{k,m}(r)$ for $r \leq 2m$. Karwe and Naus (1997) describe this recursion approach and a new recursive method that is computationally more efficient than Saperstein's methods. We summarize their description of the methods here. Extensive tables and programs are detailed in Karwe (1993). The methods are developed for the general case where the X's can take integer values $0, 1, 2, \ldots, c$. For the charge problem, $c = 2$. Note that finding the probability that the maximum moving sum of m X's $< k$, where the X's can take values $0, 1, 2$, yields the corresponding probability that the maximum moving sum of m charges $(-1, 0, 1) < k - m$.

13.5.2   Saperstein's Recursion for $G_{k,m}(2m)$

Let r denote the sum of the first m X_i's and let s denote the sum of the last m X's in the sequence of $2m$ X's.

Define the probabilities

$$b_{k,2m}(r, s) = P\{(S'_m(2m) \leq k)$$
$$\cap (Y_1(m) = r) \cap (Y_{m+1}(m) = s)\}, \qquad \max(r, s) \leq k,$$
$$= 0, \qquad r > k \text{ or } s > k, \tag{13.61}$$
$$b_{k,2m}(s) = P\{(S'_m(2m) \leq k) \cap (Y_{m+1}(m) = s)\}, \qquad s \leq k,$$
$$= 0, \qquad s > k, \tag{13.62}$$

and

$$f_m(z) = P(Y_1(m) = z). \tag{13.63}$$

For $m < i < 2m$, define

$$B_{i,k}(r, s) = P\{(S'_m(i) \leq k) \cap (Y_{m+1}(m) = r)$$
$$\cap (Y_{m+1}(m + i) = s))\}, \qquad \max(r, s) \leq k,$$
$$= 0, \quad \text{otherwise.} \tag{13.64}$$

We use the general convention here that

$$\sum_{i=a}^{b} Z_j = 0, \qquad b < a.$$

From (13.60):

$$P\{S'_m(N) \leq k\} = G_{k+1,m}(N)$$

and

$$Y_{t-m+1}(m) = \sum_{i=t-m+1}^{t} X_j.$$

Saperstein (1976) uses the following recursion formulas to find $P\{S'_m(2m) \leq k\}$:

$$P\{S'_m(2m) \leq k\} = \sum_{s=0}^{k} b_{k,2m}(s) \tag{13.65}$$

and

$$b_{k,2m}(s) = \sum_{\eta=0}^{s} \sum_{\nu=0}^{k-s+\eta} B_{2m-1,k}(\nu, s - \eta) f_1(\eta), \qquad s \leq k$$
$$= 0, \quad \text{otherwise.} \tag{13.66}$$

$B_{i,k}(r, s)$ are computed recursively by using the two relations

$$B_{m+1,k}(r, s) = \sum_{\nu=0}^{k-r} f_1(\nu) f_1(s) f_{m-1}(r), \qquad r + s \leq k,$$
$$= 0, \quad \text{otherwise,} \tag{13.67}$$

and

$$B_{i,k}(r, s) = \sum_{\eta=0}^{s} \sum_{v=0}^{k-r-s+\eta} B_{i-1,k}(r + v, s - \eta) f_1(v) f_1(\eta)$$

$$\times f_{2m-i}(r)/f_{2m-i+1}(r + n), \qquad r + s \leq k,$$

$$= 0, \qquad r + s > k. \tag{13.68}$$

From (13.67) the initial values of $B_{m+1,k}(r, s)$ for varying r and s are computed and stored in a two-dimensional array, call it $A_1(r, s)$. Then do loops on i, r, s, together with the values stored in $A_1(r, s)$ and (13.68), give values for $B_{i,k}(r, s)$, which are stored in an array $A_2(r, s)$. Then the process is iterated by setting the new $A_1(r, s) = A_2(r, s)$. The results are substituted into (13.66) and (13.65) to yield $P\{S'_m(2m) \leq k\}$.

Under the above procedure, the $B_{i,k}(r, s)$ have to be calculated anew for each new value of k or m. Karwe (1993) develops two alternative procedures that are computationally more efficient for getting $P\{S'_m(2m) \leq k\}$. The first procedure is used for generating $P\{S'_m(2m) \leq k\}$ for k and m fixed. The second procedure is used to generate tables of this probability for a range of k and m values. The reader interested in procedure two for generating extensive tables is referred to the summary in Karwe and Naus (1997) and the detailed programs in Karwe (1993). We limit our discussion here to the first procedure for generating individual values:

$$B_{2,k}(s) = \sum_{j=0}^{k} f_1(j) f_1(s), \qquad 0 \leq s \leq \min(c, k),$$

$$= 0, \quad \text{otherwise.} \tag{13.69}$$

Set $X_m = v$ and $X_{2m} = \eta$ in (13.61). For each $m \geq 2, r \leq k, s \leq k$, we have the following recursion:

$$B_{2m,k}(r, s) = \sum_{\eta=0}^{c} \sum_{v=0}^{c} B_{2m-2,k-v}(r - v, s - \eta) f_1(v) f_1(\eta). \tag{13.70}$$

Similarly, for $0 \leq s \leq k$:

$$B_{2m,k}(s) = \sum_{\eta=0}^{s} \sum_{v=0}^{k-s+\eta} B_{2m-2,k-v}(s - \eta) f_1(v) f_1(\eta). \tag{13.71}$$

The Karwe procedure for generating individual values uses (13.71) and (13.65). We start by setting up two two-dimensional arrays: $A_1(k, s)$ and $A_2(k, s)$. At the $(n + 1)$st loop, $A_1(k, s)$ stores values of $B_{2n,k}(s)$; the array $A_2(k, s)$ stores values of $B_{2(n+1),k}(s)$ that are generated using the first array's values. Then $A_2(k, s)$ becomes the new values for $A_1(k, s)$, and the process is iterated $m - 1$ times. Only the $f_1(j)$ for $j = 0, 1, 2, \ldots, c$, are needed.

13.5.3   The Case $2m < N \leq 3m$

For $2m < N$, Saperstein outlines a procedure that might be used, but it requires arrays of high dimension, and is computationally complex. Karwe (1993) develops a recursion relation that is computationally feasible for this case, and gives a computer program and tables. A summary of the relation appears in Karwe and Naus (1997). Karwe (1993) gives tables for $P\{S'_m(N) \leq k\} = G_{k+1,m}(N)$ for $m = 2(1)15$, $k = 1(1)2m - 1$ and $N = 2m - 1$, $2m$, $3m - 1$, and $3m$ and $P(X_i = 0) = .1(.1).8$, $P(X_i = 1) = .1(.1).8$; and $P(X_i = 2) = 1 - P(X_i = 0) + P(X_i = 1)$. Some values from Karwe's (1993) tables are given in the next section.

13.5.4   Approximate Results

Equation (13.48) is of the basic approximation form discussed in Chapter 3, Section 3.2:

$$G_{k,m}(T) \approx G_{k,m}(2m)\{G_{k,m}(3m)/G_{k,m}(2m)\}^{((N/m)-2)}. \qquad (13.72)$$

Glaz and Naus (1991) use this same approach to approximate the distribution of the largest net charge within a window of length m. They show simple cases where exact enumeration gives $G_{k,m}(2m)$ and $G_{k,m}(3m)$. Saperstein (1976) derives useful recursions for computing $G_{k,m}(T)$ for $T \leq 2m$, and outlines a possible but computationally complex approach for $T > 2m$. Karwe (1993) derives new recursion formulas that are computationally more efficient than Saperstein's approach for $T \leq 2m$, and computationally practical for $T = 3m - 1$ and $3m$. She developed programs and extensive tables for $G_{k,m}(T)$ for $T = 2m - 1, 2m, 3m - 1, 3m$. The results are described in the previous section. Approximation (13.72) appears highly accurate. Section 13.3 discusses bounds which when tight can be used as approximations.

13.5.5   Asymptotic Approximations

The general asymptotic results described in Deheuvels (1985a) are explicitly worked out for the Bernoulli variable case, see Section 13.4. For the charge problem, (13.57) holds, but (13.58) and (13.59) change.

Here the i.i.d. X_i's take the values $-1, 0, 1$ with respective probabilities p_{-1}, p_0, p_1. The moment generating function

$$G(t) = E(e^{xt}) = p_{-1}e^{-t} + p_0 + p_1e^t,$$
$$G'(t) = -p_{-1}e^{-t} + p_1e^t.$$

Given a value for μ, t^* is a solution of

$$\mu = (-p_{-1}e^{-t^*} + p_1e^{t^*})/(p_{-1}e^{-t^*} + p_0 + p_1e^{t^*}). \qquad (13.73)$$

Table 13.1. Approximation for $1-G_{k,14}(200)$, charge $= 0, 1, 2$.

k	$G_{k,14}(28)$	$G_{k,14}(42)$	$G_{k,14}(200)$	P(Net charge $= k$)
7	.572033	.407473	.991139	.037
8	.717681	.573306	.954551	.123
9	.831227	.730014	.831365	.212
10	.907265	.845275	.619707	.235
11	.953649	.920182	.385138	.181
12	.978603	.962307	.203826	.111
13	.990985	.983841	.093301	.055
14	.996479	.993607	.038237	.024
15	.998744	.997696	.014056	.0093
16	.999584	.999231	.004744	

Rather than solve (13.73) numerically we will, for our examples, start with a value for t^*, and compute μ from it using (13.73). We then compute $c = c(\mu)$ from

$$1/c = t^* \mu - \log\{p_{-1}e^{-t^*} + p_0 + p_1 e^{t^*}\}. \qquad (13.74)$$

Application 13.2. Let $p_{-1} = .8$, $p_0 = .1$, $p_1 = .1$, $N = 200$, and let $t^* = 1$. Then from (13.73), $\mu = -.03374$, and substituting into (13.74) gives $c = 2.68436$. $[c \log N] = 14$; $\log \log N = 1.6674$ and, from (13.56), S'_{14} is likely to be between .87 to 1.81.

The tables in Karwe (1993) give values of $G_{k,m}(2m)$ and $G_{k,m}(3m)$ for $X_i = 0, 1, 2$, and we can view the change from $-1, 0, 1$ as simply as adding a constant 1 to each X. For ease of comparison we will add 14 to S'_{14}. The asymptotic approximation (13.57) indicates that (for 0, 1, 2 variates) $(14 + S'_{14})$ would range between 14.87 to 15.81. From p. 296 in Karwe (1993), find the following values for $G_{k,14}(28)$ and $G_{k,14}(42)$. Use these in (13.72) to approximate values for $1 - G_{k,14}(200)$. The upper asymptotic limit is reasonble, but the lower asymptotic limit is not a suitable approximation. Further, the asymptotic bounds suggest that 15 is a likely value for $(14 + S'_{14})$. However, for the purposes of finding critical values, a maximum net sum of $(14 + S'_{14}) \geq 15$ is fairly unusual (at the .014 level).

13.6 Longest Run of Any Letter in a Sequence of r Letters

Suman (1994) looks at a generalization to the case where, on each of N independent trials, any of r equally likely possible letters can occur, and looks at the distribution of the longest run of any letter. On page 128, Suman relates this problem to that of the longest success run in $N - 1$ Bernoulli trials. The trick in the relationship is to observe that in the sequence of r-letter alphabets, each letter (from the second onward) is the same (success) or different (failure) as the letter that precedes it. The probability of success, $p = 1/r$. Thus, in the five-letter alphabet, the sequence

a   b   b   e   c   b   c   d   d   d   d   a   e   d   corresponds to
    f   s   f   f   f   f   f   s   s   s   f   f   s.

The longest run in the five-letter alphabet is of length 4 (dddd), corresponding to the longest success run of size 3. As an application of this relation, Suman (1994, p. 129) notes that the limiting (for N large) result for the variable τ_r = size of the longest run of any letter from an equally likely r-letter alphabet, in a sequence of N independent trials, is

$$E(\tau_r) \approx +.5 + \log_e\{(N-1)(r-1)/r)\} + \gamma)/\log_e r \qquad (13.75)$$

and

$$\mathrm{Var}(\tau_r) \approx \{(\pi^2)/2(\log_e r)^2\} + (1/12), \qquad (13.76)$$

where $\gamma = .577\ldots$ (Euler's constant).

From the above correspondence, the expected size of the longest success run in N Bernoulli trials, with probability of success $p = 1/r$, is

$$E(V_0) \approx -.5 + \log_e\{N(r-1)/r)\} + \gamma)/\log_e r, \qquad (13.77)$$

and

$$\mathrm{Var}(V_0) \approx \mathrm{Var}(\tau_r). \qquad (13.78)$$

13.7 Moments of Scan Statistics

13.7.1 The Expected Waiting Time till a Quota

Huntington (1976) derives the exact expected waiting time till a k-in-m quota. The result is expressed in terms of the ratios of determinants of matrices. Denote the expected waiting time till a k-in-m quota by $T_{k,m}$.

Naus (1982) illustrates how to use the approximate values for Q_2' and Q_3', together with (13.48), to approximate the expected waiting time. The approach is to write $E(T_{k,m})$ as an infinite sum (over N) of $P(S_m' \geq k)$, substitute in the approximation for $P(S_m' \geq k)$ based on Q_2' and Q_3', and simplify the resulting geometric sum

$$E(T_{k,m}) = \sum_{N=0}^{\infty} (1 - P(S_m' < k)) \approx 2m + Q_2'/(1 - \{Q_3'/Q_2'\}^{1/m}). \qquad (13.79)$$

Approximation (13.79) appears quite accurate. For example, $P(S_6' \geq 5)$ is 25,250 for $p = .1$, and 1025.50 for $p = .2$, both by the exact and approximate formulas.

Samuel-Cahn (1983) gives approximations and bounds for the expectation and variance of the waiting time until a cluster, and bounds for the expectation, for general point processes with i.i.d. interarrival times between the points. Details are given for the Poisson, Bernoulli, and compound Poisson processes.

We now discus Samuel-Cahns' results for the Bernoulli case. Let $Z_1, Z_2, \ldots$ denote a sequence of i.i.d. 0–1 variates, where $P(Z_i = 1) = p$. For this Bernoulli process the expected waiting times between *ones* is $1/p$.

$T_{k,m}$ denotes the total number of trials until first getting a cluster of k ones within m consecutive trials. Let $\tau_{k,m} = \tau$, and let $\tau + 1$ denote the total number of ones observed until first getting a cluster of k ones within m consecutive trials. Samuel-Cahn applies Wald's lemma, to find for the Bernoulli case

$$E(T_{k,m}) = \{1 + E(\tau_{k,m})\}/p, \tag{13.80}$$

and derives a series of approximations for $E(\tau_{k,m})$. The simplest of these is

$$E_2(\tau_{k,m}) \approx k - 1 + \{1 - P(\tau = k - 1)\}^2 / P(\tau = k), \tag{13.81}$$

where for the Bernoulli case, for $k \geq 3$ and $m \geq k - 1$:

$$P(\tau = k - 1) = p^{k-1} \sum_{j=0}^{m-k+1} \binom{j+k-2}{k-2} (1 - p)^j, \tag{13.82}$$

$$P(\tau = k) = p^{k-2} q^{m-k+2} \left\{ \binom{m-1}{k-2} \right.$$

$$\left. - \sum_{j=0}^{m-k+1} \binom{j+k-3}{k-3} (1 - p)^{m-k-j} \right\}. \tag{13.83}$$

14
Power

14.1 Introduction

Previous chapters have almost exclusively dealt with the distribution of the scan statistics under the hypothesis of uniformity. Here we will discuss the computation of power, which requires obtaining the distribution under other alternatives. Unlike other parts of the book, we will attempt to treat nearly simultaneously the cases previously discussed: unconditional scan, conditional scan, and discrete.

In this chapter, the *intensity* of an event can take on different values over *time*. For the continuous case, time is defined over $[0, T)$ (often $T = 1$). For the conditional case, the "intensity" is expressed in terms of a density $f(t)$, which integrates to 1.0 over $0 \leq t \leq T$.

For the unconditional continuous case, we shift between two descriptors. The simplest, in the context of the rest of the book, is to describe the intensity in terms of

$$e_t = E[Y_t(w)],$$

where $Y_t(w)$ is the number of events in $[t, t + w]$. Alternatively, we can superimpose a Poisson process so that

$$e_t = E[Y_t(w)] = \int_t^{t+w} \lambda(s) \, ds.$$

For the discrete case "time" takes on the integer values $1, \dots, N$ on which the binary random variables $X_1, \dots, X_N$ are defined with $P(X_t = 1) = p(t)$ and $p(t)$ takes on a series of values. For the conditional discrete case, we add the constraint $\sum p(t) = a/N$, where a is specified.

14.1.1 Step Function Alternatives

Under the null hypothesis, the intensity of the events are constant over time. For the conditional continuous case, the times of the N events are distributed according to the uniform distribution

$$f(t) = f_0, \qquad 0 \le t \le T,$$

where $f_0 = 1/T$. For the unconditional case, we either replace $f(t)$ by e_t or replace "f" by "λ", where λ is the intensity of the Poisson process. For the discrete case replace "f" by "p", and replace "$0 \le t \le T$" by "$t = 1, \ldots, N$". In subsequent development we will use ϕ to denote cases in which an equation is applicable to all cases, i.e., one can substitute for ϕ either f; λ or e; or p. The null hypothesis can be stated as

$$\phi(t) = \phi_0. \tag{14.1}$$

Almost all the exact formulas and approximations for power, and much work for the distribution under nonuniform cases, are based on a step function alternative in which, for $i = 1, \ldots, I$:

$$\phi(t) = \phi_i, \qquad t_{i-1} \le t \le t_i, \tag{14.2}$$

where for the continuous case, $t_0 = 0$ and $t_I = T$; while for the discrete case $t_0 = 1$ and $t_I = N$.

(For conditional cases additional constraints are used: for the continuous case, $\sum (t_i - t_{i-1}) f_i = 1$; and for the discrete case, $\sum p(t) = $ a.)

For power, we will frequently focus on the *pulse alternative*, characterized by a starting point b, always unknown, and a width v, often presumed to be equal to w. Specifically, the pulse alternative assumes there is a high intensity on a subinterval of width v, and a lower one elsewhere

$$\phi(t) = \phi_H, \qquad b \le t < b + v,$$
$$= \phi_L, \qquad \text{otherwise.} \tag{14.3}$$

For computational purposes, we will frequently limit attention to the case $b = iw$, i an integer. For the unconditional continuous case, this translates into two Poisson intensities: a (high) one, λ_H on a subinterval of length v; and a lower one λ_L on the rest of the interval. For the discrete case, we have two probabilities of success: a (high) one, p_H, for v consecutive trials; and a lower one, p_L, for all other trials.

For the conditional continuous case, since the densities must integrate to one,

$$f(t) = f_H = \theta/[1 - v + v\theta], \qquad b \le t \le b + v;$$
$$= f_L = 1/[1 - v + v\theta], \qquad \text{otherwise,} \tag{14.4}$$

$\theta > 1$. A subtle difference between the conditional and unconditional cases arises in interpreting the low intensity. For the unconditional case, one sets $\lambda_L = \lambda_0$, while for the conditional case, $f_L < f_0$. (The zero subscript indicates the null hypothesis.)

The power of the test based on the scan statistic is the probability that the scan statistic exceeds the critical value k (which depends on N, w, and α). For the continuous case, the power is given by

$$P(S_w \geq k \mid H_A),$$

where $S_w = \sup_t Y_t(w)$, and H_A is some alternative, often of the form (14.2). For the discrete case, the power is given by

$$P(S_m \geq k \mid H_A),$$

where $S_m = \max Y_t(m)$, and $Y_t(m)$ is the number of successes in trials $[t, t + 1, \ldots, t + m - 1]$.

Naus (1966b) showed that the test that rejects the null hypothesis for large values of the scan statistic is a generalized likelihood ratio test against a special case of (14.4), with $v = w$. The proof of this assertion will be given in Chapter 15, where we will give a slight generalization. For the circle, Cressie (1977b) shows that the scan statistic is a most powerful invariant test for distant alternatives.

As noted, the remainder of this chapter stresses pulse alternatives, which is natural since the scan has optimal properties for such alternatives. Sahu, Bender, and Sison (1993) simulate both pulse (rectangular) and triangular alternatives, which may be a more realistic description of environmental contamination. These results are helpful to obtain a feeling for power, but since the uses of the scan are so broad, generalizations for a particular application are difficult to develop.

These calculations of power have practical applications. For example, Cressie (1977b) concludes that it is better to choose a window size that is (slightly) less than the size of the true pulse than one that is slightly too large.

Cressie (1977a) discusses the distribution of spacings (r-scan statistics in the nomenclature of Chapter 17) and gives (Theorem 3.2) the exact distribution. He also gives, apparently, the only asymptotic result for a pulse alternative in his Theorem 4.1. Cressie's simulation results indicate that some caution is required in applying this asymptotic result, which mirrors the caution we have previously expressed to these results for the distribution under the null.

Fu and Curnow (1990), using a different approach than that used here, find the null and alternative distributions for the discrete scan statistic and relate it to a change point problem. Most of the derivations of results in the remainder of this chapter follow the approach of Wallenstein, Naus, and Glaz (1993, 1994, 1995).

Section 4.2 of this chapter gives, for the investigator interested primarily in applications, a very simple approximation to power whose derivation is the result of successive cruder approximations to be described in this chapter. Section 14.3 gives exact results, similar in spirit to exact results for the distribution of the scan under the null hypothesis. Section 14.4 extends the Markovian Q_2/Q_3 approximation in Naus (1982) previously used in Section 10.6. Section 14.5 gives explicit formulas for the extensions of Q_2/Q_3 required in these applications. Section 14.6 derives the simple approximations previously illustrated in Section 14.2, while Section 14.7 briefly discusses power for other alternatives.

14.2   Very Simple Approximations

The very simplest approximation developed in Section 14.6 indicates that, in all three cases, to detect a θ-fold increase in rates, $\theta \gg 1$, for the pulse alternative in (14.3) with $v = w$, and $w \le b \le T - 2w$:

$$\text{Power} = P_A(S_w \ge k) \approx P_A[Y_b(w) \ge k] + \frac{2P_A[Y_b(w) = k]}{(\theta - 1)}$$
$$- \frac{P_A[Y_b(w) = k + 1]}{\theta^2}, \tag{14.5}$$

where $P_A(E)$ is the probability of the event E under the (pulse) alternative and $Y_b(w)$ is the number of events in the interval of increased *risk*, b to $b + w$. (For the discrete case, m takes on the role of w.)

Specifically, for the conditional continuous case, $Y_b(w) \sim \text{Bin}(N, \theta w/[1 - w + w\theta])$, where θ is the ratio of the two densities, so that setting $\omega = \theta w/[1 - w + w\theta]$:

$$P_A(S_w \ge k \mid w < b < T - w) \approx G_b(k, N, \omega) + \frac{2b(k, N, \omega)}{(\theta - 1)} - \frac{b(k + 1, N, \omega)}{\theta^2}. \tag{14.6}$$

For the unconditional, $Y_b(w) \sim \text{Poisson}(w\theta\lambda_L)$, so that

$$\text{Power} \approx G_p(k, w\theta\lambda_L) + \frac{2p(k, w\theta\lambda_L)}{(\theta - 1)} - \frac{p(k + 1, w\theta\lambda_L)}{\theta^2}. \tag{14.7}$$

For the discrete unconditional case, θ is the odds ratio, and $Y_b(m) \sim \text{Bin}(m, p_H)$, so that

$$\text{Power} \equiv P_A(S'_m \ge k) \approx G_b(k, m, p_H) + \frac{2b(k, m, p_H)}{(\theta - 1)} - \frac{b(k + 1, m, p_H)}{\theta^2}.$$

The documentation of the adequacy of these approximations is based on assuming that α is small, $\theta \gg 1$, and additionally (but less importantly) that w is small or k large. The approximation is for the case $v = w$, i.e., the width of the window is equal to the width of the pulse, and the pulse is not too close to either end. A similar simple approximation, when the pulse is at the end, is given in Section 14.8. We will now illustrate the application of (14.5) for three cases:

14.2.1   Conditional Case

When $N = 80$ and $w = 1/8$, the critical value at $\alpha = .05$ is $k = 21$, since $P(21; 80, 0.125) = .038$. To find power against a pulse alternative with $\theta = 2.5$, we first compute $\omega = \theta w/[1 - w + w\theta] = .263$. Thus since $G_b(21, 80, .263)$ $= .85479$, $b(21, 80, .263) = .1009$, and $G_b(22, 80, .263) = .0966$, the power of detecting a 2.5-fold increase of the risk on an interval of length 1/8 at $\alpha = .05$ is approximately

$$\text{Power} \approx .5479 + 2(0.1009)/1.5 - 0.966/[2.5^2] = .6670.$$

The power based on the much more complicated equation (14.13) is .6671, as is the simulated value.

14.2.2 Unconditional Case

Consider nearly the same case: $w = 1/8$, and under the null

$$E_0[Y_t(1/8)] \equiv e_t = w\lambda_L = 10 \qquad \text{for all } t,$$

while under the alternative of a pulse at $[b, b + w)$ with a 2.5 relative risk

$$E_A[Y_t(1/8)] \equiv e_b = \theta w\lambda_L = 10(2.5) = 25.$$

For this case, the critical value at $\alpha = .05$ is given by $k = 22$. Under the alternative, $Y_b(w)$ has a Poisson distribution with the expected value $\lambda_H = 10(2.5) = 25$. Noting that

$$P_A[Y_b(w) = 22] = p(22, 25) = e^{-25}(22)^{25}/25! = 0.07023,$$

$p(23, 25) = .0766$, and $G_p(22, 25) = 0.7257$, (14.7) yields

$$\text{Power} \approx .7257 + 2(.0702)/1.5 - .0766/2.5^2 = .834.$$

The estimate of power based on 300,000 simulations is .8357.

14.2.3 Discrete

Consider the case $N = 100$, $m = 20$, $p_L = .5$, $p_H = 0.9$. The odds ratio is $\theta = [.5 \times .9]/[.9 \times .1]$. Thus $Y_b(m) \sim \text{Bin}(20, 0.9)$, $G_b(17, 20, .9) = .8670$, $b(17, 20, .9) = .1901$, and $b(18, 20, .9) = .2852$, so that

$$\text{Power} \approx .8670 + 2(.1901)/8 - .2852/9^2 = .911.$$

The exact power is .9122.

14.3 Exact Results

Cressie (1977b) gives exact formulas for power of the conditional test against a pulse alternative, and the result is easily extended to the unconditional case.

His approach is based on the theorem of Karlin and McGregor (1959) which we discussed in detail under exact results in Chapter 8, Section 8.5. We derive the result for the relatively simple case that $w = 1/L$, L an integer, and also, without loss of generality, set $T = 1$. The reader is referred to Cressie (1977a) for the more general case which is an extension of the results of Huntington and Naus (1975) discussed in Chapter 8.

The computation of power is based on the conditional distribution based on cell occupancy numbers $n_1, \ldots, n_L$ where $n_i = Y_{(i-1)w}(w)$. This conditional distribution is thus the same whether one is calculating the distribution under the null, or calculating power. In all cases (equation (8.23)):

$$P(S_w \leq k \mid Y_{(i-1)w}(w) = n_i, i = 1, \ldots, L) = \det |1/c_{ij}!| \prod_{i=1}^{L} n_i!,$$

where the $L \times L$ matrix C is given following (8.22). To find the operating characteristic curve (i.e., either the type I error, or type II error) multiply the conditional probability above by $P(\{n_i\})$, which varies depending on application, and sum over the distribution of $\{n_i\}$ of interest.

We first describe results for the conditional continuous case under the general case of a step function rather than the more restricted case of a pulse alternative, so that

$$f(t) = \tilde{f}_i, \qquad (i-1)w \leq t \leq iw.$$

Then since

$$P\{n_i\} = P\{Y_{(i-1)w}(w) = n_i\} = w^N N! \prod_{i=1}^{L} \frac{\tilde{f}_i^{n_i}}{n_i!}, \qquad (14.8)$$

the type II error is

$$P(S_w < k) = w^N N! \sum_{\{n_1, \ldots, n_L\}} \det |1/c_{ij}!| \prod_{i=1}^{L} \tilde{f}_i^{n_i}, \qquad (14.9)$$

where the summation is over $n_i < k$, with the constraint that $\sum n_i = N$. (This would reduce to (8.22), the probability under the null, if we replaced $\tilde{f}_i$ by 1, so the product disappears.)

Next we restrict ourselves to the pulse alternative where $\tilde{f}_i$ takes on only two values: a high one, f_H, on the interval $[b, b + w)$, and a low one elsewhere. For example, if the pulse were at the start ($b = 0$), and the pulse of width $v = w$:

$$P(S_w < k) = w^N N! \sum_{\{n_1, \ldots, n_L\}} \det |1/c_{ij}!| f_H^{n_1} f_L^{N-n_1}$$

$$= [w/(1 - w + w\theta)]^N N! \sum_{\{n_1, \ldots, n_L\}} \det |1/c_{ij}!| \theta^{n_1}. \quad (14.10)$$

For the unconditional case, we can perform two conditionings: first on the total number of events $\sum n_i$, then to the individual components $\{n_i\}$. The sum $\sum n_i$

has a Poisson distribution and the individual components, conditional on their sum, a multinomial, as in (14.8), with wf_i replaced by $e_i / \sum e_i = e_i / E(N)$. The formulas for power are conceptually similar in the discrete case.

Cressie (1984, p. 95) notes, in the context of the conditional continuous scan, that the type of results presented above are difficult to implement for moderate or large samples, except in specialized cases, because they involve summation over many large determinants.

Fu and Curnow (1990) show that the discrete scan statistic can be derived based on the log likelihood ratio for testing for a changed segment in a series of Bernoulli trials. They use a recurrence relationship to derive the null and alternative distributions. Numerical results are given for segment lengths up to size $m = 20$. Beyond this point, space limitations apparently limit application of the method.

14.4 Markovian Approximations for a Pulse of Width w

Conceptually, it appears possible to apply many of the approximations or, for that matter, the bounds developed for finding the null distribution to power. We will focus on extending the Markov-type approximation of Naus (1982). We begin by considering a special case of (14.2) that the alternative is a step function with (possible) steps at $t_i = (i - 1)w$. In practice, this "special case" is not at all restrictive. In the second part of the section, we will make the more restrictive assumption that $v = w$, i.e., the (unknown) width of the pulse coincides with the window of the scan statistic. This section approximates the power in terms of quantities that are extensions of Q_2 and Q_3 of Chapter 10. Section 14.5 gives formulas for these intermediate terms. Section 14.7 outlines how power can be computed when v differs from w.

14.4.1 Approximation Applied in the General Context

Calculations are simplified for $w = 1/L$, L an integer. Recall that for the continuous case (Chapter 10, Section 10.5), we defined E_i as the event that no interval of length $w = 1/L$, overlapping the ith and $(i + 1)$st intervals, contains k or more points, i.e.,

$$E_i = \left\{ \sup_{(i-1)w \le t \le iw} Y_t(w) < k \right\}. \tag{14.11}$$

For the discrete case,

$$E_i = \left\{ \sup Y_t(m) < k, (i - 1)m \le t \le im \right\}.$$

The Markov-type approximation is based on

$$P(E_j \mid E_1, E_2, \ldots, E_{j-1}) \approx P(E_j \mid E_{j-1})$$

which, as given in (10.24), implies that

$$P\left(\bigcap_i E_i\right) \approx \prod_{i=2}^{L-1} P(E_{i-1} \cap E_i) \bigg/ \prod_{i=2}^{L-2} P(E_i). \qquad (14.12)$$

Thus, approximating the operating characteristic curve requires only computing the simple probability of the E_i's and the two-way intersections. We follow the same steps as in the previous chapter, by first finding the conditional probabilities. For the continuous case, we condition on the number of events in the ith and $(i + 1)$st intervals of length w, whereas for the discrete case we condition on the number of successes in the ith and $(i + 1)$ series of m trials. We let n_i and n_{i+1} be the number of such events. As was the case when we found the exact distribution, the conditional distribution of E_i given n_{i-1} and n_i does not depend on whether we are sampling under the null or alternative hypothesis. These conditional probabilities have all been given previously and all we have to do is multiply them by the probability of various cell occupancy numbers, which are either three-way multinomials or the two- or three-way products of Poisson probabilities, and then sum over the cell occupancy numbers. Specifically,

$$P(E_i) = \sum_{n_i, n_{i+1}} P\big(E_i \mid Y_{(i-1)w} = n_i, Y_{iw} = n_{i+1}\big) P\big(Y_{(i-1)w} = n_i, Y_{iw} = n_{i+1}\big),$$

$$(14.13)$$

with an analogous expression for $P(E_i \cap E_{i+1})$.

Thus the problem is conceptually solved and involves a two-to-three-way summation for $P(E_i)$ and a three-to-four-way summation for $P(E_i \cap E_{i+1})$. However, some further notation is helpful to simplify the expressions and indicate how power varies with the placement of the pulse (as well as the width of the pulse). For $P(E_i)$, there are at most four possibilities of interest depending on whether n_i and n_{i+1} are evaluated under low or high intensities. Let Q_{LH} denote the case that one cell occupancy number, n_i, is evaluated under a low intensity, and the other, n_{i+1}, under a high intensity. Let Q_{LL} denote the probability $P(E_i)$ where both are evaluated under the low density. (For the unconditional case, Q_{LL} is the same as Q_2; however, for the conditional case, the two differ.) Note that we could define Q_{HL} but it is identical to Q_{LH}. Also by analogy, though not of immediate application, Q_{HH} is $P(E_i)$ where both cell occupancy numbers are evaluated under the high density.

Similarly there are at most 2^3 possible values for $P(E_{i-1} \cap E_i)$ depending on whether each cell has a "high" or "low" intensity. For example, Q_{LHL} is the probability where the intensity is low in the first and third cells but high in the second cell.

14.4.2 Power when the Width of the Pulse and Window are Identical

We now recalculate power for the simple pulse alternative in (14.3) when the width of the pulse v is identical to the window of the scan statitic, w. (Power for the more general case is discussed in Section 14.7.) When $w = v$, there are three different possibilities depending on whether the cluster starts at the end of the interval [$b = 0$ or $b = (L-1)w$], very close to the end [$b = w$ or $b = (L-2)w$], or in the middle ($2w \le b \le T - 3w$).

(A) For the case in (14.3) with $b = 0$, $P(E_1) = Q_{HL}$, and for $i > 1$, $P(E_i) = Q_{LL}$. Similarly, $P(E_1 \cap E_2) = Q_{HLL}$ and $P(E_i \cap E_{i+1}) = Q_{LLL}, i > 1$. Substituting these expressions into (14.12) yields:

$$P_A(S_w < k \mid b = 0) \approx Q_{HL}(Q_{HLL}/Q_{HL})(Q_{LLL}/Q_{LL})^{L-3}$$
$$= Q_{HLL}(Q_{LLL}/Q_{LL})^{L-3}. \tag{14.14}$$

(B) For the case in (14.3) with $b = w$, $P(E_1) = Q_{LH}$, $P(E_2) = Q_{HL}$, $P(E_i) = Q_{LL}$ otherwise. Similarly, $P(E_1 \cap E_2) = Q_{LHL}$, $P(E_2 \cap E_3) = Q_{HLL}$), $P(E_i \cap E_{i+1}) = Q_{LLL}$, otherwise. Substituting these expressions into (14.12):

$$P_A(S_w < k \mid b = w) \approx Q_{LH}(Q_{LHL}/Q_{LH})(Q_{HLL}/Q_{HL})(Q_{LLL}/Q_{LL})^{L-4}$$
$$= Q_{LHL}(Q_{HLL}/Q_{HL})(Q_{LLL}/Q_{LL})^{L-4}. \tag{14.15}$$

(C) For the case in (14.3) with $b = 2w$, and by implication for $w < b < T - 3w$, $P(E_1) = Q_{LL}$, $P(E_2) = Q_{LH}$, $P(E_3) = Q_{HL}$, and $P(E_i) = Q_{LL}$ otherwise. For two-way intersections, $P(E_1 \cap E_2) = Q_{LLH}$, $P(E_2 \cap E_3) = Q_{LHL}$, $P(E_3 \cap E_4) = Q_{HLL}$, $P(E_i \cap E_{i+1}) = Q_{LLL}$, otherwise, so that

$$P_A(S_w < k \mid b = 2w) \approx Q_{LL}(Q_{LLH}/Q_{LL})(Q_{LHL}/Q_{LH})$$
$$\times (Q_{HLL}/Q_{HL})(Q_{LLL}/Q_{LL})^{L-5} \tag{14.16}$$
$$= Q_{LHL}(Q_{HLL}/Q_{HL})^2(Q_{LLL}/Q_{LL})^{L-5}.$$

The probabilities required will be given in Section 14.5. Before giving these, we indicate a slight simplification that will enable us to avoid calculating one of the more complicated terms.

14.4.3 A Further Simplification

Heuristically, we would not expect power to vary much if the pulse started at $b = w$ or at $b = 2w$. Fu and Curnow (1990, p. 300) utilize this fact in constructing their tables, and note that numerical results indicate differences, at most, in the third decimal place between a cluster starting at position w, and ones starting at the center. This suggests that the approximations in (14.15) and (14.16) are nearly identical or that

$$Q_{HLL} \approx Q_{LHL}Q_{LH}/Q_{LL}. \qquad (14.17)$$

Applying (14.17) to (14.14)–(14.16) indicates that there are only two approximations for power. For cases where the pulse begins at the end ($b = 0$ or $b = (L-2)w$):

$$P_A(S_w \geq k \mid b = 0) \approx 1 - Q_{LH}(Q_{LLL}/Q_{LL})^{1/w-2}, \qquad (14.18)$$

and for $w < b < T - 2w$:

$$P_A(S_w \geq k \mid w < b < T - w) \approx 1 - Q_{LHL}(Q_{LLL}/Q_{LL})^{1/w-3}. \qquad (14.19)$$

In addition to simplifying the expression, this further approximation obviates the need to calculate the somewhat cumbersome Q_{LLH}.

14.5   Intermediate Calculations: Exact Power when $w/T = 1/2$ or $1/3$

In this section, we evaluate the expressions Q_{LH} and Q_{LHL} needed to approximate power in (14.18) and (14.19).

14.5.1   One-Way Probabilities

14.5.1.1   Continuous Case

As noted in (10.18), for the continuous case (both conditional and unconditional):

$$P(E_1 \mid n_2, n_2) = 1 - \frac{n_1! \, n_2!}{k! \, (n_1 + n_2 - k)!}, \qquad n_1 < k, \, n_2 < k,$$
$$= 0, \qquad\qquad\qquad \text{otherwise.}$$

What varies in the different cases is $P(n_1, n_2)$. For the conditional case, $(n_1, n_2) \sim \text{MULT}(N, \phi, \phi')$, i.e.,

$$P(n_1 = a, n_2 = b) = \binom{N}{a, b}\phi^a \phi'^b (1 - \phi - \phi')^{N-a-b}, \qquad (14.20)$$

where ϕ and ϕ' could each denote either

$$\phi_L = w f_L = w/(1 - w + w\theta)$$

or

$$\phi_H = \theta \phi_L = w f_H = \theta w/(1 - w + w\theta).$$

Combining the two formulas and using the convention $1/x! = 0$ for $x < 0$:

$$Q_{LH} = \sum \sum \left[1 - \frac{a! \, b!}{k! \, (a+b-k)!} \right] \binom{N}{a, b} \phi_L^a \phi_H^b (1 - \phi_L - \phi_H)^{N-a-b},$$

(14.21)

where the summation is over $a < k, b < k$.

Wallenstein, Naus, and Glaz (1993) replace the two-way summation by a one-way summation of cumulative probabilities to find, for the conditional case,

$$Q_{LH} = \sum_{j=0}^{k-1} b(j, N, \phi_H) F_b \left(k - 1, N - j, \frac{\phi_L}{1 - \phi_H} \right) - b(k, N, \phi_H)$$

$$\times \sum_{i=1}^{k-1} \theta^{-i} F_b \left(k - i - 1, N - k, \frac{\phi_L}{1 - \phi_H} \right), \qquad (14.22)$$

where $F_b(j, N, \phi)$ is the cumulative binomial. Q_2 and Q_{LL} can be evaluated in a similar way

$$Q_{LL} = \sum_{j=0}^{k-1} b(j; N, \phi_L) F_b \left(k - 1, N - j, \frac{\phi_L}{1 - \phi_L} \right)$$

$$- b(k; N, \phi_L) \sum_{i=1}^{k-1} F_b \left(k - i - 1, N - k, \frac{\phi_L}{1 - \phi_L} \right), \qquad (14.23)$$

$$Q_2 = \sum_{j=0}^{k-1} b(j; N, w) F_b \left(k - 1, N - j, \frac{w}{1 - w} \right)$$

$$- b(k; N, w) \sum_{i=1}^{k-1} F_b \left(k - i - 1, N - k, \frac{w}{1 - w} \right). \qquad (14.24)$$

For computing Q_{LH} for the unconditional case, the argument is the same except that (14.20) is replaced by

$$P(n_1 = a, n_2 = b) = p(a, w\lambda_L) p(b, w\lambda_H),$$

where $p(i, \phi) = e^{-\phi} \phi^i / i!$.

Arguments, given in more detail in the Appendix of Wallestein, Naus, and Glaz (1993), yield that for the unconditional case

$$Q_{LH} = F_p(k - 1, w\lambda_H) F_p(k - 1, w\lambda_L) - p(k, w\lambda_H) \{ F_p(k - 1, w\lambda_L)$$

$$- \theta^{1-k} \exp(w\lambda_H - w\lambda_L) F_p(k - 1, w\lambda_H) \} / (\theta - 1), \qquad (14.25)$$

where

$$F_p(k - 1, \phi) = \sum_{i=0}^{k-1} p(i, \phi).$$

Q_2 can be viewed as a special case of the above and is given by (11.3).

For the discrete case, $P(E_1)$ is given in Corollary 1 of Naus (1974). As indicated in Wallenstein, Naus, and Glaz (1993):

$$Q_{LH} = F_b(k-1, m, \phi_L) F_b(k-1, m, \phi_H)$$
$$-b(k; m, \phi_H) \sum_{i=1}^{k-1} \theta^{-i} F_b(k-i-1, m, \phi_L), \qquad (14.26)$$

where ϕ_L and ϕ_H are the probabilities of success under the low and under the high intensities, and θ is the odds ratio $\theta = \phi_H(1 - \phi_L)/(1 - \phi_H)\phi_L$. Q_2 can be evaluated by setting $\theta = 1$, and replacing ϕ_H by ϕ_L.

14.5.2 Joint Probabilities

To compute $P(E_i \cap E_{i+1})$, we will condition on the number of events in "cells" $i, i+1, i+2$. Without loss of generality, we can focus on the first three cells.

14.5.2.1 Continuous Case

For the continuous case, the conditional probabilities are given in (9.21) and (10.21). What varies in the different cases is $P(n_1, n_2, n_3)$. For the conditional case, $n_1, n_2, n_3 \sim \text{MULTN}(N, \phi, \phi', \phi'')$ where ϕ and ϕ' and ϕ'' can each denote either ϕ_L or ϕ_H:

$$P(n_1 = a, n_2 = b, n_3 = c) = \binom{N}{a, b, c} \phi^a \phi'^b \phi''^c (1 - \phi - \phi' - \phi'')^{N-a-b-c}.$$
$$(14.27)$$

Multiplying the conditional probability $P(E_1 \cap E_2 \mid n_1, n_2, n_3)$ by the probability in (14.27) and summing, Wallenstein, Naus, and Glaz (1993) show that

$$Q_{LHL} = \sum_{j=0}^{k-1} b(j; N, \phi_H) \sum_{i=0}^{k-1} b\left(i; N-j, \frac{\phi_L}{1-\phi_H}\right)$$
$$\times F_b\left(k-1, N-i-j, \frac{\phi_L}{1-\phi_L-\phi_H}\right)$$
$$-2\sum_{j=0}^{k-1} b(j; N, \phi_L) b\left(k; N-j, \frac{\phi_H}{1-\phi_L}\right) \sum_{i=1}^{k-1} \theta^{-i}$$
$$\times F_b\left(k-i-1, N-k-j, \frac{\phi_L}{1-\phi_L-\phi_H}\right)$$
$$+\sum_{j=1}^{k-1} b(k+j; N, \phi_H)\theta^{-2j} \sum_{i=0}^{k-1-j} b\left(i; N-j-k, \frac{\phi_L}{1-\phi_H}\right)$$

$$\times F_b \left(k - 1 - j, N - j - i - k, \frac{\phi_L}{1 - \phi_L - \phi_H} \right)$$

$$+ \sum_{j=1}^{k-2} \left\{ b(k; N, \phi_L) b \left(k; N - k, \frac{\phi_H}{1 - \phi_L} \right) \theta^{-j} \right.$$

$$- b(k + j; N, \phi_L) b \left(k - j; N - k - j, \frac{\phi_H}{1 - \phi_L} \right) \right\}$$

$$\times \sum_{i=0}^{k-j-2} F_b \left(i, N - 2k, \frac{\phi_L}{1 - \phi_L - \phi_H} \right). \tag{14.28}$$

Q_{LLL} can be evaluated by setting $\theta = 1$ in the above expressions and changing ϕ_H to ϕ_L, while Q_3 can be evaluated by setting $\theta = 1$ and changing ϕ_L to w.

For computing Q_{LHL} for the unconditional case, the argument is the same except that

$$P(n_1 = a, n_2 = b, n_3 = c) = p(a, w\lambda_L) p(b; w\lambda_H) p(c, w\lambda_L),$$

with analogous expressions for other combinations of intensities. The arguments, given in more detail in the Appendix of Wallestein, Naus, and Glaz (1993), yield

$$Q_{LHL} = F_p(k - 1, w\lambda_H) F_p^2(k - 1, w\lambda_L) - 2F_p(k - 1, w\lambda_L) p(k, w\lambda_H)$$

$$\times \left\{ F_p(k - 1, w\lambda_L) - \theta^{1-k} \exp(w\lambda_H - w\lambda_L) F_p(k - 1, w\lambda_H) \right\} / (\theta - 1)$$

$$+ \sum_{j=1}^{k-1} p(k + j, w\lambda_H) \theta^{-2j} F_p^2(k - j - 1, w\lambda_L)$$

$$+ \sum_{j=1}^{k-2} [F_p(k - j - 2, w\lambda_L)(k - j - 1 - w\lambda_L)$$

$$+ w\lambda_L p(k - j - 2, w\lambda_L)][p(k, w\lambda_L) p(k, w\lambda_H) \theta^{-j}$$

$$- p(k + j, w\lambda_L) p(k - j, w\lambda_H)]. \tag{14.29}$$

In this unconditional case, Q_3 and Q_{LLL} are equivalent and can be viewed as special cases of the above when $\theta = 1$, and are explicitly given by (11.4).

For the discrete case, Wallenstein, Naus, and Glaz (1994) have developed an explicit formula for any combination of three different intensities, i.e., $P(E_1 \cap E_2)$ given three arbitrary values for $E(n_i)$, $i = 1, 2,$ and 3. For example, for pulse alternative where the probability of success is high ($p(t) = p_H$) for the middle string of m events, and low ($p(t) = p_L$) elsewhere:

$$Q_{\text{LHL}} = F_b^2(k-1, m, p_{\text{L}}) F_b(k-1, m, p_{\text{H}})$$

$$- 2b(k; m, p_{\text{H}}) F_b(k-1, m, p_{\text{L}}) \sum_{j=1}^{k-1} \theta^{-j} F_b(k-j-1, m, p_{\text{L}})$$

$$+ \sum_{j=1}^{\min(k-1, m-k)} b(k+j; m, p_{\text{H}}) \theta^{-2j} F_b^2(k-j-1, m, p_{\text{L}})$$

$$+ \sum_{j=1}^{k-2} \{b(k; m, p_{\text{L}}) b(k, m, p_{\text{H}}) \theta^{-j} - b(k+j; m, p_{\text{L}})$$

$$\times b(k-j; m, p_{\text{H}})\} \sum_{g=0}^{k-j-2} (k-g-j-1) b(g; m, p_{\text{L}}). \qquad (14.30)$$

14.6 Simple, Somewhat ad hoc Approximation for Power

Equation (14.5) gave an exceedingly simple approximation to power. The previous section gave a rigorous approximation, based on three-to-four-way summations, which does not involve excessive computation, but would require considerable programming time. This section develops an intermediate level formula not requiring any summation. The formal derivation of these approximations is based on assuming that α is small, $\theta \gg 1$, and additionally (but less importantly) that w is small or λ large. The derivation is somewhat similar to that given for the approximation to the type I error as described in Chapter 10, Section 10.7.

We begin by considering the unconditional continuous case, since the conditional continuous case uses a further simplification.

14.6.1 A Very Simple Approximation to Power: Unconditional Case

Using methods similar to that invoked in Section 10.7 of Chapter 10 and, in addition, deleting terms of the forms θ^{-j} for $j > 3$, Wallenstein, Naus, and Glaz (1993) approximate the expressions in (14.22) and (14.29) above by

$$Q_{\text{LH}} \approx F_p(k-1, w\theta\lambda_{\text{L}}) - p(k, w\theta\lambda_{\text{L}})/(\theta-1), \qquad (14.31)$$

$$Q_{\text{LHL}} \approx F_p(k-1, w\theta\lambda_{\text{L}}) - \frac{2p(k, w\theta\lambda_{\text{L}})}{(\theta-1)} + \frac{p(k+1, w\theta\lambda_{\text{L}})}{\theta^2[1 - w\lambda_{\text{H}}/(\theta k + \theta)]} \quad (14.32)$$

An intermediate-level approximation would combine these approximations with those for Q_2 and Q_3 derived prior to (10.31), and substitute results back into (14.18) and (14.19). The resulting expression is fairly straightforward. However, an even simpler approximation to power given in Wallenstein, Naus, and Glaz (1995) sets the ratio $(Q_3/Q_2) = Q_{LLL}/Q_{LL}$ to 1.0 to yield the approximation (14.5).

14.6.2 Conditional Continuous Case

For the unconditional case, we went to the effort of calculating the ratio of Q_3 to Q_2 and raising it to a power, even though the resulting expression was close to 1, and would be bounded by $1 - \alpha$. In the conditional case, the ratio Q_{LLL}/Q_{LL} would be even closer to one than Q_3/Q_2. Thus the power is approximated by $1 - Q_{LHL}$. Using methods similar to those above, Wallenstein, Naus, and Glaz (1993) suggest the approximation for a pulse of width $w = v$ starting at $w \leq t \leq T - w$:

$$P_A(S_w \geq k \mid w < b < T - w) \approx G_b(k, N, \omega) + \frac{2b(k, N, \omega)}{(\theta - 1)} - \frac{b(k+1, N, \omega)}{\theta^2(1 - \varepsilon)},$$
$$(14.33)$$

where, as in (14.6), $\omega = \theta w/[1 - w + w\theta])$ and $\varepsilon = (N - k - 1)w/[\theta(k+2)(1 - \omega)(1 - w + w\theta)]$. Dropping the $1 - \varepsilon$ term yields (14.5).

14.6.3 Power for a Pulse Starting at $b < w$

As noted in (14.18), the formula for a pulse starting at 0 or at $T - w$ ($b = 0$ or $b = T - w$ in (14.3)) is simpler than the case discussed above and only involves Q_{LH}. Simplifying Q_{LH} further yields the cruder somewhat ad hoc approximation analogous to (14.5). Specifically, the power for a pulse at the end of the interval is given by

$$P_A(S_w \geq k \mid b = 0) \approx P_A[Y_b(w) \geq k + 1] + P_A[Y_b(w) = k]/(\theta - 1).$$

Power for the case where the pulse starts at $u, 0 \leq u \leq w$, could be approximated by interpolation

$$P_A(S_w \geq k \mid b = u) \approx w^{-1}[(w - u)P_A(S_w \geq k \mid b = 0)$$
$$+ u P_A(S_w \geq k \mid b = w)].$$

14.6.4 Accuracy of Approximations

Wallenstein, Naus, and Glaz (1993), (1994) indicate that the first series of approximations ((14.8), (14.9)), based on exact values of the Q's in Section 15.4, yields approximations accurate to three–four places for a range of usual values. A fairly extensive evaluation of results appears to suggest three place accuracy, even for the simple approximations in Section 14.6. Lastly, the ultrasimple approximation (14.6), has a larger error, of perhaps .01–.02.

14.7 Power for Other Alternatives

As noted, the Markovian approximation derived in (14.12) is applicable in a general context. In the last few sections, we limited attention to the case where $v = w$, so that the size of the window is equivalent to the width of the pulse. In this section, we calculate power for a single pulse of width $2w$ ($v = 2w$), and then briefly indicate how results can be extended to a window of width Iw. Power for $v = 2w$ would enable the investigator to calculate the power of the test for the case where the investigator mistakenly chooses a scan statistic with a width that is only half of the true pulse. These results were presented by Wallenstein, Naus, and Glaz (1994) for the discrete cases, but are easily extended to the general case.

In analogy to results leading to (14.14)–(14.16), the Markovian approximation, (14.12), for power for the case of $v = 2w$ and $b = 2w$ requires the calculation of one- and two-way probabilities for the events E_i. For this case, $P(E_1) = Q_{LL}$, $P(E_2) = Q_{LH}$, $P(E_3) = Q_{HH}$, $P(E_4) = Q_{HL}$, and $P(E_i) = Q_{LL}$ otherwise. For three-way intersections, $P(E_1 \cap E_2) = Q_{LLH}$, $P(E_2 \cap E_3) = Q_{LHH}$, $P(E_3 \cap E_4) = Q_{HHL}$, $P(E_4 \cap E_5) = Q_{HLL}$, and for $i > 4$, $P(E_i \cap E_{i+1}) = Q_{LLL}$. Thus applying (14.12) yields

$$
\begin{aligned}
P_A(S_w &< k \mid b = 2w, v = 2w) \\
&\approx Q_{LL}(Q_{LLH}/Q_{LH})(Q_{LHH}/Q_{HH})(Q_{HHL}/Q_{HL}) \\
&\quad \times (Q_{HLL}/Q_{LL})/(Q_{LLL}/Q_{LL})^{L-6} \\
&= Q_{LHL}(Q_{HLL}/Q_{HL})^2(Q_{LLL}/Q_{LL})^{L-5}.
\end{aligned}
$$

By construction, these results should hold for any pulse beginning at $2w \le b \le 1 - 3w$.

In general, for a pulse of width $v = Iw$, Wallenstein, Naus, and Glaz (1994) show that for $IW \le b \le T - (I+1)w$:

$$
P(S_w < k \mid v = Iw) \approx Q_{HHL}^2 \left[\frac{Q_{HLL}^2}{Q_{HH}Q_{LH}^2} \right] \left[\frac{Q_{HHH}}{Q_{HH}} \right]^{I-2} \left[\frac{Q_{LLL}}{Q_{LL}} \right]^{L-I-4}.
$$

Aproximation of power would then require Q_{HHL} or its mirror image Q_{LLH}. These probabilities could be calculated as described in Section 14.4.1, requiring a four-fold summation. However, a computationally simpler expression for these terms is available only for the discrete case.

14.8 Practical Implementation of Power: Conditional Case

For conditional tests, calculation of power is associated with a conceptual problem since N, the total number of cases for the continuous case, or a, the total number of successes for the discrete case, is not generally known beforehand.

The investigator prefers to use a conditional, rather than an unconditional test, so that if the null hypothesis is rejected, it is because of a pattern of "clustering" and not due to an error in specifying the expected value of N. In this context, the investigator would stipulate the distribution of N—a Poisson distribution would be a common assumption. The computation of power is much more complicated and would, strictly speaking, involve finding conditional power for each N and then averaging over the distribution. At least a crude approximation to power can be obtained by simply replacing N by the investigator's conjecture of the expected value of N.

15
Testing for Clustering Superimposed on a Nonuniform Density and Related Generalizations of Ballot Problems

15.1 Introduction

The scan statistics presented until now test the null hypothesis of uniformity again a pulse alternative. In this chapter, we modify the scan statistics to detect a cluster superimposed on temporal or seasonal trends. Attention will be focused on the conditional continuous case, but similar procedures could be used for the discrete statistic.

Such trends occur frequently in surveillance; for example, Edmonds and James (1993) note that cardiovascular birth defects increased dramatically in the 1980s and ascribe the trend to either true increases in births, higher survival rates of seriously sick babies with these defects, increased recognition of mild or asymptomatic defects, or technical changes in reporting based on provisional diagnoses.

Suppose that the null hypothesis postulates that events occur in time $[0, T)$ with

$$H_0: E[Y_t(w)] = E_0[Y_t(w)], \qquad 0 \leq t < T, \qquad (15.1)$$

where, for now, we consider $E_0[Y_t(w)]$ to be known. Alternatively, especially for the conditional case, it may be worthwhile to define the null hypothesis via the density

$$H_0: f(t) = f_0(t), \qquad 0 \leq t \leq T, \qquad (15.2)$$

and then generate $E_0[Y_t(w)]$ by

$$E_0[Y_t(w)] = N \int_{s=t}^{t+w} f_0(s)\, ds.$$

The postulated density could be linearly increasing in time or, for detecting clusters of diseases superimposed on a seasonal pattern, be given by a sine curve. We propose to test H_0 against some alternative suggesting of clustering, as will be presented in (15.3) or (15.4).

For the analogous problem for the discrete statistic, the scan statistic is the sum of m consecutive X_i's, and the X_i's are not necessarily identically distributed, or perhaps nonindependent.

There are at least four approaches to this problem. Possibly the most obvious, but the least practical, is a problem in probability: compute the distribution of the usual single critical value scan statistic, even though intuitively it does not even approximate an optimal statistic. Naus (1963) gives some exact results for the distribution of the range under $F(t) = t^2$. David and Kinyon (1983) derive $P(N - 1, N, w)$ and $P(N - 2, N, w)$ for any distribution of interarrival times. Newell (1964) derives asymptotic results for more general random variables. Fu and Lou (1999) use the finite Markov chain embedding approach of Fu and Koutras (1994b), applied in a similar context by Lou (1996), to find the exact distribution of the discrete scan statistic when the observations are not independent and identically distributed (i.i.d.).

The second approach, suggested by Weinstock (1981), used by at least some cancer registries and described in Section 15.2, shrinks or stretches time so that on a revised time scale, the risk is common. The two remaining approaches keep the window fixed but change the critical value. Kulldorff and coworkers find the optimal statistic, given in (15.5), but rely on simulation to find the critical value. The fourth approach, described in Section 15.4, describes a suboptimal but heuristically meaningful statistic that has a simple distribution. Section 15.5 discusses possible approaches to be used when the density under the null must be estimated from the data. Derivations of probabilities related to this work will be given in Section 15.6.

15.2   Weinstock's Approach

Weinstock (1981) modifies the scan statistic to be applicable for time trends by stretching or contracting the window so that it is of variable width $\omega^*(t)$, and always contains w/T percent of the observations. Formally, his statistic is $\max_t Y_t(\omega^*(t))$, where $\omega^*(t)$ is defined by

$$w = \int_{s=t}^{t+\omega^*(t)} f_0(s)\, ds.$$

As can be seen by extending the arguments in Naus (1966b) or in Section 15.2, Weinstock's statistic is a likelihood ratio test for the alternative of a cluster in a stretched window of length $\omega^*(b)$:

$$f(t) = \theta f_0(t)/[1 + (\theta - 1)w], \qquad b \leq t < b + \omega^*(b),$$
$$f(t) = f_0(t)/[1 + (\theta - 1)w], \qquad \text{otherwise}, \qquad (15.3)$$

where $\theta > 1$ and b are unknown. This alternative is not likely to be one that an investigator would specify a priori. In addition, there are often temporal trends, such as effects due to days of the week, that could be balanced out using an m-week window. A variable width window would not allow for such balance. The statistic, however, does have the major advantage of relatively simple calculation of p-values based on the conventional scan statistic, and has been frequently used by disease registries.

15.3 An Optimal Test Statistic

The natural extension of the pulse alternative in (14.3) is that over the interval $[b, b + w)$, unknown b, the density is a θ-fold multiple of that postulated by the null. Integrating $f(t)$ to 1.0 we can formally express this generalized pulse alternative as

$$f(t) = \theta f_0(t), \qquad b \leq t < b + w,$$
$$f(t) = f_0(t)[N - \theta E_0[Y_b(w)]]/[N - E_0[Y_b(w)]], \qquad \text{otherwise}, \qquad (15.4)$$

where b $(0 \leq b \leq T - w)$ and $\theta > 1$ are unknown.

Theorem 15.1. *Let* $0 \leq t_1 \leq t_2 \leq \cdots \leq t_N \leq T$ *be the ordered times of the observations. The generalized likelihood ratio test for testing the null hypothesis in (15.2) against the alternative in (15.4) rejects H_0 for large values of*

$$S = \max_{j=1,\ldots,N} \mathcal{L}\{Y_{t_j}(w), E[Y_{t_j}(w)]\}, \qquad (15.5)$$

$t_j < T - w$, *where*

$$\mathcal{L}[O, E] = O \ln(O/E) + (N - O) \ln[(N - O)/(N - E)], \qquad O > E$$
$$\mathcal{L}[O, E] = 0, \qquad \qquad \text{otherwise.}$$

This statistic, and the proof of the theorem, is implicit in various papers of Kulldorff and coworkers, see, for example, Kulldorff, Martin, and Nagarwalla (1995), except that they consider a more general case involving geographical clustering.

Proof. The generalized likelihood ratio test rejects H_0 for small values of

$$\prod_{i=1}^{N} f_0(t_i) / \max \prod_{i=1}^{N} f(t_i). \qquad (15.6)$$

Use Y_b as an abbreviation for $Y_b(w)$. Since

$$\prod_{i=1}^{N} f(t_i) = g(b, \theta) \prod_{i=1}^{N} f_0(t_i),$$

where

$$g(b, \theta) = \theta^{Y_b}\{[N - \theta E_0(Y_b)]/[N - E_0(Y_b)]\}^{N - Y_b},$$

the expression in (15.6) is maximized by finding estimates of b and θ that maximize $g(b, \theta)$. Setting $\gamma(\theta, b) = \theta Y_b/N$:

$$\max_{b,\theta} g(b, \theta) = N^N \max_{b}\{[E_0(Y_b)^{Y_b}(N - E_0(Y_b))^{N - Y_b}]^{-1}$$

$$\times \max_{\theta} \gamma(\theta, b)^{Y_b}[1 - \gamma(\theta, b)]^{N - Y_b}\}.$$

As noted by Naus (1966b), the maximization over θ occurs for $\gamma(\theta, b) = Y_b/N$, so that

$$\max_{b,\theta} g(b, \theta) = N^N \max_{b}[Y_b/E_0(Y_b)]^{Y_b(w)}\{[(N - Y_b(w))]/[N - E_0(Y_b)]\}^{N - Y_b}$$

$$= N^N \max_{t} \exp[\mathcal{L}(Y_t(w), E_0(Y_b(w)))],$$

and therefore the theorem is proven that the generalized likelihood ratio test rejects H_0 for large values of the statistic S in (15.5).

To make S look more like a scan statistic, we can express it as follows: Fix α, and let L_α be the critical value for S, so that under H_0:

$$P\left[\max_{0 \le t \le T} \mathcal{L}(Y_t(w), E_0(Y_b(w)) < L_\alpha\right] = \alpha. \tag{15.7}$$

Then, we reject H_0 if for any $0 \le t \le T$:

$$Y_t(w) \ge k_\alpha(t),$$

where $k_\alpha(t)$ is the smallest integer so that

$$\mathcal{L}(k_\alpha(t), E[Y_t(w)]) \le L_\alpha. \tag{15.8}$$

The probability problem is thus to evaluate

$$P_{f(t)}[Y_t(w) < k_\alpha(t), \ 0 \le t \le T], \tag{15.9}$$

where $k_\alpha(t)$ is a known function based on (15.8) that would produce a level-α test for the optimal test statistic, and $P_{f(t)}\{F\}$ denotes the probability of F evaluated under the density $f(t)$.

We know of no way to evaluate $P(S \le s)$ in the general case, especially for the continuous case.

Kulldorff, Martin, and Nagarwalla (1995) evaluate the p-value based on simulation. To implement such a procedure, one would generate a set of N random variables, $t_1, t_2, \ldots, t_N$, under H_0, calculate $\mathcal{L}\big(Y_{t_j}(w), E[Y_t(w)]\big)$ for $j = 1, \ldots, N$, and find the maximum. (The upper value of j would have to be constrained by $t_j + w < T$.) The procedure is repeated M times, M fairly large, and we take as our estimate of the p-value, the percentage of the M trials in which this maximum is greater than or equal to s', where s' is the maximum value under (15.4).

Wallenstein (1999) evaluates $P(S \leq s)$ exactly when $f(t)$ and $k(t)$ are both step functions with jumps at $w, 2w, \ldots, Lw$. Below we approximate this probability using a corollary to this result, together with a generalization of the approximation of Naus (1982).

15.3.1 Derivation of Approximate Significance Level

To derive an approximation for the probability in (15.9), we will assume for simplicity that $T/w = L$ is an integer, but the approximation should be applicable with minor modification for the arbitrary case. The derivation of the approximation will assume that $E[Y_t(w)]$ will increase slowly over two to three consecutive intervals, each of width w.

Extending the definition of E_i and of Q_2 and Q_3 given in previous chapters, e.g., (9.2), let

$$E_i = \{Y_t(w) < k_\alpha(t),\ (i-1)w \leq t < iw\}. \tag{15.10}$$

Applying the Markovian approximation of Naus (1982, Chapter 9):

$$P[Y_t(w) < k_\alpha(t),\ 0 \leq t \leq T] = P\left(\bigcap_{i=1,2,\ldots,L-1} E_i\right)$$
$$= P(E_1)P(E_2 \mid E_1)P(E_3 \mid E_2 \cap E_1)$$
$$\ldots P(E_{L-1} \mid E_{L-2} \cap E_{L-3} \cap \cdots \cap E_1)$$
$$\approx P(E_1)P(E_2 \mid E_1)P(E_3 \mid E_2)P(E_{L-1} \mid E_{L-2}). \tag{15.11}$$

The probabilities $P(E_i \mid E_{i-1})$ (involving $P(E_i)$ and $P(E_i \cap E_{i-1})$) are much simpler than $P[Y_t(w) < k(t),\ 0 \leq t \leq T]$, but analytic results for these probabilities are still elusive if we use (15.8) to consider rejection regions since, among other problems:

(i) it is conceivable that at different points in the interval, $(i-1)w \leq t \leq iw$, different critical values would be used; and

(ii) nearly all known formulas for $P(E_i)$ and $P(E_i \cap E_{i-1})$ assume at least a step-function for the underlying density.

We will approximate $P(E_i)$ and $P(E_i \cap E_{i-1})$ under an arbitrary density with the probability under a step function SF where $P_{\mathrm{SF}}\{E\}$ denotes the probability of the arbitrary event E when the density is a step function with values $f(t) = \tilde{f}_i$ for $(i - 1)w \leq t < iw$. (We defer, for now, selecting the best step function.) We will also assume that w is sufficiently small so we can replace the probability of exceeding a variable critical value that depends on a variable density, with a probability of exceeding a constant critical value given a step function density.

Thus formally, for $i = 1, \ldots, L$, we set k_i to be the critical value at the midpoint

$$k_i = k_\alpha((i - 0.5)w).$$

We then propose to approximate

$$P_{f(t)}(E_i) = P_{f(t)}[Y_t(w) < k_\alpha(t), \ (i - 1)w \leq t < iw]$$

by

$$Q_2(i) = P_{SF}\{Y_t(w) < k_i, \ (i - 1)w \leq t < iw\}, \qquad (15.12)$$

and similarly to replace

$$P_{f(t)}(E_i \cap E_{i+1}) = P_{f(t)}[Y_t(w) < k_\alpha(t), \ (i - 1)w \leq t < (i + 1)w]$$

by

$$Q_3(i) = P_{SF}\{[Y_t(w) < k_i, \ (i - 1)w \leq t < iw]$$
$$\cap [Y_t(w) < k_{i+1}, \ iw \leq t < (i + 1)w]\}. \qquad (15.13)$$

Substituting these expressions into (15.11), we propose to approximate the distribution of the generalized scan statistic by

$$P[Y_t(w) < k_\alpha(t), \ 0 \leq t \leq T] \approx Q_2(1) \frac{Q_3(1)Q_3(2)Q_3(3)}{Q_2(1)Q_2(2)Q_2(3)} \cdots \frac{Q_3(L - 1)}{Q_2(L - 1)}.$$
$$(15.14)$$

Computing $Q_2(i)$ requires some minor modification of the similar expressions given in Chapters 9 and 10, and $Q_3(i)$ requires some new methodological development. The extension of the generalized ballot problem yielding $Q_3(i)$ is given in Section 15.6 below, and values of $Q_2(i)$ and $Q_3(i)$ are given in (15.22) and (15.23), respectively, for the conditional case. The values for the unconditional case are derived similarly.

Thus, in summary, to use this approximation to evaluate the probabilities in (15.9), we first replace the arbitrary density by a step function taking L steps in such a way that π_i, the probability of an event being in $(i - 1)w \leq t < iw$, is unchanged. Next, solve for $i = 1, \ldots, L$ the equation

$$\mathcal{L}(k_i, N\pi_i) \leq s', \qquad (15.15)$$

where s' is the value of the statistic based on the optimal test in (15.5), i.e., k_i is the largest integer so that the above equation holds. Then compute $Q_2(i)$ and

$Q_3(i)$ based on these values of k_i by the results in Section 15.6, and substitute into (15.14) to calculate the approximate p-value.

By construction, we conjecture that this approximation is applicable if $E[Y_t(w)]$ is not too rapidly increasing, perhaps for $E[Y_{(i+1)w}(w)] - E[Y_{iw}(w)] < 1.5$. In the next section, we present an approximation that, based on construction, would require that the density be even more slowly increasing, perhaps $E[Y_{i+1)w}(w)] - E[Y_{(i-1)w}(w)] < 0.5$. On the other hand, we have made two different assumptions that may cancel each other out, even when $E[Y_t(w)]$ is more rapidly increasing than above.

There is some ambiguity due to discreteness. One could argue that a better solution is to set k_i to be the smallest integer so that $\mathcal{L}(k_i, N\pi_i) \geq s'$; or that getting both p-values and taking the average would be best.

15.4   A Reasonable, but Nonoptimal Statistic

When $w \ll t$, that is, the window size is small relative to the whole period (say a window of a week within a year), and where variation in base rates over the year due to seasonality or trends changes gradually relative to the window size, the following nonoptimal, but hopefully close to optimal, test statistic is suggested:

At each point in time, t, observe the number of cases, $Y_t(w)$, that have occurred in $(t, t + w)$. At each observation, compute the observed significance level of $Y_t(w)$ using the appropriate conditional or unconditional scan probability, assuming that the rate in the interval of interest would hold over the entire range. Specifically, reject H_0 in the unconditional case, if for any t:

$$P^*(Y_t(w), TE[Y_t(w)]/w, w/T) \leq \alpha, \tag{15.16}$$

and reject H_0 in the conditional case if for any t:

$$P(Y_t(w), TE[Y_t(w)]/w, w/T) \geq \alpha.$$

We will now indicate, in a somewhat ad hoc manner, that the test described in (15.16) has approximate size α.

15.4.1   Proof of Approximation

To approximate the distribution of the statistic defined via (15.16), we assume that $E[Y_w(t)]$ is very slowly changing so that for $i = 1, \ldots, L$:

$$P(E_i) \approx Q_2(i) \approx \tilde{Q}_2(i)$$

and

$$P(E_i \cap E_{i+1}) \approx Q_3(i) \approx \tilde{Q}_3(i),$$

where $\widetilde{Q_2}(i)$ and $\widetilde{Q}_3(i)$ are similar to $Q_3(i)$ and $Q_2(i)$ defined in (15.12) and (15.13), but differ in that they are evaluated under a constant density, and constant critical value. Specifically,

$$\widetilde{Q}_2(i) = P_0[Y_t(w) < k_i, \ (i-1)w \le t < iw].$$

The subscript zero indicates that this expression differs from $Q_2(i)$ in that it is evaluated under a constant density with $f(t) = w(\pi_i + \pi_{i+1})/2$ for $(i-1) \le t < (i+1)w$. Similarly,

$$\widetilde{Q}_3(i) = P_0[Y_t(w) < k_i, \ (i-1)w \le t < (i+1)w],$$

where the subscript zero indicates that this expression is evaluated under a constant density with $f(t) = w(\pi_i + \pi_{i+1} + \pi_{i+2})/3$ for $(i-1) \le t \le (i+2)w$.

In these expressions, we choose $k_1, k_2, \ldots, k_{L-1}$ to be the critical value for the nonoptimal test, i.e., the smallest integer values satisfying (15.16). Thus the approximation in (15.14) becomes

$$P[Y_t(w) < k_\alpha(t), \ 0 \le t \le T] \approx \widetilde{Q}_2(1) \frac{\widetilde{Q}_3(1)\widetilde{Q}_3(2)\widetilde{Q}_3(3)}{\widetilde{Q}_2(1)\widetilde{Q}_2(2)\widetilde{Q}_2(3)} \cdots \frac{\widetilde{Q}_3(L-2)}{\widetilde{Q}_2(L-2)}. \tag{15.17}$$

On the other hand, by the Markovian approximation in Chapter 9, if k_i is the critical value for the test in (15.16):

$$1 - \alpha = 1 - P(k_i, \ TE[Y_{t_i}(w)]/w, \ w/T) \approx \widetilde{Q}_2(i)\big[\widetilde{Q}_3(i)/\widetilde{Q}_2(i)\big]^{L-2},$$

so that

$$\widetilde{Q}_3(i)/\widetilde{Q}_2(i) \approx \big[(1-\alpha)/\widetilde{Q}_2(i)\big]^{1/L-2}. \tag{15.18}$$

Substituting (15.18) into (15.17) indicates that when $k_\alpha(t)$ is a step function with values $k_1, k_2, \ldots, k_{L-1}$ constructed to satisfy (15.16):

$$P[Y_t(w) < k_\alpha(t), \ 0 \le t \le T] \approx (1-\alpha)\delta,$$

where $\delta = \widetilde{Q}_2(1)/\big\{\widetilde{Q}_2(1)\widetilde{Q}_2(2)\ldots\widetilde{Q}_2(L-2)\big\}^{1/L-2}$, which we might approximate as

$$\delta \approx \widetilde{Q}_2(1)/\text{median}_i \, \widetilde{Q}_2(i).$$

Since for applied problems (L large, α small) these $\widetilde{Q}_2(i)$'s are all extremely close to one, setting $\delta = 1$ will not introduce much error and will complete the proof that the approximate size of the test based on (15.16) is about α.

Thus, in summary, to simply approximate the p-value for the nonoptimal test, find the most noteworthy cluster using

$$p = \min_{0 \le t \le T} P(Y_t(w), \ TE[Y_t(w)]/w, \ w/T),$$

where any of the approximations in Chapter 10 is used.

As noted above, the primary purpose for suggesting this test is the simplicity of getting the p-value. Alternatively, with much more computation, we could view this procedure as a way to generate a test with nominal value α, but with actual value that could be more accurately approximated using the methods in the previous section, and basing the approximation on the presumably more accurate (15.14), rather than (15.17).

15.5 Practical Implementation: Estimating $f_0(t)$

Often, $f_0(t)$ or $E_0[Y_t(w)]$ will not be known. In some scenarios, a known proxy variable exists, and the lack of knowledge concerning $f_0(t)$ will not be a major problem. For example, $Y_t(w)$ could indicate birth defects in $[t, t + w)$ and we could assume that the density is proportional to the number of births in $[t, t + w)$, which could be available from vital statistical data.

In other cases, it would be required to estimate the density from available data. We will have to assume some smooth function for $f_0(t)$, with unknown parameters, for example, a trigonometric model for seasonality or a monotone increasing trend for time. We would then use the observed data to estimate the parameters. In other applications, the expected number of events in a small time interval can be predicted by a multiple regression. For example, monthly admissions to emergency rooms for asthma could be modeled by including maximum temperature in the month, air quality, and related variables, and indicator variables for the month and year.

The simplest suggestion in the nonideal case is to estimate the density under H_0 and then proceed as above, replacing the unknown parameters by their estimates. However, it could be argued that the fitting might decrease the power since outlying points are influential observations. For example, if we used standard regression and if the pulse were at the upper end of the interval, the fitted regression line would gravitate toward the pulse. The problem of influential observations is not as great here as in some other contexts since the observations are at least regularly spaced.

Nevertheless, the best solution to the problem is apparently an unsolved problem: Suppose there is an unknown density function with a specified form, and we superimpose on it a pulse of width w. Find the optimal estimate of the underlying density that is unbiased, or at least yields consistent estimates of the parameters of the underlying density under both H_0 and H_a.

In the absence of theoretical work available for this purpose, one can attempt to minimize the possible problem of diminished power by using methods of estimating under H_0 that are less sensitive to outliers, or by specifically constructing somewhat ad hoc estimates that are consistent. We discuss this for the linear case below.

15.5.1 Linearly Changing Density

We will assume that the density is linear:

$$f_0(t) = a + bt, \qquad 0 \le t < T.$$

Since the density integrates to 1, $a = 1/T - bT/2$, and we would actually fit the equation with a single parameter

$$f_0(t) = T^{-1} + b(t - T/2).$$

In this case, $E[Y_t(w)]$ is also linearly increasing:

$$E[Y_t(w)] = N(aw + bw^2/2) + Nbwt, \qquad (15.19)$$

or, equivalently, $E[Y_t(w)] = \alpha + \beta t$, where $\beta = Nbw$ and $\alpha = Nw/T - 0.5\beta(T - w)$.

Thus, estimation involves a single parameter, a fact that will be very useful in constructing estimates insensitive to a pulse. In particular, if we wanted to minimize the possible bias, and w were very small, we could delete two intervals of width w which were most influential in each direction: whose deletions are associated with the largest and smallest values. Given that one is constraining on N, there is reason to believe, especially at points not near an end, that the expected values are somewhat insensitive to the method of estimation.

Note that (15.19) is not a conventional model for count data, and that the more conventional model uses the log link, $\log E[Y_t(w)] = \alpha + \beta t$. For our model, one must check, after the preliminary fit, that the density is never negative.

15.6   Exact Distribution of a Statistic with Critical Values Changing on Each Interval of Length w

In this section, we find $P_{f(t)}[Y_t(w) < k(t), 0 \le t < T - w]$ when the functions f and k are constant over intervals of widths w, so that for $(i - 1)w \le t < iw$:

$$f(t) = \tilde{f}_i, \quad i = 1, \dots, L, \qquad k(t) = k_i, \quad i = 1, \dots, L - 1.$$

Thus there are $L = T/w$ cells, each of width w, on which the density is constant. For simplicity of notation, especially in the sequel, let, for $i = 1, \dots, L$, $n_i = Y_{(i-1)w}(w)$ (the number of events in each cell), and let π_i denote the probability that an observation is in $[(i - 1)w, iw)$ so that

$$(n_1, n_2, \dots, n_L) \sim \text{Mult}(N; \pi_1, \pi_2, \dots, \pi_L),$$

where $\sum \pi_i = 1$. (Note that $\pi_i = w\tilde{f}_i$.)

Under these conditions

$$P_{f(t)}[Y_t(w) < k(t), \text{ all } 0 \le t < T - w] = P_{SF}\left(\bigcap_{i=1,\ldots,L-1} E_i\right)$$

$$= P_{SF}\left[\bigcap_{i=1,\ldots,L-1}\left\{\sup_{0 \le s \le w} Y_{(i-1)w+s}(w) < k_i\right\}\right],$$

where SF indicates a step function. Wallenstein (1999) proves the following theorem:

Theorem 15.2. *Let G be a square matrix with L rows, and elements* $1/g_{ij}!$ *where*

$$g_{ij} = k_i + \sum_{u=i+1}^{j-1}(k_u - n_u), \qquad i < j - 1,$$

$$= k_i, \qquad\qquad\qquad i = j - 1,$$

$$= n_i, \qquad\qquad\qquad i = j,$$

$$= n_i + \sum_{u=j}^{i-1}(n_u - k_u), \qquad i > j, \qquad\qquad (15.20)$$

where $1/x! = 0$ *if* $x < 0$. *Then*

$$P_{SF}\left[\bigcap_{i=1,\ldots,L-1}\left\{\sup_{0 \le s \le w} Y_{(i-1)w+s}(w) < k_i\right\}\right] = N! \sum_{v_L(N)} \det G \prod_{i=1}^{L} \pi_i^{n_i},$$

$$(15.21)$$

where $v_L(N)$ *is the set of* $\{n_1, \ldots, n_L\}$ *such that* $\sum_{i=1}^{L} n_i = N$ *and* $n_i < \min(k_i, k_{i-1})$, $i = 1, \ldots, L$. *(For consistency, set* $k_0 = k_1, k_L = k_{L-1}$*).*

The proof of the theorem given in Wallenstein (1999) is an extension of the proof required for the case when there is a single critical value, and is based on the same ballot problem solved by Karlin and McGregor (1959) that was cited in Chapter 8.

Corollary 15.1 (Conditional Case).

$$Q_2(i) = P_{SF}(E_i) = N! \sum_{n_i} \sum_{n_{i+1}}\left[\frac{1}{n_i!\, n_{i+1}!} - \frac{1}{k_i!\,(n_i + n_{i+1} - k_i)!}\right]$$

$$\times \frac{(1 - \pi_i - \pi_{i+1})^{N-M}}{(N - M)!}\pi_i^{n_i}\pi_{i+1}^{n_{i+1}}, \qquad (15.22)$$

where $M = n_i + n_{i+1}$, *and the pair of summations is over* $0 \le n_i, n_{i+1} < k$, $n_i + n_{i+1} \le N$. *Similarly, set*

$$G(3) = \begin{pmatrix} 1/n_i! & 1/k_i! & 1/(k_i + k_{i+1} - n_{i+1})! \\ 1/(n_i + n_{i+1} - k_i)! & 1/n_{i+1}! & 1/k_{i+1}! \\ 1/(M - k_i - k_{i+1})! & 1/(n_{i+1} + n_{i+2} - k_{i+1})! & 1/n_{i+2}! \end{pmatrix}$$

where $1/x! = 0$ if $x < 0$ and $M = n_i + n_{i+1} + n_{i+2}$. Then

$$Q_3(i) = P_{SF}(E_i \cap E_{i+1})N! \sum_{n_i} \sum_{n_{i+1}} \sum_{n_{i+2}} \det G(3)$$

$$\times \frac{(1 - \pi_i - \pi_{i+1} - \pi_{i+2}))^{N-M}}{(N-M)!} \pi_i^{n_i} \pi_{i+1}^{n_{i+1}} \pi_{i+2}^{n_{i+2}}, \qquad (15.23)$$

where, for $j = i, i+1, i+2$, the summations are over $0 \le n_j < k_j$, and where $n_i + n_{i+1} + n_{i+2} \le N$.

16
Two-Dimensional Scan Statistics

16.1 A Discrete Scan Statistic

Let $[0, T_1] \times [0, T_2]$ be a rectangular region. Let $h_i = T_i/N_i > 0$, where N_i are positive integers, $i = 1, 2$. In many applications the exact locations of the observed events in the rectangular region are unknown. What is usually available are the counts in small rectangular subregions. For $1 \leq i \leq N_1$ and $1 \leq j \leq N_2$, let X_{ij} be the number of events that have been observed in the rectangular subregion $[(i - 1)h_1, ih_1] \times [(j - 1)h_2, jh_2]$. We are interested in detecting unusual clustering of these events under the null hypothesis that X_{ij} are independent and identically distributed (i.i.d.) nonnegative integer valued random variables from a specified distribution. For $1 \leq i_1 \leq N_1 - m_1 + 1$ and $1 \leq i_2 \leq N_2 - m_2 + 1$ define

$$Y_{i_1,i_2} = \sum_{j=i_2}^{i_2+m_2-1} \sum_{j=i_1}^{i_1+m_1-1} X_{ij} \qquad (16.1)$$

to be the number of events in a rectangular region comprised of $m_1 \times m_2$ adjacent rectangular subregions with area $h_1 h_2$ and the southwest corner located at the point $((i_i - 1)/h_1, (i_2 - 1)h_2)$. If Y_{i_1,i_2} exceeds a preassigned value of k, we will say that k events are clustered within the inspected region. We define a *two-dimensional discrete scan statistic* as the largest number of events in any $m_1 \times m_2$ adjacent rectangular subregions with area $h_1 h_2$ and the southwest corner located at the point $((i_1 - 1)h_1, (i_2 - 1)h_2)$:

$$S'_{m_1,m_2} = \max\{Y_{i_1,i_2}; 1 \leq i_1 \leq N_1 - m_1 + 1, 1 \leq i_2 \leq N_2 - m_2 + 1\}. \quad (16.2)$$

S'_{m_1,m_2} can be viewed as an extension of the one-dimensional discrete scan statistic discussed in Chapter 13. We are interested in evaluating $P(S'_{m_1,m_2} \geq k)$.

A special interesting case is when X_{ij} are i.i.d. Bernoulli random variables and $k = m_1 m_2$. In this case we are evaluating the probability that an $m_1 \times m_2$ rectangular grid has all ones. This extends the notion of a run of ones to two dimensions. Approximations, and inequalities for $P(S'_{m_1,m_2} = m_1 m_2)$ presented below are based on Sheng and Naus (1996). Earlier work on this problem includes: Darling and Waterman (1985, 1986) and Nemetz and Kusolitsch (1982).

S'_{m_1,m_2} is used for testing the null hypothesis of randomness that assumes the X_{ij}'s are i.i.d. binomial random variables with parameters n_0 and $0 < p_0 < 1$ or i.i.d. Poisson random variables with mean $\theta_0 > 0$, respectively. For the alternative hypothesis of clustering we specify a rectangular subregion

$$R(i_1, i_2) = [(i_1 - 1)h_1, (i_1 + m_1 - 1)h_1] \times [(i_2 - 1)h_2, (i_2 + m_2 - 1)h_2]$$

such that for any $i_1 \leq i \leq i_1 + m_1 - 1$ and $i_2 \leq j \leq i_2 + m_2 - 1$, X_{ij} has a binomial distribution with parameters n_0 and p_1, where $p_1 > p_0$ or a Poisson distribution with mean θ_1 where $\theta_1 > \theta_0$, respectively. For $(i, j) \notin [i_1, i_1 + m_1 - 1] \times [i_2, i_2 + m_2 - 1]$, X_{ij} is distributed according to the distribution specified by the null hypothesis. It is routine to verify that the generalized likelihood ratio test rejects the null hypothesis in favor of the alternative hypothesis whenever S'_{m_1,m_2} exceeds the value k, where k is determined from a specified significance level of the testing procedure. To implement this two-dimensional scan statistic, accurate approximations for $P(S'_{m_1,m_2} \geq k)$ are needed. There are no exact results available for $P(S'_{m_1,m_2} \geq k)$.

The use of S'_{m_1,m_2} for testing the null hypothesis of randomness specified above is of interest in following areas of applications: astronomy (Darling and Waterman (1986)), computer science (Pfaltz (1983)), ecology (Cressie (1991) and Koen (1991)), epidemiology (Cressie (1991) and Kulldorff (1999)), image analysis (Rosenfeld (1978)), pattern recognition (Panayirci and Dubes (1983)), and minefield detection via remote sensing (Glaz (1996)).

Another area of applications where approximations for $P(S'_{m_1,m_2} \geq k)$ are of interest is reliability theory. Consider a system of $N_1 N_2$ components arranged on a rectangular grid of size $N_1 \times N_2$. This system fails if and only if there exists at least one rectangular subregion of the entire system of size $m_1 \times m_2$ with k or more failed components. In the reliability theory literature this system is referred to as a *two-dimensional k-within-consecutive-$m_1 \times m_2$-out-of-$N_1 \times N_2$ F: system* (Barbour, Chryssaphinou, and Roos (1996), Boutsikas and Koutras (2000), Fu and Koutras (1994a), Koutras, Papadopoulos, and Papastavridis (1993), Malinowski and Preuss (1996), Salvia and Lasher (1990), Yamamoto and Miyakawa (1995), and Zuo (1993)). For $1 \leq i \leq N_1$ and $1 \leq j \leq N_2$, let $X_{ij} = 1$ if the ijth component is functioning and $X_{ij} = 0$ if the ijth component has failed. Assume that $P(X_{ij} = 1) = p_{ij}$ and $P(X_{ij} = 1) = 1 - p_{ij}$, where $0 < p_{ij} < 1$. For the special case of identical components $p_{ij} = p$. If X_{ij} are independent random variables, $P(S'_{m_1,m_2} \leq k - 1)$ is the reliability of a *two-dimensional k-within-consecutive-$m_1 \times m_2$-out-of-$N_1 \times F_2$ F: system.*

16.1.1 Approximations and Inequalities for $P(S'_{m_1,m_2} = m_1 m_2)$ for i.i.d. Bernoulli Trials

Let $X_{i,j}$ be i.i.d. Bernoulli random variables, with $P(X_{i,j} = 1) = p = 1 - P(X_{i,j} = 0), 0 < p < 1$. Then,

$$P(m_1, m_2 \mid N_1, N_2) = P(S'_{m_1,m_2} = m_1 m_2)$$

$$= P\left\{ \bigcup_{i_1=1}^{N_1-m_1+1} \bigcup_{i_2=1}^{N_2-m_2+1} \left[\bigcap_{i=i_1}^{i_1+m_1-1} \bigcap_{j=i_2}^{i_2+m_2-1} (X_{i,j} = 1) \right] \right\}$$

$$= P\left\{ \bigcup_{i_1=1}^{N_1-m_1+1} \bigcup_{i_2=1}^{N_2-m_2+1} (Y_{i_1,i_2} = m_1 m_2) \right\}, \qquad (16.3)$$

where Y_{i_1,i_2} is defined in (16.1). Denote by

$$Q(m_1, m_2 \mid N_1, N_2) = 1 - P(m_1, m_2 \mid N_1, N_2).$$

For $1 \le i_1 \le N_1 - m_1 + 1$, let

$$E_{i_1} = \left(\bigcap_{i_2=1}^{N_2-m_2+1} (Y_{i_1,i_2} < m_1 m_2) \right).$$

The product-type approximations in Sheng and Naus (1996) are based on the representation

$$Q(m_1, m_2 \mid N_1, N_2) = P\left(\bigcap_{i_1=1}^{N_1-m_1+1} E_{i_1} \right)$$

$$= P\left(\bigcap_{i_1=1}^{r} E_{i_1} \right) \prod_{j=r+1}^{N_1-m_1+1} \left[\frac{P(\bigcap_{i_1=1}^{j} E_{i_1})}{P(\bigcap_{i=1}^{j-1} E_{i_1})} \right], \qquad (16.4)$$

the stationarity of E_{i_1}'s and a *Markov-like* approximation of order $r, r = 1, 2$, for the terms in (16.4):

$$\frac{P(\bigcap_{i_1=1}^{j} E_{i_1})}{P(\bigcap_{i_1=1}^{j-1} E_{i_1})} \approx \frac{P(\bigcap_{i_1=j-r}^{j} E_{i_1})}{P(\bigcap_{i_1=j-r}^{j-1} E_{i_1})} = \frac{P(\bigcap_{i_1=1}^{r+1} E_{i_1})}{P(\bigcap_{i_1=1}^{r} E_{i_1})}, \qquad (16.5)$$

for $r + 1 \le j \le N_1 - m_1 + 1$. Substituting (16.5) into (16.4) yields the product approximations

$$P(m_1, m_2 \mid N_1, N_2) \approx 1 - P(E_1 \cap E_2) \left[\frac{P(E_1 \cap E_2)}{P(E_1)} \right]^{N_1-m_1-1}, \qquad (16.6)$$

for $r = 1$, and

$$P(m_1, m_2 \mid N_1, N_2) \approx 1 - P(E_1 \cap E_2 \cap E_3) \left[\frac{P(E_1 \cap E_2 \cap E_3)}{P(E_1 \cap E_2)} \right]^{N_1-m_1-2}, \qquad (16.7)$$

for $r = 2$.

The Bonferroni-type upper bounds for $P(m_1, m_2 \mid N_1, N_2)$ are obtained from (7.10) for $r = 1, 2$:

$$P(m_1, m_2 \mid N_1, N_2) \le 1 - (N_1 - m_1 - r + 1) P \left(\bigcap_{i=1}^{r+1} E_i \right)$$

$$+ (N_1 - m_1 - r) P \left(\bigcap_{i=1}^{r} E_i \right). \tag{16.8}$$

To evaluate the approximations and inequalities for $P(m_1, m_2 \mid N_1, N_2)$, Sheng and Naus (1996) derive recursive formulas for $P(\bigcap_{i=1}^{r} E_i)$, $i = 1, 2, 3$. We present here the formulas for $P(E_1)$ and $P(E_1 \cap E_2)$. The formula for $P(E_1 \cap E_2 \cap E_3)$ is lengthy and approximation (16.6) and inequality (16.8) for $r = 1$ is quite accurate.

To evaluate $P(E_1) = P(m_1, m_2 \mid m_1, N_2)$, let $\mathbf{X}_j$ denote an $m_1 \times 1$ column vector whose elements are $X_{1,j}, X_{2,j}, \ldots, X_{m_1,j}$. Let $\mathbf{1}$ denote an $m_1 \times 1$ column vector all of whose elements are ones. For $1 \le j \le N_2$, let $I_j = 1$ if $\mathbf{X}_j = \mathbf{1}$, and $I_j = 0$, otherwise. Then, $I_1, \ldots, I_{N_2}$ are i.i.d. Bernoulli trials with $P(I_j = 1) = p^{m_1}$. E_1 occurs if there exists a run of ones of length m_2, or longer, in the I_j sequence. Therefore,

$$P(E_1) = \sum_{j=1}^{[N_2/m_2]} (-1)^j \left[p^{m_1} + (N_2 - jm_2 + 1)(1 - p^{m_1})/j \right]$$

$$\times \binom{N_2 - jm_2}{j - 1} p^{jm_1m_2}(1 - p^{m_1})^{j-1}$$

(Bateman, 1948). A recursion formula for $P(E_1)$ is obtained by writing

$$P(E_1) = P(m_1, m_2 \mid m_1, N_2)$$

$$= P((\mathbf{X}_1 \neq \mathbf{1}) \cap E_1) + \sum_{j=1}^{m_2-1} P \left\{ \left[\bigcap_{i=1}^{j} (\mathbf{X}_i = \mathbf{1}) \right] \right.$$

$$\left. \cap (\mathbf{X}_{j+1} \neq \mathbf{1}) \cap E_1) \right\} + p^{m_1m_2}$$

$$= p^{m_1m_2} + (1 - p^{m_1}) P(m_1, m_2 \mid m_1, N_2 - 1)$$

$$+ \sum_{j=1}^{m_2-1} (1 - p^{m_1}) p^{jm_1} P(m_1, m_2 \mid m_1, N_2 - 1 - j)$$

$$= p^{m_1m_2} + \sum_{j=0}^{m_2-1} (1 - p^{m_1}) p^{jm_1} P(m_1, m_2 \mid m_1, N_2 - 1 - j). \tag{16.9}$$

The initial conditions for the recursive formula in (16.9) are

$$P(m_1, m_2 \mid m_1, j) = 0, \qquad 1 \le j \le k - 1.$$

To derive a recursion for $P(E_1 \cap E_2) = P(m_1, m_2 \mid m_1 + 1, N_2)$, denote by $(0, 1)$ an $(m_1 + 1) \times 1$ column vector with first element zero and the remaining elements ones, $(1, 0)$ an $(m_1 + 1) \times 1$ column vector with first m_1 elements one and the last element zero, $(1, 1)$ an $(m_1 + 1) \times 1$ column vector all of ones. Let $q = 1 - p$, $p^* = p^{m_1 - 1}$ and $q^* = 1 - p^*$. Let $\mathbf{X}_j$ denote now an $(m_1 + 1) \times 1$ column vector whose elements are $X_{1,j}, X_{2,j}, \ldots, X_{m_1+1,j}$, $G_j = \cap_{i=1}^{j}[\mathbf{X}_i = (1, 0)]$, and $H_j = \cap_{i=1}^{j}[\mathbf{X}_i = (1, 1)]$. Define $A_j(N_2) = P(E_1 \cap E_2 \mid G_j)$ and $B_j(N_2) = P(E_1 \cap E_2 \mid H_j)$. Since $\mathbf{X}_1 = (0, 1), (1, 0), (1, 1)$ or none of these we get

$$
\begin{aligned}
P(E_1 \cap E_2) &= P(m_1, m_2 \mid m_1 + 1, N_2) \\
&= 2qp^* p A_1(N_2) + p^* p^2 B_1(N_2) \\
&\quad + (1 - 2qp^* p - p^* p^2) P(m_1, m_2 \mid m_1 + 1, N_2 - 1) \\
&= 2qp^* p A_1(N_2) + p^* p^2 B_1(N_2) \\
&\quad + (q^* + q^2 p^*) P(m_1, m_2 \mid m_1 + 1, N_2 - 1).
\end{aligned}
\tag{16.10}
$$

To find a recursion for $A_j(N_2)$ note that after a string of j $(1, 0)$'s there are for some $0 \le i \le m_2 - j$, exactly i $(1, 1)$'s followed by either $(1, 0)$ or $(0, 1)$, or none of $(0, 1)$, $(1, 0)$, or $(1, 1)$. It follows that

$$
\begin{aligned}
A_j(N_2) &= \sum_{i=0}^{m_2-j-1} (p^2 p^*)^i [qpp^*(A_{j+i+1}(N_2) + A_{i+1}(N_2 - j)) \\
&\quad + (q^* + q^2 p^*) P(m_1, m_2 \mid m_1 + 1, N_2 - j - i - 1)] \\
&\quad + (p^2 p^*)^{m_2-j}.
\end{aligned}
\tag{16.11}
$$

A similar approach yields a recursion for $B_j(N_2)$:

$$
\begin{aligned}
B_j(N_2) &= p^2 p^* B_{j+1}(N_2) + 2qp^* p A_{j+1}(N_2) \\
&\quad + P(m_1, m_2 \mid m_1 + 1, N_2 - j - 1).
\end{aligned}
\tag{16.12}
$$

To evaluate recursively $P(E_1 \cap E_2) = P(m_1, m_2 \mid m_1 + 1, N_2)$ the following initial conditions have to be set:

$$
\begin{aligned}
P(m_1, m_2 \mid m_1 + 1, N_2) = 0, &\qquad 0 \le N_2 \le m_2 - 1, \\
A_j(N_2) = B_j(N_2) = 0, &\qquad 1 \le j \le N_2 \le m_2 - 1,
\end{aligned}
$$

and

$$
A_j(N_2) = B_j(N_2) = 1, \qquad N_2 \ge m_2.
$$

16.1.2 A Product-Type Approximation

Let $X_{i,j}$ be i.i.d. binomial random variables with parameters n_0 and $0 < p_0 < 1$ or i.i.d. Poisson random variables with mean $\theta_0 > 0$, respectively. For $1 \le i_1 \le$

$N_1 - m_1 + 1$ and $1 \leq i_2 \leq N_2 - m_2 + 1$ define the events

$$A_{i_1,i_2} = \sum_{i=i_1}^{i_1+m_1-1} \sum_{j=i_2}^{i_2+m_2-1} X_{i,j} \geq k. \tag{16.13}$$

Then,

$$P(S'_{m_1,m_2} \leq k - 1) = P\left(\bigcap_{i_1=1}^{N_1-m_1+1} \bigcap_{i_2=1}^{N_2-m_2-1} A^c_{i_1,i_2}\right). \tag{16.14}$$

To simplify the presentation of the results, we will discuss here only the case of $N_1 = N_2 = N$ and $m_1 = m_2 = m$. For fixed values of $1 \leq i_1 \leq N - m + 1$, one can approximate accurately $P(\bigcap_{i_2=1}^{N-m+1} A^c_{i_1,i_2})$ using a product-type approximation discussed in Glaz and Naus (1991):

$$P\left(\bigcap_{i_2=1}^{N-m+1} A^c_{i_1,i_2}\right) = P\left(\bigcap_{i_2=1}^{m+1} A^c_{i_1,i_2}\right) \prod_{i_2=m+2}^{N-m+1} \left[\frac{P(\bigcap_{j=1}^{i_2} A^c_{i_1,j})}{P(\bigcap_{j=1}^{i_2-1} A^c_{i_1,j})}\right]$$

$$\approx P\left(\bigcap_{i_2=1}^{m+1} A^c_{i_1,i_2}\right) \prod_{i_2=m+2}^{N-m+1} \left[\frac{P(\bigcap_{j=i_2-m}^{i_2} A^c_{i_1,j})}{P(\bigcap_{j=i_2-m}^{i_2-1} A^c_{i_1,j})}\right]$$

$$\approx q_{m,2m} \left(\frac{q_{m,2m}}{q_{m,2m-1}}\right)^{N-2m}, \tag{16.15}$$

where

$$q_{m,m+l-1} = P\left(A^c_{1,1} \cap A^c_{1,2} \cap \cdots \cap A^c_{1,l}\right) \tag{16.16}$$

for $1 \leq l \leq N - m + 1$. The quantities $q_{m,m+l-1}$ can be evaluated via an algorithm in Saperstein (1976), extended to moving sums of discrete random variables in Glaz and Naus (1991) or via an algorithm in Karwe and Naus (1997). Since we have to scan $N - m + 1$ rectangular $m \times N$ adjacent regions we recommend the following product-type approximation (Chen and Glaz (1996)):

$$P(S'_{m,m} \leq k - 1) \approx \left[q_{m,2m} \left(\frac{q_{m,2m}}{q_{m,2m-1}}\right)^{N-2m}\right]$$

$$\times \left[\left(\frac{q_{m,2m}}{q_{m,2m-1}}\right)\left(\frac{q_{m,2m}}{q_{m,2m-1}}\right)^{N-2m}\right]^{N-m}$$

$$= q_{m,2m-1} \left(\frac{q_{m,2m}}{q_{m,2m-1}}\right)^{(N-2m+1)(N-m+1)}. \tag{16.17}$$

Equation (16.17) is using approximation (16.15) for $i_1 = 1$, and for $2 \leq i_1 \leq N - m + 1$, it uses an adjusted approximation based on (16.15), with $q_{m,2m}$ replaced by $q_{m,2m}/q_{m,2m-1}$, to account for the dependence of the events $\{A^c_{i_1,i_2};$

Table 16.1. Comparison of four approximations and an upper bound to $P(S_{m,m} \geq k)$ for the i.i.d. binomial $(5, p)$ model for the two-dimensional case.

N	m	p	k	$\hat{P}(S'_{m,m} \geq k)$	(16.18)	(16.24)	(16.28)	(16.21)
25	5	.05	15	.2420	.2830	.4853	.2954	.4305
			16	.1068	.1170	.2077	.1232	.1613
			17	.0383	.0423	.0734	.0446	.0559
			18	.0132	.0138	.0232	.0146	.0181
			19	.0052	.0042	.0067	.0044	.0054
	10	.05	40	.1259	.1155	.4991	.1289	.3065
			41	.0814	.0715	.3267	.0805	.1849
			42	.0495	.0428	.1983	.0484	.1085
			43	.0297	.0247	.1135	.0281	.0620
			44	.0200	.0139	.0622	.0158	.0345
			45	.0100	.0076	.0329	.0086	.0187
			46	.0064	.0040	.0169	.0046	.0099
100	5	.05	19	.0843	.1022	.1326	.1032	.1137
			20	.0252	.0300	.0383	.0304	.0322
			21	.0071	.0080	.0098	.0082	.0086
			22	.0014	.0020	.0022	.0021	.0022
	10	.05	47	.0862	.1337	.2396	.1351	.1626
			48	.0476	.0698	.1248	.0706	.0819
			49	.0249	.0349	.0617	.0354	.0402
			50	.0119	.0170	.0291	.0172	.0193

$\hat{P}(S'_{m,m} \geq k)$ is a simulated value of $P(S'_{m,m} \geq k)$ based on 10,000 trials.

$i_2 = 1, \ldots, N - m + 1\}$, for different values of i_1. Equation (16.17) yields

$$P(S'_{m,m} \geq k) \approx 1 - q_{m,2m-1} \left(\frac{q_{m,2m}}{q_{m,2m-1}} \right)^{(N-2m+1)(N-m+1)}. \qquad (16.18)$$

In Tables 16.1 and 16.2, we evaluate the performance of this product-type approximation for selected values of N, m, and k and the parameters of binomial and Poisson distributions, respectively. Based on the numerical results it is evident that approximation (16.18) is the most accurate approximation for the binomial and Poisson models.

16.1.3   A Bonferroni-Type Inequality

To derive a Bonferroni-type inequality for $P(S'_{m,m} \geq k)$ we use the lexicographic listing of the $(N - m + 1)^2$ events A_{i_1,i_2}, $1 \leq i_1, i_2 \leq N - m + 1$. Consider the representation

$$P(S'_{m,m} \geq k) = P \left(\bigcup_{i_1=1}^{N-m+1} \bigcup_{i_2=1}^{N-m+1} A_{i_1,i_2} \right). \qquad (16.19)$$

Table 16.2. Comparison of four approximations and an upper bound to $P(S_{m,m} \geq k)$ for the i.i.d. Poisson model for the two-dimensional case.

N	m	μ	k	$\hat{P}(S'_{m,m} \geq k)$	(16.18)	(16.24)	(16.28)	(16.21)
25	5	.25	14	.5350	.6382	.8960	.6526	1.0000
			15	.2970	.3556	.5966	.3698	.5683
			16	.1404	.1626	.2905	.1708	.2300
			17	.0598	.0649	.1154	.0686	.0870
			18	.0217	.0236	.0407	.0250	.0309
			19	.0070	.0080	.0133	.0084	.0104
			20	.0023	.0025	.0041	.0027	.0033
25	5	.50	26	.1122	.1241	.2176	.1306	.1717
			27	.0579	.0603	.1046	.0637	.0807
			28	.0255	.0277	.0470	.0293	.0364
			29	.0170	.0122	.0200	.0129	.0159
			30	.0066	.0051	.0082	.0054	.0067
100	5	.50	30	.1039	.1233	.1589	.1246	.1388
			31	.0464	.0520	.0661	.0525	.0563
			32	.0184	.0207	.0259	.0209	.0221
			33	.0077	.0079	.0097	.0080	.0084

$\hat{P}(S'_{m,m} \geq k)$ is a simulated value of $P(S'_{m,m} \geq k)$ based on 10,000 trials.

The following Bonferroni-type inequality or order $r \geq 3$ is valid here (Glaz (1990) and Hoover (1990)):

$$P(S'_{m,m} \geq k) \leq \sum_{i_1=1}^{N-m+1} \sum_{i_2=1}^{N-m+1} P(A_{i_1,i_2}) - \sum_{i_1=1}^{N-m+1} \sum_{i_2=1}^{N-m} P\left(A_{i_1,i_2} \cap A_{i_1,i_2+1}\right)$$

$$- \sum_{i_1=1}^{N-m} P\left(A_{i_1,1} \cap A_{i_1+1,1}\right)$$

$$- \sum_{i_1=1}^{N-m+1} \sum_{l=2}^{r-1} \sum_{i_2=1}^{N-m+1-l} P\left(A_{i_1,i_2} \cap A^c_{i_1,i_2+1}\right.$$

$$\left. \cap \cdots \cap A^c_{i_1,i_2+l-1} \cap A_{i_1,i_2+l}\right). \tag{16.20}$$

Since the main purpose for deriving this upper bound is to evaluate the approximations for $P(S^*_{m,m} \geq k)$, and very little improvement is gained for $r \geq 5$ (Chen and Glaz (1996)), only the case $r = 4$ is presented here. For a fixed value of i_1 (respectively, i_2) the events A_{i_1,i_2}, $1 \leq i_2$ (respectively, i_1) $\leq N - m + 1$, are stationary. For $r = 4$, inequality (16.20) simplifies to

$$P(S'_{m,m} \geq k) \leq 1 + 2(N - m)q_{m,m} - (N - m)q_{m,m+1}$$
$$+ (N - m - 3)(N - m + 1)q_{m,m+2}$$
$$- (N - m - 2)(N - m + 1)q_{m,m+3}, \tag{16.21}$$

where $q_{m,m+l}$ for $1 \leq l \leq m + 1$ are defined in (16.16).

In Tables 16.1 and 16.2, we evaluate this Bonferroni-type inequality for selected values of N, m, and k and the parameters of binomial and Poisson distributions, respectively.

16.1.4 Poisson-Type Approximations

Let $\Gamma = \{(i_1, i_2); 1 \leq i_1, i_2 \leq N - m + 1\}$, denote the index set of a collection
of the integer valued random variables $\{I_\alpha; \alpha \in \Gamma\}$, where

$$I_\alpha = \begin{cases} 1 & \text{if } Y_\alpha \geq k, \\ 0 & \text{otherwise,} \end{cases} \tag{16.22}$$

and Y_α is defined in (16.1). Then

$$P(S'_{m,m} \geq k) = 1 - P\left(\sum_{\alpha \in \Gamma} I_\alpha = 0\right). \tag{16.23}$$

Under quite general conditions the distribution of $\sum_{\alpha \in \Gamma} I_\alpha$ converges to a Poisson
distribution with mean λ_2, where

$$\lambda_2 = E\left(\sum_{\alpha \in \Gamma} I_\alpha\right) = (N - m + 1)^2 (1 - q_{m,m})$$

and $q_{m,m} = P(A^c_{1,1})$ (Darling and Waterman (1986)). Poisson approximations
for this problem for the special case of $k = m^2$ have been discussed in Barbour, Chryssaphinou, and Roos (1996), Koutras, Papadopoulos, and Papastavridis
(1993), and Roos (1994). In Tables 16.1 and 16.2, we evaluate the performance
of the following Poisson approximation:

$$P(S'_{m,m} \geq k) \approx 1 - \exp(-\lambda_2), \tag{16.24}$$

for selected values of N, m, and k and the parameters of binomial and Poisson
distributions, respectively.

Poisson approximation (16.4) is not expected to perform well when $k < m^2$,
since the events $\{(Y_\alpha \geq k); \alpha \in \Gamma\}$ tend to clump. We consider an improved
Poisson approximation (Chen and Glaz (1996)), utilizing the idea of declumping
put forward in Arratia, Goldstein, and Gordon (1990) in their investigation of the
distribution of the largest run of ones for a sequence of i.i.d. Bernoulli trials. Let
$B_\alpha \subset \Gamma$, defined as follows:

$$B_\alpha = \{\beta \in \Gamma; \beta \geq \alpha \text{ and } I_\alpha \text{ and } I_\beta \text{ are dependent}\},$$

where $\geq$ is the lexicographic ordering on Γ. To utilize the full declumping approach one has to evaluate an approximate mean of an asymptotic Poisson distribution given by

$$\sum_{\alpha \in \Gamma} P\left\{A\alpha \cap \left(\bigcap_{\beta \in B_\alpha} A^c_\beta\right)\right\}.$$

The computational complexity of the problem at hand renders the full declumping
approach as nonfeasible. We proceed to describe a local declumping approach

investigated in Glaz, Naus, Roos, and Wallenstein (1994). Let $\Gamma_{N-m+1} = \{(N - m + 1, i_2); 1 \le i_2 \le N - m + 1\}$. It follows that

$$\sum_{\alpha \in \Gamma_{n-m+1}} P\left\{A_\alpha \cap \left(\bigcap_{\beta \in B_\alpha} A_\beta^c\right)\right\}$$

$$= \sum_{j=1}^{N-2m+1} P\left\{A_{N-m+1,j} \cap \left(\bigcap_{i_2=j+1}^{m+j-1} A_{N-m+1,i_2}^c\right)\right\}$$

$$+ P\left\{A_{N-m+1,j} \cap \left(\bigcap_{i_2=j+1}^{\min(m+j-1,N-m+1)} A_{N-m+1,i_2}^c\right)\right\}$$

$$+ P(A_{N-m+1,N-m+1})$$

$$= (N - 2m + 2)(q_{m,2m-2} - q_{m,2m-1}) + (1 - q_{m,2m-2}). \quad (16.25)$$

For $1 \le j \le n - m$, we employ the following approximation:

$$\sum_{\alpha \in \Gamma_j} P\left\{A_\alpha \cap \left(\bigcap_{\beta \in B_\alpha} A_\beta^c\right)\right\} \approx (n - 2m + 2)(q_{m,2m-2} - q_{m,2m-1}). \quad (16.26)$$

Approximation (16.26) was obtained from (16.25) by replacing $(1 - q_{m,2m-2})$ with $(q_{m,2m-2} - q_{m,2m-1})$ to account for the dependence of the sequences of indicator random variables $\{I_\alpha; \alpha \in \Gamma_j\}$ for different values of j. This results in the following approximate mean for the asymptotic Poisson distribution:

$$\lambda_2^* = 1 - q_{m,2m-2} + (N - 2m + 2)(N - m + 1)(q_{m,2m-2} - q_{m,2m-1}). \quad (16.27)$$

In Tables 16.1 and 16.2, we present numerical results for the following improved Poisson approximation:

$$P(S'_{m,m} \ge k) \approx 1 - \exp(-\lambda_2^*), \quad (16.28)$$

for selected values of N, m, and k and the parameters of binomial and Poisson distributions, respectively.

16.1.5 A Compound Poisson Approximation

For the Bernoulli model, the compound Poisson approximations for $P(S'_{m,m} \ge k)$ presented below is based on Roos (1993b, 1994). In Roos (1993b) it is recommended to approximate the distribution of $\sum_{\alpha \in \Gamma} I_\alpha$ by the compound Poisson distribution of $M = \sum_{i=1}^\infty i M_i$, where M_i are independent Poisson random variables with mean λ_i. A discussion about this particular representation of a compound Poisson distribution is given in Feller (1968, Chap. XII, Sect. 2). The constants λ_i, for the special case of $k = m^2$, have been evaluated in Roos (1993b).

Based on the Roos (1993b) approach, Chen and Glaz (1996) evaluated the constants λ_i for $k < m^2$:

$$\lambda_i = \frac{1}{i} P(S'(1, 1) \geq k)\{4\mu_{1,i} + 4(N - m - 1)\mu_{2,i} + (N - m + 1)^2 \mu_{3,i}\},$$

(16.29)

where for $1 \leq i \leq 5$:

$$\mu_{1,i} = P\{I_{1,2} + I_{2,1} = i - 1 \mid I_{1,1} = 1\},$$
$$\mu_{2,i} = P\{I_{1,1} + I_{2,2} + I_{3,1} = i - 1 \mid I_{2,1} = 1\},$$

and

$$\mu_{3,i} = P\{I_{1,2} + I_{2,1} + I_{2,3} + I_{3,2} = i - 1 \mid I_{2,2} = 1\}.$$

It is tedious but routine to evaluate $\mu_{1,i}$, $\mu_{2,i}$, and $\mu_{3,i}$; and therefore their derivation, which is quite lengthy and given in Chen (1998), will not be presented here. Chen and Glaz (1996, Table 1) evaluate the performance of the following compound Poisson approximation:

$$P(S'_{m,m} \geq k) \approx 1 - \exp\left(-\sum_{i=1}^{5} \lambda_i\right),$$

(16.30)

for selected values of N, m, and k and for selected values of p for the Bernoulli distribution.

16.1.6   A Markov Chain Embedding Method for the Bernoulli Model

Let $1 \leq m_i \leq N_i$, $i = 1, 2$, and $0 \leq k \leq m_1 m_2$ be integers. Recently, for the special case of i.i.d. Bernoulli trials, Boutsikas and Koutras (2000) employed a *finite Markov chain embedding* method to derive accurate approximations for $P(S'_{m_1,m_2} \geq k)$, that can be easily computed for all values of N_1, N_2, m_1, m_2, and k. This method has been developed in a series of articles by Fu (1986), Fu and Hu (1987), Fu and Koutras (1994), Koutras and Alexandrou (1995), and Koutras (1996). We present here a brief account of the approximations given in Boutsikas and Koutras (2000).

For $1 \leq i \leq N_1$ and $1 \leq j \leq N_2$, let X_{ij} be i.i.d. Bernoulli trials with $P(X_{ij} = 1) = p$ and $P(X_{ij} = 0) = 1 - p$, $0 < p < 1$. For $N_i^* \leq N_i$, $i = 1, 2$, define

$$S'_{m_1,m_2}(N_1^*, N_2^*) = \max\{Y_{i_1,i_2}; 1 \leq i_j \leq N_j^* - m_j + 1, j = 1, 2\}, \quad (16.31)$$

to be the discrete scan statistic on the rectangular region of dimension $N_1^* \times N_2^*$. For $N_i^* = N_i$, $i = 1, 2$, $S'_{m_1,m_2}(N_1, N_2) = S'_{m_1,m_2}$, given in (16.1) and (16.2). The following is potentially the most accurate approximation for $P(S'_{m_1,m_2} \geq k - 1)$:

$$P(S'_{m_1,m_2} \geq k) \approx 1 - \frac{\left[P\{S'_{m_1,m_2}(j_2, N_2) \leq k - 1\}\right]^{(N_1-j_1)/(j_2-j_1)}}{\left[P\{S'_{m_1,m_2}(j_1, N_2) \leq k - 1\}\right]^{(N_1-j_2)/(j_2-j_1)}}, \quad (16.32)$$

where $m_1 \leq j_1 < j_2 < \min(N_1, N_2)$. For the special case of $k = m_1 m_2$, when one selects $j_1 = m_1$ and $j_2 = m_1 + 1$, the approximation (16.32) reduces to approximation (16.6). For $j_1 = m_1 + 1$ and $j_2 = m_1 + 2$, approximation (16.32) reduces to approximation (16.7). For $k < m_1 m_2$, approximation (16.31) is computationally impractical for large values of N_1, N_2, m_1, m_2, and k. Boutsikas and Koutras (2000) derive the following simple approximation for $P(S'_{m_1,m_2} \leq k-1)$:

$$P(S'_{m_1,m_2} \leq k - 1)$$
$$\approx \frac{\left[P\{S'_{m_1,m_2}(j_1, l_1) \leq k - 1\}\right]^{(N_1-j_2)(N_2-l_2)/(j_2-j_1)(l_2-l_1)}}{\left[P\{S'_{m_1,m_2}(j_1, l_2) \leq k - 1\}\right]^{(N_1-j_2)(N_2-l_1)/(j_2-j_1)(l_2-l_1)}}$$
$$\times \frac{\left[P\{S'_{m_1,m_2}(j_2, h_2) \leq k - 1\}\right]^{(N_1-j_1)(N_2-h_1)/(j_2-j_1)(h_2-h_1)}}{\left[P\{S'_{m_1,m_2}(j_2, h_1) \leq k - 1\}\right]^{(N_1-j_1)(N_2-h_2)/(j_2-j_1)(h_2-h_1)}} (16.33)$$

where $m_1 \leq j_1 < j_2 < \min(N_1, N_2)$, $m_2 \leq h_1 < h_2 < \min(N_1, N_2)$ and $m_2 \leq l_1 < l_2 < \min(N_1, N_2)$. For $j_1 = m_1, j_2 = m_1+1, h_1 = m_2, h_2 = m_2+1$, and $l = m_2, l_2 = m_2 + 1$, this approximation simplifies further to

$$P(S'_{m_1,m_2} \leq k - 1) \approx \frac{\left[P\{S'_{m_1,m_2}(m_1, m_2) \leq k - 1\}\right]^{(N_1-m_1-1)(N_2-m_2-1)}}{\left[P\{S'_{m_1,m_2}(m_1, m_2 + 1) \leq k - 1\}\right]^{(N_1-m_1-1)(N_2-m_2)}}$$
$$\times \frac{\left[P\{S'_{m_1,m_2}(m_1 + 1, m_2 + 1) \leq k - 1\}\right]^{(N_1-m_1)(N_2-m_2)}}{\left[P\{S'_{m_1,m_2}(m_1 + 1, m_2) \leq k - 1\}\right]^{(N_1-m_1)(N_2-m_2-1)}}. \quad (16.34)$$

Approximation (16.34) is readily evaluated with the following formulas:

$$P\{S'_{m_1,m_2}(m_1, m_2) \leq k - 1\} = F_b(k - 1; m_1, m_2, p),$$
$$P\{S'_{m_1,m_2}(m_1, m_2 + 1) \leq k - 1\}$$
$$= \sum_{s=0}^{k-1} F_b^2(k - 1 - s; m_1, p)b(s; m_1(m_2 - 1), p),$$
$$P\{S'_{m_1,m_2}(m_1 + 1, m_2) \leq k - 1\}$$

$$= \sum_{s=0}^{k-1} F_b^2(k-1-s; m_2, p)b(s; (m_1-1)m_2, p),$$

$$P\{S'_{m_1,m_2}(m_1+1, m_2+1) \leq k-1\}$$

$$= \sum_{s_1,s_2=0}^{k-1} \sum_{t_1,t_2=0}^{k-1} \sum_{i_j=0, 1 \leq j \leq 4}^{i} b_1(s_1)b_1(s_2)b_2(t_1)b_2(t_2)$$

$$\times p^{\sum_{j=1}^{4} i_j}(1-p)^{4-\sum_{j=1}^{4} i_j} F_b((x; (m_1-1)(m_2-1), p),$$

where for $i = 1, 2$, $b_1(s_i) = b(s_i; m_1-1, p)$ and $b_2(t_i) = b(t_i; m_2-1, p)$,
$x = \min\{k-1-s_1-t_1-i_1, k-1-s_2-t_1-i_2, k-1-s_1-t_2-i_3, k-1-s_2-t_2-i_4\}$,
$b(j; N, w) = \binom{N}{j}w^j(1-w)^{N-j}$ and $F_b(i; N, w) = \sum_{j=0}^{i} b(j; N, w)$.

For $N_1 = N_2 = N$ and $m_1 = m_2 = m$ approximation (16.34) reduces to

$$P(S'_{m,m} \leq k-1) \approx \left[\frac{\left[P\{S'_{m,m}(m, m) \leq k-1\} \right]^{(N-m-1)^2}}{\left[P\{S'_{m,m}(m, m+1) \leq k-1\} \right]^{2(N-m-1)(N-m)}} \right]$$

$$\times \left[P\{S'_{m,m}(m+1, m+1) \leq k-1\} \right]^{(N-m)^2}. \quad (16.35)$$

Boutsikas and Koutras (2000) noted that for some values of the parameters N, m, k, and p, approximation (16.35) is more accurate than approximation (16.17).

We now present another accurate approximation for $P(S'_{m_1,m_2} \leq k-1)$. It follows from Sheng and Naus (1996) and from (16.32) for $j_1 = m_1$ and $j_2 = m_1 + 1$ that

$$P(S'_{m_1,m_2} \leq k-1) \approx \frac{\left[P\{S'_{m_1,m_2}(m_1+1, N_2) \leq k-1\} \right]^{N_1-m_1}}{\left[P\{S'_{m_1,m_2}(m_1, N_2) \leq k-1\} \right]^{N_1-m_1-1}}. \quad (16.36)$$

For $N_1 = N_2$ and $m_1 = m_2$ approximation (16.36) reduces to

$$P(S'_{m,m} \leq k-1) \approx \frac{\left[P\{S'_{m,m}(m+1, N) \leq k-1\} \right]^{N-m}}{\left[P\{S'_{m,m}(m, N) \leq k-1\} \right]^{N-m-1}}. \quad (16.37)$$

Approximate

$$P\{S'_{m,m}(m, N) \leq k-1\} \approx \frac{(q_{m,2m})^{(N-2m+1)}}{(q_{m,2m-1})^{(N-2m)}} \quad (16.38)$$

(Glaz and Naus (1991) and Chen and Glaz (1996)), where $q_{m,2m-1}$ and $q_{m,2m}$ are given in (16.16). To approximate $P\{S'_{m,m}(m+1, N) \leq k-1\}$ one can employ a simple Markov-like approximation:

$$P\{S'_{m,m}(m+1, N) \leq k-1\} \approx \frac{\left[P\{S'_{m,m}(m+1, m+1) \leq k-1\} \right]^{N-m}}{\left[P\{S'_{m,m}(m+1, m) \leq k-1\} \right]^{N-m-1}}. \quad (16.39)$$

Table 16.3. Approximations for the expected value and standard deviation for the binomial $(5, p)$ model, $N = 25$, $m = 5$.

p	$\hat{E}(S'_{m,m})$	(16.18)	(16.28)	$\widehat{SD}(S'_{m,m})$	(16.18)	(16.28)
.05	13.53	13.85	13.89	1.57	1.40	1.42
.10	22.20	22.58	22.64	1.97	1.75	1.77

$\hat{E}(S'_{m,m})$ and $\widehat{SD}(S'_{m,m})$ based on a simulation with 10,000 trials.

Substitute approximations (16.38) and (16.39) into (16.37) to obtain the following approximation:

$$P(S'_{m,m} \leq k - 1) \approx \frac{\left[P\{S'_{m,m}(m + 1, m + 1) \leq k - 1\}\right]^{(N-m)^2}}{\left[P\{S'_{m,m}(m + 1, m) \leq k - 1\}\right]^{(N-m-1)(N-m)}}$$
$$\times \frac{(q_{m,2m-1})^{(N-2m)(N-m-1)}}{q_{m,2m})^{(N-2m+1)(N-m-1)}} . \tag{16.40}$$

Approximation (16.40) is a member of a class of approximations in Boutsikas and Koutras (2000), given in (16.33), for the special case of $N_1 = N_2 = N$, $m_1 = m_2 = m$, $h_1 = m$, $h_2 = m + 1$, $j_1 = m$, $j_2 = m + 1$, $l_1 = 2m - 1$, and $l_2 = 2m$.

16.1.7   Approximations for the Expected Size and Standard Deviation

Since $S'_{m,m}$ is a discrete random variable,

$$E(S'_{m,m}) = \sum_{k=1}^{m^2} P(S'_{m,m} \geq k) \tag{16.41}$$

and

$$\text{Var}(S'_{m,m}) = 2 \sum_{k=1}^{m^2} k P(S'_{m,m} \geq k) - E(S'_{m,m})\left[1 + E(S'_{mm})\right]. \tag{16.42}$$

Therefore, approximations for $P(S'_{m,m} \geq k)$ will yield approximations for $E(S'_{m,m})$ and $\text{Var}(S'_{m,m})$. In Tables 16.3 and 16.4, we present approximate values for $E(S'_{m,m})$ and $SD = [\text{Var}(S'_{m,m})]^{1/2}$ based on the product-type approximation (16.18) and improved Poisson approximation (16.28), for selected values of the parameters for the binomial and Poisson models. To evaluate the performance of these approximations we present simulated values for $E(S'_{m,m})$ and $SD(S'_{m,m})$, denoted by $\hat{E}(S'_{m,m})$ and $\widehat{SD}(S'_{m,m})$, respectively, based on 10,000 trials.

Table 16.4. Approximations for the expected value and standard deviation for the Poisson (μ) model, $N = 25$, $m = 5$.

μ	$\hat{E}(S'_{m.m})$	(16.18)	(16.28)	$\widehat{SD}(S'_{m.m})$	(16.18)	(16.28)
.25	13.79	14.13	14.18	1.65	1.48	1.49
.50	22.85	23.30	23.36	2.16	1.93	1.94

$\hat{E}(S'_{m.m})$ and $\widehat{SD}(S'_{m.m})$ based on a simulation with 10,000 trials.

16.1.8   A Multiple Scan Statistic

A two-dimensional discrete multiple scan statistic is defined as

$$\xi' = \sum_{i_1=1}^{N-m+1} \sum_{i_2=1}^{N-m+1} I_{i_1,i_2}, \tag{16.43}$$

where I_{i_1,i_2} is defined in (16.22). This multiple scan statistic counts the number of $m \times m$ rectangular windows containing k or more events. Note that the multiple scan statistic defined in (16.43) is related to the scan statistic in (16.2) via the following identity:

$$P(\xi' \geq 1) = P(S'_{m.m} \geq k).$$

A product-type approximation for this statistic is extremely complex and of limited value. Poisson approximations give poor results for $P(\xi^* \geq c)$, $c \geq 2$. Based on the compound Poisson approximation for $P(S^*_{m,m} \geq k)$, a compound Poisson approximation for the multiple scan statistics is given by

$$P(\xi' \geq c) \approx 1 - \sum_{j=0}^{c-1} \left(\sum_{\beta_1+2\beta_2+3\beta_3+4\beta_4+5\beta_5=j} \prod_{i=1}^{5} \frac{\lambda_i^{\beta_i}}{\beta_i!} \right) \exp\left(-\sum_{i=1}^{5} \lambda_i \right),$$

$$\tag{16.44}$$

where β_i are nonnegative integers and λ_i are given in (16.28). In Table 16.5, we present numerical results for this compound Poisson approximation for selected values of N, m, and k for selected values of p for the Bernoulli distribution.

16.2   A Conditional Discrete Scan Statistic

In this section we are interested in approximations for the distribution of the two-dimensional discrete scan statistic, conditioned on the number of events that have occurred in the rectangular region $[0, T_1] \times [0, T_2]$. In what follows, we derive product-type, Poisson, and compound Poisson approximations for the distribution of the conditional scan statistic. We also derive Bonferroni-type inequalities. These approximations and inequalities yield approximations and inequalities for the expected size and standard deviation of the conditional scan statistic. These approximations and inequalities are based on simulation algorithms, described in Section 16.3, for binomial and Poisson models. Numerical results are presented in Tables 16.6–16.10.

Table 16.5. A compound Poisson approximation to $P(\xi^* \geq l)$ for a Bernoulli model for the two-dimensional case.

$N = 25$						$N = 100$					
m	p	k	l	$\hat{P}(\xi^* \geq l)$	(16.44)	m	p	k	l	$\hat{P}(\xi^* \geq l)$	(16.44)
5	.05	6	2	.1180	.1637	5	.05	7	2	.3436	.4203
			3	.0720	.0807				3	.2227	.2528
			4	.0486	.0327				4	.1559	.1429
			5	.0317	.0131				5	.0103	.0778
		7	2	.0168	.0228			8	2	.0420	.0516
			3	.0071	.0076				3	.0178	.0158
			4	.0061	.0017				4	.0116	.0039
			5	.0027	.0003				5	.0053	.0010
	.10	9	2	.0459	.0600		.10	10	2	.1743	.2064
			3	.0250	.0217				3	.0971	.0906
			4	.0152	.0062				4	.0588	.0369
			5	.0104	.0017				5	.0320	.0145
		10	2	.0090	.0095			11	2	.0210	.0272
			3	.0032	.0025				3	.0100	.0065
10	.05	12	2	.1224	.2912	10	.05	15	2	.1632	.3071
			3	.0978	.2026				3	.1187	.1942
			4	.0780	.1200				4	.0988	.1092
			5	.0671	.0644				5	.0738	.0586
		13	2	.0500	.1122			16	2	.0520	.0936
			3	.0398	.0678				3	.0346	.0478
			4	.0323	.0323				4	.0282	.0197
			5	.0229	.0127				5	.0198	.0071

$\hat{p}(\xi^* \geq l)$ is a simulated value of $p(\xi^* \geq l)$ based on 10,000 trials.

16.2.1   Product-Type Approximations

Let $X_{i,j}$, $1 \leq i \leq N_1$, $1 \leq j \leq N_2$, be i.i.d. nonnegative integer valued random variables. If the total number of events that have occurred in the two-dimensional rectangular region is known to be a, then the scan statistic defined in Section 16.1, (16.2), is referred to as the *conditional* two-dimensional discrete scan statistic. We are interested in approximations for

$$P(S'_{m_1,m_2}(a) \geq k) = P\left(S'_{m_1,m_2} \geq k \,\Big|\, \sum_{j=1}^{N_2} \sum_{i=1}^{N_1} X_{i,j} = a \right). \qquad (16.45)$$

To simplify the presentation of the results, we assume that $N_1 = N_2 = N$ and $m_1 = m_2 = m$. For $1 \leq i_1, i_2 \leq N - m + 1$, define

$$A_{i_1,i_2} = (Y_{i_1,i_2} \geq k)$$

and

$$B = \left(\sum_{j=1}^{N} \sum_{i=1}^{N} X_{i,j} = a \right). \tag{16.46}$$

Then,

$$P\left(S'_{m,m}(a) \geq k\right) = P\left(\bigcup_{i_1=1}^{N-m+1} \bigcup_{i_2=1}^{N-m+1} A_{i_2,i_2} \,\middle|\, B \right). \tag{16.47}$$

In Section 16.1, the following product-type approximation for $P(S'_{m,m} \geq k)$ has been discussed:

$$P(S'_{m,m} \geq k) \approx 1 - q_{m,2m-1} \left(\frac{q_{m,2m}}{q_{m,2m-1}} \right)^{(N-2m+1)(N-m+1)}, \tag{16.48}$$

where $q_{m,2m-1}$ and $q_{m,2m}$ are defined in (16.16). This approximation was at times not accurate (Chen and Glaz, 1996), since we were not able to obtain an accurate approximation for

$$P(E_i \cap E_{i_1+1}),$$

where

$$P(E_{i_1}) = P\left(\bigcap_{i_2=1}^{N-m+1} A^c_{i_1,i_2} \right) \tag{16.49}$$

and $1 \leq i_1 \leq N - m$. Therefore, we will not pursue this approximation here.

In this section, we present a simulation-based method, introduced in Chen and Glaz (2000), for approximating the distribution of this conditional scan statistic. This method is based on the representation

$$P\left(S'_{m,m}(a) \leq k - 1\right) = P\left(\bigcap_{i_1=1}^{N-m+1} E_{i_1} \,\middle|\, B \right)$$

$$= P\left(\bigcap_{i=1}^{r} E_i \,\middle|\, B \right) \prod_{i_1=r+1}^{N-m+1} \left[\frac{P(\bigcap_{j=1}^{i_1} E_i \mid B)}{P(\bigcap_{j=1}^{i_1-1} E_i \mid B)} \right], \tag{16.50}$$

and a *Markov-like* approximation

$$\frac{P(\bigcap_{j=1}^{i_1} E_i \mid B)}{P(\bigcap_{j=1}^{i_1-1} E_i \mid B)} \approx \frac{P(\bigcap_{j=i_1-r}^{i_1} E_i \mid B)}{P(\bigcap_{j=i_1-r}^{i_1-1} E_i \mid B)} = \frac{P(\bigcap_{j=1}^{r+1} E_i \mid B)}{P(\bigcap_{j=1}^{r} E_i \mid B)},$$

where $r = 1$ or 2. This yields product-type approximations

$$P\left(S'_{m,m}(a) \leq k - 1\right) \approx \frac{[P(E_1 \cap E_2 \mid B)]^{N-m}}{[P(E_1 \mid B)]^{N-m-1}} \tag{16.51}$$

and

$$P\left(S'_{m,m}(a) \leq k - 1\right) \approx \frac{[P(E_1 \cap E_2 \cap E_3 \mid B)]^{N-m-1}}{[P(E_1 \cap E_2 \mid B)]^{N-m-2}}, \tag{16.52}$$

Table 16.6. Comparison of five approximations to $P(S_{m,m}(a) \geq k)$ for a Bernoulli model, $N = 100$, $m = 10$.

k	a	(16.52)	(16.54)	(16.56)	(16.57)	(16.59)	Simulation
5	80	0.6612	0.9628	0.6384	0.7861	1.0000	0.6793
	90	0.8165	0.9948	0.8289	0.9193	1.0000	0.8464
	100	0.9267	0.9997	0.9178	0.9763	1.0000	0.9412
	110	0.9773	1.0000	0.9662	0.9950	1.0000	0.9851
	120	0.9932	1.0000	0.9861	0.9991	1.0000	0.9975
6	80	0.1611	0.3759	0.1714	0.2170	0.1742	0.1709
	90	0.2862	0.5968	0.2939	0.3706	0.3320	0.2918
	100	0.4524	0.7739	0.4415	0.5361	0.5870	0.4411
	110	0.5993	0.9046	0.5953	0.6974	0.8784	0.5962
	120	0.7454	9.9714	0.7475	0.8356	1.0000	0.7503
7	80	0.0249	0.0524	0.0263	0.0301	0.0252	0.0242
	90	0.0561	0.0991	0.0574	0.0624	0.0576	0.0506
	100	0.0903	0.1968	0.1092	0.1225	0.0943	0.0932
	110	0.1672	0.3471	0.1565	0.2003	0.1816	0.1609
	120	0.2587	0.4855	0.2590	0.3060	0.2958	0.2512
8	80	0.0034	0.0057	0.0036	0.0037	0.0034	0.0029
	90	0.0070	0.0136	0.0046	0.0070	0.0071	0.0074
	100	0.0147	0.0293	0.0123	0.0156	0.0148	0.0140
	110	0.0257	0.0489	0.0255	0.0293	0.0260	0.0271
	120	0.0514	0.1089	0.0422	0.0576	0.0527	0.0499

The simulation is based on 10,000 trials.

respectively. To implement these approximations, efficient algorithms for simulating $P(E_1 \cap E_2 \cap E_3 \mid B)$, $P(E_1 \cap E_2 \mid B)$, and $P(E_1 \mid B)$ are needed. If m and N are not too large, it is a feasible task. Moreover, one gains significant savings over simulating $P(S'_{m,m}(a) \leq k-1)$ on the entire rectangular region. The algorithms for simulating $P(E_1 \cap E_2 \cap E_3 \mid B)$, $P(E_1 \cap E_2 \mid B)$, and $P(E_1 \mid B)$ are given below. Numerical results for this approximation are presented in Tables 16.6–16.8.

16.2.2 Poisson Approximations

For $1 \leq j \leq N - m + 1$, let I_j be a Bernoulli random variable with

$$P(I_j = 1) = P(E_j^c \mid B) = 1 - P(I_j = 0), \qquad (16.53)$$

where E_j and B are defined in (16.49) and (16.46), respectively. Then

$$P(S'_{m,m}(a) \geq k) = 1 - P\left(\sum_{j=1}^{N-m+1} I_j\right).$$

The distribution of $\sum_{j=1}^{N-m+1} I_j$ can be approximated by a Poisson distribution with mean λ, where

$$\lambda = E\left(\sum_{j=1}^{N-m+1} I_j\right) = (N - m + 1)(1 - P(E_1 \mid B)).$$

Poisson approximations for the unconditional case have been discussed in Barbour, Chryssaphinou, and Roos (1996), Chen and Glaz (1996), Darling and Waterman (1986), Koutras, Papadopoulos, and Papastavridis (1993), and Roos (1993b). In Tables 16.6 and 16.7, we present numerical results for the following Poisson approximation:

$$P(S'_{m,m}(a) \geq k) \approx 1 - \exp(-\lambda), \tag{16.54}$$

for the binomial and Poisson models for selected values of N, m, k, and a.

The Poisson approximation (16.54) is not expected to perform well when $k < m^2$, since the events $\{(I_j = 1); 1 \leq j \leq N - m + 1\}$ tend to clump. We propose to employ a local declumping approach discussed in Chen and Glaz (1996), for the unconditional case, to obtain a more accurate Poisson approximation. For $1 \leq j \leq N - m$, let I_j^* be a Bernoulli random variable with

$$P(I_j^* = 1) = P(E_j^c \cap E_{j+1} \mid B) = 1 - P(I_j^* = 0) \tag{16.55}$$

and

$$P(I_{N-m+1}^* = 1) = P(E_{N-m+1}^c \mid B) = 1 - P(I_{N-m+1}^* = 0).$$

The improved Poisson approximation is given by

$$P(S'_{m,m}(a) \geq k) \approx 1 - \exp(-\lambda^*), \tag{16.56}$$

where

$$\lambda^* = 1 - P(E_1 \mid B) + (N - m)[P(E_1 \mid B) - P(E_1 \cap E_1 \mid B)].$$

In Tables 16.6–16.8, we present numerical results for the improved Poisson approximation (16.56) for selected values of N, m, k, and a, and for the binomial and Poisson models.

16.2.3 A Compound Poisson Approximation

The following compound Poisson approximation for $P(S'_{m,m}(a) \geq k)$ is based on the approach in Roos (1993b, 1994):

$$P(S'_{m,m}(a) \geq k) \approx 1 - \exp\left(-\sum_{i=1}^{3} \lambda_i\right). \tag{16.57}$$

The constants λ_i are evaluated by extending the method in Roos (1993b):

$$\lambda_i = \frac{1}{i}\{2\pi_{1,i} + (N - m - 1)\pi_{2,i}\}, \qquad i = 1, 2, 3,$$

where

$$\pi_{1,1} = P\{I_1 = 1, I_2 = 0\} = P(E_1 \mid B) - P(E_1 \cap E_2 \mid B),$$
$$\pi_{1,2} = P\{I_1 = 1, I_2 = 1\} = 1 - 2P(E_1 \mid B) + P(E_1 \cap E_2 \mid B),$$
$$\pi_{2,1} = P\{I_1 + I_3 = 0, I_2 = 1\}$$
$$= P(E_1 \cap E_3 \mid B) - P(E_1 \cap E_2 \cap E_3 \mid B),$$
$$\pi_{2,2} = P\{I_1 + I_3 = 1, I_2 = 1\}$$
$$= 2[P(E_1 \mid B) - P(E_1 \cap E_2 \mid B) - P(E_1 \cap E_3 \mid B)$$
$$+ P(E_1 \cap E_2 \cap E_3 \mid B)],$$

and

$$\pi_{2,3} = P\{I_1 + I_3 = 2, I_3 = 1\}$$
$$= 1 - 3P(E_1 \mid B) + 2P(E_1 \cap E_2 \mid B) + P(E_1 \cap E_3 \mid B)$$
$$- P(E_1 \cap E_2 \cap E_3 \mid B),$$

where I_j is defined in (16.53). The algorithms for evaluating these terms are presented below. In Tables 16.6–16.8, we evaluate this compound Poisson approximation for selected values of N, m, k, and a, and for the binomial and Poisson models.

16.2.4   Bonferroni-Type Inequalities

From (16.50) we have

$$P(S'_{m,m}(a) \geq k) = P\left(\bigcup_{i_1=1}^{N-m+1} E_{i_1}^c \mid B\right).$$

It follows from (7.4), (7.5), (7.8), and (7.10), that second- and third-order upper Bonferroni-type inequalities are given by

$$P(S'_{m,m}(a) \geq k) \leq (N - m + 1)P(E_1^c \mid B) - (N - m)P(E_1^c \cap E_2^c \mid B)$$
$$= 1 + (N - m - 1)P(E_1 \mid B)$$
$$- (N - m)P(E_1 \cap E_2 \mid B) \qquad (16.58)$$

and

$$P(S'_{m,m}(a) \geq k) \leq 1 + (N - m - 2)P(E_1 \cap E_2 \mid B)$$
$$- (N - m - 1)P(E_1 \cap E_2 \cap E_3 \mid B), \qquad (16.59)$$

respectively. In Tables 16.6–16.8, we evaluate these Bonferroni-type inequalities for selected values of N, m, k, and a, and for the binomial and Poisson models.

Table 16.7. Comparison of five approximations to $P(S_{m,m}(a) \geq k)$ for a binomial model, $n = 5$.

N	m	a	k	(16.52)	(16.54)	(16.56)	(16.57)	(16.59)	Simulation
25	5	25	5	0.3109	0.4795	0.3055	0.3013	0.3531	0.3159
			6	0.0620	0.0936	0.0552	0.0611	0.0635	0.0631
		50	6	0.8072	0.9510	0.7620	0.8190	1.2863	0.8534
			7	0.3944	0.5677	0.3949	0.4202	0.4673	0.4130
			8	0.1188	0.1786	0.1318	0.1341	0.1242	0.1177
			9	0.0274	0.0384	0.0291	0.0296	0.0276	0.0271
			10	0.0051	0.0063	0.0054	0.0052	0.0051	0.0040
		150	13	0.6211	0.7928	0.5988	0.6342	0.8478	0.6432
			14	0.3397	0.4706	0.3402	0.3562	0.3925	0.3560
			15	0.1418	0.2067	0.1524	0.1573	0.1497	0.1460
			16	0.0530	0.0725	0.0563	0.0575	0.0541	0.0566
			17	0.0175	0.0233	0.0199	0.0197	0.0176	0.0172
			18	0.0052	0.0058	0.0057	0.0054	0.0052	0.0053
	10	50	15	0.3601	0.6202	0.3587	0.4193	0.4077	0.3497
			16	0.1879	0.3427	0.1951	0.2213	0.1999	0.1808
			17	0.0838	0.1485	0.0858	0.0956	0.0861	0.0784
			18	0.0332	0.0544	0.0332	0.0358	0.0335	0.0316
		150	36	0.2849	0.5052	0.2934	0.3378	0.3136	0.2919
			37	0.1858	0.3406	0.1930	0.2212	0.1974	0.1790
			38	0.1146	0.2038	0.1172	0.1317	0.1190	0.1053
			39	0.0668	0.1154	0.0688	0.0762	0.0682	0.0619
			40	0.0374	0.0626	0.0402	0.0430	0.0378	0.0336
			41	0.0202	0.0316	0.0205	0.0219	0.0203	0.0185
			42	0.0103	0.0160	0.0099	0.0110	0.0103	0.0095
			43	0.0042	0.0065	0.0040	0.0044	0.0042	0.0042
50	5	100	5	0.8544	0.9670	0.8330	0.8682	1.6847	0.8661
			6	0.3162	0.4491	0.3228	0.3322	0.3708	0.3009
			7	0.0622	0.0808	0.0624	0.0617	0.0640	0.0533
			8	0.0100	0.0097	0.0079	0.0078	0.0100	0.0078
	10	150	14	0.5396	0.8377	0.5588	0.6353	0.7222	0.5814
			15	0.2864	0.5159	0.3106	0.3497	0.3276	0.3138
			16	0.1295	0.2302	0.1302	0.1478	0.1372	0.1375
			17	0.0493	0.0835	0.0438	0.0513	0.0504	0.0548
			18	0.0156	0.0247	0.0160	0.0171	0.0157	0.0184
			19	0.0060	0.0074	0.0051	0.0053	0.0060	0.0060

The simulation is based on 10,000 trials.

16.2.5 Approximations and Inequalities for the Expected Size and Standard Deviation

Since $S'_{m,m}(a)$ is a discrete random variable,

$$E(S'_{m,m}(a)) = \sum_{k=1}^{m^2} P(S'_{m,m}(a) \geq k) \qquad (16.60)$$

Table 16.8. Comparison of five approximations to $P(S_{m,m}(a) \geq k)$ for a Poisson model.

N	m	a	k	(16.52)	(16.54)	(16.56)	(16.57)	(16.59)	Simulation
25	5	150	12	0.8952	0.9813	0.8518	0.8968	1.0000	0.9374
			13	0.6784	0.8514	0.6571	0.6963	0.9646	0.7142
			14	0.4006	0.5575	0.4014	0.4215	0.4769	0.4159
			15	0.1895	0.2792	0.1977	0.2071	0.2042	0.1939
			16	0.0794	0.1123	0.0860	0.0871	0.0818	0.0787
			17	0.0278	0.0388	0.0309	0.0312	0.0281	0.0282
			18	0.0100	0.0133	0.0108	0.0107	0.0100	0.0096
			19	0.0027	0.0039	0.0031	0.0032	0.0027	0.0030
		300	20	0.9193	0.9863	0.0866	0.9118	1.0000	0.9504
			21	0.7766	0.9190	0.7423	0.7846	1.0000	0.8119
			22	0.5761	0.7491	0.5684	0.5947	0.7616	0.5937
			23	0.3747	0.5103	0.3726	0.3898	0.4408	0.3790
			24	0.2137	0.2974	0.2173	0.2251	0.2329	0.2128
			25	0.1097	0.1514	0.1172	0.1187	0.1144	0.1087
			26	0.0521	0.0703	0.0579	0.0574	0.0532	0.0500
			27	0.0252	0.0311	0.0264	0.0260	0.0255	0.0239
			28	0.0104	0.0126	0.0108	0.0107	0.0104	0.0103
			29	0.0044	0.0050	0.0042	0.0042	0.0044	0.0044
100	5	1000	9	0.9784	0.9981	0.9737	0.9820	1.0000	0.9846
			10	0.6718	0.8178	0.6708	0.6943	1.0000	0.6879
			11	0.2506	0.3411	0.2379	0.2544	0.2860	0.2662
			12	0.0626	0.0833	0.0683	0.0682	0.0668	0.0703
			13	0.0172	0.0200	0.0134	0.0146	0.0174	0.0173
			14	0.0021	0.0047	0.0034	0.0036	0.0021	0.0041
	10	1000	23	0.4359	0.6801	0.4416	0.4960	0.5602	0.4248
			24	0.2235	0.3842	0.2332	0.2615	0.2506	0.2192
			25	0.1097	0.1802	0.1118	0.1225	0.1157	0.1028
			26	0.0456	0.0758	0.0491	0.0527	0.0466	0.0438
			27	0.0169	0.0295	0.0199	0.0215	0.0170	0.0178

The simulation is based on 10,000 trials.

and

$$\mathrm{Var}(S'_{m,m}(a)) = 2\sum_{k=1}^{m^2} k P(S'_{m,m}(a) \geq k) - E(S'_{m,m}(a))\left[1 + E(S'_{m,m}(a))\right].$$

$$(16.61)$$

Approximations and inequalities for $P(S'_{m,m}(a) \geq k)$ yield approximations and inequalities, respectively, for $E(S'_{m,m}(a))$ and $\mathrm{Var}(S'_{m,m}(a))$. In Tables 16.9 and 16.10, we present approximations and inequalities for $E(S'_{m,m}(a))$ based on a product-type approximation (16.51), improved Poisson approximation (16.56), compound Poisson approximation (16.57), and Bonferroni-type inequality (16.59), for selected values of the parameters for the binomial and Poisson models. To

Table 16.9. Approximations for $E(S_{m,m}(a))$ for a Bernoulli model, $m = 5$.

N	a	(16.52)	(16.56)	(16.57)	(16.59)	Simulation
25	10	2.4501	2.3347	2.4913	2.5676	2.5079
	25	4.0977	3.9965	4.1247	4.3464	4.1815
100	25	1.9362	1.9208	2.0095	2.0580	2.0124
	100	3.2330	3.2369	3.2869	3.2899	3.2697

The simulation is based on 10,000 trials.

Table 16.10. Approximations for $E(S_{m,m}(a))$ for a Poisson model, $m = 5$.

N	a	(16.52)	(16.56)	(16.57)	(16.59)	Simulation
25	50	6.4108	6.2669	6.4506	6.7003	6.4868
	150	13.2705	13.1387	13.3196	13.7694	13.3924
100	250	4.9380	4.9186	4.9741	5.2053	4.9529
	1000	9.9831	9.9681	10.0186	10.3705	10.0340

The simulation is based on 10,000 trials.

evaluate the performance of these approximations we present simulated values for $E(S'_{m,m}(a))$ based on 10,000 trials.

16.2.6 Simulation Algorithms

16.2.6.1 Binomial Model

We proceed to describe an algorithm for evaluating $P(E_1 \mid B)$, $P(E_1 \cap E_2 \mid B)$, $P(E_1 \cap E_3 \mid B)$, and $P(E_1 \cap E_2 \cap E_3 \mid B)$, for the binomial model. Let $X_{i,j}$, $1 \le i, j \le N$, be i.i.d. binomial random variables with parameters $n \ge 1$ and $0 < p < 1$. The joint distribution of $X_{i,j}$, $1 \le i, j \le N$, conditional on B, is a multivariate hypergeometric distribution given by

$$P(X_{1,1} = x_{1,1}, \ldots, X_{N,N} = x_{N,N} \mid B) = \frac{\binom{n}{x_{1,1}} \cdots \binom{n}{x_{N,N}}}{\binom{N^2 n}{a}}, \quad (16.62)$$

where $0 \le x_{i,j}$ and $0 \le x_{N,N} = a - \sum_{j=1}^{N-1} \sum_{i=1}^{N} x_{i,j}$ are integers. Let $V_{1,1}, \ldots, V_{N,N}$ be a sequence of random variables with the multivariate hypergeometric distribution given in (16.62). For $1 \le t \le 3$, it follows that

$$P\left(\bigcap_{s=1}^{t} E_s \mid B\right) = P\left\{\bigcap_{s=1}^{t} \bigcap_{i_2=1}^{N-m+1} \left(\sum_{i=t}^{m+t-1} \sum_{j=i_2}^{i_2+m-1} V_{i,j} \le k-1\right)\right\} \quad (16.63)$$

and

$$P(E_1 \cap E_3 \mid B) = P\left\{\bigcap_{t=1,3} \bigcap_{i_2=1}^{N-m+1} \left(\sum_{i=t}^{m+t-1} \sum_{j=i_2}^{i_2+m-1} V_{i,j} \le k-1\right)\right\}. \quad (16.64)$$

To evaluate the probabilities given in (16.63) and (16.64) we use the algorithm in Patefield (1981) for simulating the multivariate hypergeometric distribution for

$V_{1,1}, \ldots, V_{m+2,N}$, given by

$$P(V_{1,1} = v_{1,1}, \ldots, V_{m+2,N} = v_{m+2,N})$$

$$= \frac{\binom{n}{v_{1,1}} \cdots \binom{n}{v_{m+2,N}} \binom{N(N-m-2)n}{a - \sum_{i=1}^{m+2} \sum_{j=1}^{N} v_{i,j}}}{\binom{N^2 n}{a}}.$$

The results of this simulation are arranged in an $(m+2) \times N$ matrix. This process is repeated 10,000 times to obtain simulated values of the probabilities given in (16.63) and (16.64).

16.2.6.2 Poisson Model

Let $X_{i,j}, 1 \leq i, j \leq N$, be i.i.d. Poisson random variables with mean μ. The joint distribution of $X_{i,j}, 1 \leq i, j \leq N$, conditional on B, is a multinomial distribution given by

$$P(X_{1,1} = x_{1,1}, \ldots, X_{N,N} = x_{N,N} \mid B) = \binom{a}{x_{1,1}, \ldots, x_{N,N}} \left(\frac{1}{N^2}\right)^a,$$

$$(16.65)$$

where $0 \leq x_{i,j}$ and $0 \leq x_{N,N} = a - \sum_{j=1}^{N-1} \sum_{i=1}^{N} x_{i,j}$ are integers. Let $W_{1,1}, \ldots,$ $W_{N,N}$ be a sequence of random variables with the multinomial distribution given in (16.65). For $1 \leq t \leq 3$, it follows that

$$P\left(\bigcap_{s=1}^{t} E_s \mid B\right) = P\left\{\bigcap_{s=1}^{t} \bigcap_{i_2=1}^{N-m+1} \left(\sum_{i=t}^{m+t-1} \sum_{j=i_2}^{i_2+m-1} W_{i,j} \leq k - 1\right)\right\} \quad (16.66)$$

and

$$P(E_1 \cap E_3 \mid B) = P\left\{\bigcap_{t=1,3} \bigcap_{i_2=1}^{N-m+1} \left(\sum_{i=t}^{m+t-1} \sum_{j=i_2}^{i_2+m-1} W_{i,j} \leq k - 1\right)\right\}. \quad (16.67)$$

To evaluate the probabilities given in (16.66) and (16.67), we use the Fortran IMSL library for simulating the multinomial distribution for $W_{1,1}, \ldots, W_{m+2,N}$, given by

$$P(W_{1,1} = w_{1,1}, \ldots, W_{m+2,N} = w_{m+2,N})$$

$$= \binom{a}{w_{1,1}, \ldots, w_{m+2,N}, w^*} \left(\frac{1}{N^2}\right)^{\sum_{i=1}^{m+2} \sum_{j=1}^{N} w_{i,j}} \left(1 - \frac{(m+2)N}{N^2}\right)^{a-w^*},$$

where $w^* = a - \sum_{i=1}^{m+2} \sum_{j=1}^{N} w_{i,j}$. The results of this simulation are arranged in an $(m+2) \times N$ matrix. This process is repeated 10,000 times to obtain simulated values of the probabilities given in (16.66) and (16.67).

16.3 A Scan Statistic for a Two-Dimensional Poisson Process

Let $\{X(s, t); 0 \leq s, t < \infty\}$ be a two-dimensional homogeneous Poisson process with intensity λ. For $0 \leq s, t < \infty$ and $0 \leq u, v < \infty$, let $Y_{s,t}(u, v)$ be the number of points in the rectangle $[s, s + u) \times [t, t + v)$, of dimension $u \times v$ with a southwest location at s, t. For $0 < u < T_1 < \infty$ and $0 < v < T_2 < \infty$, the two-dimensional *scan statistic*

$$S_{u,v} = S_{u,v}(\lambda, T_1, T_2) = \max_{\substack{0 \leq s < T_1 - u \\ 0 \leq t \leq T_2 - v}} Y_{s,t}(u, v), \qquad (16.68)$$

denotes the largest number of points in any rectangle of dimension $u \times v$ within $[0, T_1) \times [0, T_2)$. The approximations for the distribution of $S_{u,v}$ presented here are based on the results in Alm (1997, 1999).

To approximate the distribution of $S_{u,v}$, fix a value of t and scan the rectangular strip $[0, T_1) \times [t, t + v)$ with a rectangle of dimension $u \times v$. For a fixed value of $0 \leq t < \infty$, $X^{(1)}(s) = X_t^{(1)}(s) = X(s, t)$ is a one-dimensional Poisson process with intensity λv. For $0 < u < T_1 < \infty$, let $Y_{t,s}^{(1)}(u) = X^{(1)}(s + u) - X^{(1)}(s)$, be the number of points in the rectangle $[s, s+u) \times [t, t+v)$, of dimension $u \times v$ with a southwest location at s, t. $Y_{s,t}^{(1)}(u)$ is the scanning process associated with the one-dimensional Poisson process $X_t^{(1)}(s)$ in the rectangular strip $[0, T_1) \times [t, t + v)$. For the Poisson process $X_t^{(1)}(s)$ and its associated scanning process $Y_{s,t}^{(1)}(u)$, we can define the scan statistic

$$S_u^{(1)} = S_u^{(1)}(t) = \max_{0 \leq s \leq T_1 - u} Y_{s,t}^{(1)}(u). \qquad (16.69)$$

For a fixed value of t, it follows from (11.52) that

$$P\left(S_u^{(1)} < k\right) \approx F_p(k - 1; \lambda uv)e^{-(1-(\lambda uv/k))\lambda v(T_1 - u)p(k-1, \lambda uv)}$$

$$= F_p(k - 1; \lambda^*)e^{-(1-(\lambda^*/k))\lambda^*(T_1^* - 1)p(k-1, \lambda^*)}, \qquad (16.70)$$

where $\lambda^* = \lambda uv$, $T_1^* = T_1/u$, and $T_2^* = T_2/v$. In fact, three parameters are sufficient here.

Now, $\{S_u^{(1)}(t), 0 \leq t \leq T_2 - v\}$ is also a one-dimensional stationary stochastic process. It follows that

$$\max_{0 \leq t \leq T_2 - v} S_u^{(1)}(t) = \max_{0 \leq t \leq T_2 - v} \left(\max_{0 \leq s \leq T_1 - u} Y_{s,t}^{(1)}(u) \right)$$

$$= \max_{0 \leq t \leq T_2 - v} \left(\max_{0 \leq s \leq T_1 - u} X^{(1)}(s + u) - X^{(1)}(s) \right)$$

$$= \max_{0 \leq t \leq T_2 - v} \left(\max_{0 \leq s \leq T_1 - u} Y_{s,t}(u, v) \right)$$

$$= \max_{\substack{0 \leq s \leq T_1 - u \\ 0 \leq t \leq T_2 - v}} Y_{s,t}(u, v) = S_{u,v}(\lambda, T_1, T_2). \qquad (16.71)$$

Therefore, the two-dimensional scan statistic $S_{u,v}$ can be viewed as a scan statistic associated with a one-dimensional scanning process $\{S_u^{(1)}(t), 0 \leq t \leq T_2 - v\}$. Employing the approach used in the one-dimensional case, Alm (1997) obtains

$$P(S_{u,v} < k) \approx P(S_u^{(1)} < k)e^{-\gamma_k}, \qquad (16.72)$$

where an approximation for $P(S_u^{(1)} < k)$ is given in (16.70) and γ_k is the expected number of primary $k - 1$ upcrossings of the scanning process $\{S_u^{(1)}(t), 0 \leq t \leq T_2 - v\}$. The *primary* upcrossings occur almost independently of each other, while the *secondary* upcrossings are the ones that follow closely after the primary upcrossings (Alm, 1997). γ_k can be approximated using the same approach that leads to the approximation in (16.70) to get

$$\gamma_k \approx \gamma_k^{(1)} = \left(1 - \frac{\lambda uv}{k-1}\right) \lambda uv \left(\frac{T_2}{v} - 1\right) P(S_u^{(1)} = k - 2)$$
$$= \left(1 - \frac{\lambda^*}{k-1}\right) \lambda^*(T_2^* - 1)P(S_u^{(1)} = k - 2), \qquad (16.73)$$

where $P(S_u^{(1)} = k - 2)$ can be approximated from (16.70). Substitute (16.73) into (16.72) to obtain an approximation for $P(S_{u,v} < k)$:

$$P(S_{u,v} < k) \approx P(S_u^{(1)} < k)e^{-\gamma_k^{(1)}}, \qquad (16.74)$$

where an approximation for $P(S_u^{(1)} < k)$ is given in (16.70).

Approximation (16.74) for $P(S_{u,v} < k)$ does not take into account the possiblity of having several primary or secondary upcrossings of level $k - 1$ by the scanning process $\{S_u^{(1)}(t), 0 \leq t \leq T_2 - v\}$. Alm (1997, 1999) argues that the effect of the multiple secondary upcrossings is negligible and proposes an improved approximation for γ_k that takes into account multiple primary upcrossings. It is based on the following approximation for γ_k:

$$\gamma_k \approx \gamma_k^{(2)} = \left(1 - \frac{\lambda uv}{k}\right) \lambda uv \left(\frac{T_2}{v} - 1\right) (\mu_{k-1} - \mu_k)e^{-\mu_k}$$
$$= \left(1 - \frac{\lambda^*}{k}\right) \lambda^*(T_2^* - 1)(\mu_{k-1} - \mu_k)e^{-\mu_k}, \qquad (16.75)$$

where

$$\mu_k \approx \left(1 - \frac{\lambda uv}{k-1}\right) \lambda uv \left(\frac{T_1}{u} - 1\right) p(k - 2; \lambda uv)$$
$$= \left(1 - \frac{\lambda^*}{k-1}\right) \lambda^*(T_1^* - 1)p(k - 2; \lambda^*). \qquad (16.76)$$

Substitute (16.74) and (16.75) into (16.72) to obtain

$$P(S_{u,v} < k) \approx P(S_u^{(1)} < k)e^{-\gamma_k^{(2)}}, \qquad (16.77)$$

where an approximation for $P\left(S_u^{(1)} < k\right)$ is given in (16.70). Based on numerical results in Alm (1997, 1999), approximation (16.77) is more accurate than approximation (16.74) for small or moderate values of k, if $T_1^* = T_2^*$. For $T_1^* \neq T_2^*$, Alm (1999) recommends to reparametrize so that $T_1^* < T_2^*$, and use approximation (16.74).

16.4 A Scan Statistic for N Points Uniformly Distributed in a Two-Dimensional Rectangular Region

Let $X_{1,1}, \ldots, X_{1,N}$ and $X_{2,1}, \ldots, X_{2,N}$ be i.i.d. observations from a uniform distribution on the interval $[0, 1)$. For $1 \leq i \leq N$, let $\mathbf{X}_i = (X_{1,i}, X_{2,i})$. Then $\mathbf{X}_1, \ldots, \mathbf{X}_N$ can be viewed as N random points in the unit square $[0, 1) \times [0, 1)$. For $0 < u, v < 1$, $0 \leq s < 1 - u$, and $0 \leq t < 1 - v$, let $Y_{s,t}(u, v)$ be the number of points in the rectangle $[s, s + u) \times [t, t + v)$, of dimension $u \times v$ with a southwest location at s, t. The conditional two-dimensional *scan statistic*

$$S_{u,v} = \max_{0 \leq s \leq 1-u, 0 \leq t \leq 1-v} Y_{s,t}(u, v), \qquad (16.78)$$

is the largest number of points in any rectangle of dimension $u \times v$ within the unit square $[0, 1) \times [0, 1)$. For simplicity, we have chosen to present here the results for the unit square. The results are valid for any bounded rectangular region. We are interested in deriving approximations and inequalities for

$$P(k; N, u, v) = P(S_{u,v} \geq k). \qquad (16.79)$$

Exact results for $P(k; N, u, v)$ for $k = N - 1$, N are given in Chapter 5. The inequalities for $P(k; N, u, v)$ derived below are based on Naus (1965b). An upper bound for $P(k; N, u, v)$ follows immediately from the fact that if we have a rectangle of dimension $u \times v$ with at least k points, then there are at least k points among $X_{1,1}, \ldots, X_{1,N}$ and among $X_{2,1}, \ldots, X_{2,N}$, respectively, that are within an interval of length u and v, respectively. Since these observations are i.i.d. from the uniform distribution on $[0, 1)$, we obtain

$$P(k; N, u, v) \leq P(k; N, u)P(k; N, v), \qquad (16.80)$$

where $P(k; N, u)$ and $P(k; N, v)$ are the one-dimensional scan statistic probabilities discussed in Chapters 8–10. Now, k or more points are contained in a rectangle of dimension $u \times v$ if at least k of the first coordinates of $\mathbf{X}_1, \ldots, \mathbf{X}_N$ are contained within an interval of length u, and if at least k of the second coordinates of $\mathbf{X}_1, \ldots, \mathbf{X}_N$, corresponding to those first coordinates, are contained within an interval of length v. This implies that

$$P(k; N, u)P(k; k, v) \leq P(k; N, u, v). \qquad (16.81)$$

Since inequality (16.81) is symmetric in u and v we get

$$\max\{P(k; N, u)P(k; k, v), P(k; k, u)P(k; N, v)\} \leq P(k; N, u, v). \quad (16.82)$$

Naus (1965b, Theorem 2) showed that for $k > N/2$, as u and v approach zero, the ratio of the upper bound in (16.81) to the lower bound in (16.82), is given by $\binom{N}{k}$. The following upper bound (Naus, 1965b, Theorem 3) converges to the lower bound (16.82) for $k > N/2$, as u and v approach zero:

$$P(k; N, u, v) \leq P(k; N, u)P(k; N, v)$$

$$- \left(1 - \binom{N}{k}^{-1}\right) P(1 : k; N, u, 1)P(1 : k; N, 1, v) \quad (16.83)$$

where $P(1 : k; N, u, 1)$ ($P(1 : k; N, 1, v)$ resp.) is the probability that there exists only one set of k first (second, resp.) coordinates of the N random points contained in an interval of length u (v, resp.) and there are no intervals of length u (v, resp.) that contain more than k of the first (second, resp.) coordinates.

As a consequence of this improved upper bound (Naus, 1965b, Theorem 4) obtains an asymptotic expression for $P(k; N, u, v)$ when $k > N/2$, as u and v approach zero:

$$P(k; N, u, v) = k^2 \binom{N}{k}(uv)^{k-1} + o([uv]^{k-1}). \quad (16.84)$$

Based on this result the use of the lower bound in (16.82) as an approximation for $P(k; N, u, v)$ is recommended in Naus (1965b).

We now present an approximation for $P(k; N, u, v)$ based on Loader (1991, Theorem 3.1). The approach used in Loader (1991) is based on methods of large deviation theory. Let u, v, and $\varepsilon > 0$. Assume that $uv(1 + \varepsilon)$ is a rational number and $N \to \infty$ with $k = Nuv(1 + \varepsilon)$ being an integer. Then, for large N:

$$P(k; N, u, v) \approx \frac{N^2 uv(1 - u)(1 - v)\varepsilon^3}{(1 - uv)^3(1 + \varepsilon)} b(k; N, uv)$$

$$+ \left[\frac{Nv(1 - u)\varepsilon}{1 - uv} + \frac{Nu(1 - v)\varepsilon^2}{(1 + \varepsilon)(1 - uv)^2} \right.$$

$$\left. + \frac{(1 + \varepsilon)(1 - uv)}{\varepsilon} \right] b(k; N, uv). \quad (16.85)$$

The first line in approximation (16.85) is a first-order approximation given in Loader (1991, Theorem 3.1). The terms on the second and third line of approximation (16.85) are second-order terms that improve significantly on the first-order approximation. Based on the numerical results presented in Loader (1991) for $u = v = .5$, approximation (16.85) performed quite well.

17
Number of Clusters: Ordered Spacings

17.1 Notation and Introduction

Let $X_{(1)} \leq X_{(2)} \leq \cdots \leq X_{(N)}$ be the ordered values of the X's where N could be fixed or random. Define the event A_j to occur if the distance between $r + 1$ consecutive observations is less than or equal to w, that is,

$$A_j = \{X_{(j+r)} - X_{(j)} \leq w\}.$$

Note that A_j is the event that the sum of r-spacings is less than w. The terminology r-scan has become standard in this field and we use that term consistently in this chapter, rather than focusing attention on the $r + 1$ (or k) points in the cluster. The indicator variable associated with A_j is

$$I_j = 1 \qquad \text{if } X_{(j+r)} - X_{(j)} \leq w, \qquad (17.1)$$
$$= 0 \qquad \text{otherwise.}$$

As noted in (10.1):

$$P(A_1) = \sum_{i=r}^{N} b(i; N, w) \quad \text{conditional case,}$$

$$= \sum_{i=r}^{\infty} p(i, w\lambda) \quad \text{unconditional case} \qquad (17.2)$$

where λ is the expected number of events per unit time, and where $b(i, N, w)$ and $p(i, \mu)$ denote $P(Y = i)$, where Y has a BIN(N, w) distribution in the former case, and a POSN(μ) distribution in the latter case.

Berman and Eagelson (1985) show that for the conditional case

$$P(A_2^c \cap A_1) = P(A_1^c \cap A_2) = \sum_{i=r}^{N}(-1)^{i-r}b(i; N, w). \qquad (17.3)$$

Su and Wallenstein (2000) modify this result for the unconditional case to find

$$P(A_2^c \cap A_1) = \sum_{i=r}^{\infty}(-1)^{i-r}p(i, w\lambda).$$

Define the number of nonoverlapping clusters by

$$\xi = \sum I_j,$$

and note that, in both the conditional and unconditional cases,

$$E(\xi) = (E(N) - r)P(A_1). \qquad (17.4)$$

Dembo and Karlin (1992) define a nonoverlapping cluster recursively by setting the indicator variable back to zero if a nonoverlapping cluster starts in one of the previous $r - 1$ events, that is, the indicator variable for the start of a nonoverlapping cluster is

$$I_j'(w) = I_j(w) \prod_{i=1}^{r-1}[1 - I_j'(w)], \qquad (17.5)$$

where $I_j'(w) = 0$ for $i \leq 0$.

Define the number of nonoverlapping clusters as

$$\eta_r(w) = \sum I_j'(w). \qquad (17.6)$$

(We shall generally drop the subscript and the argument w, until Section 17.8.)

Dembo and Karlin (1992) argue that if N increases and w approaches zero as $O(1/N^{1+1/r})$, the distribution of both ξ and η is a Poisson distribution with mean $E(\xi) = (N - r)P(A_1)$ (or possibly an asymptotic limit thereof), so that

$$P(\xi \geq m) \approx \sum_{i=m}^{\infty} \exp\{-E(\xi)\}E(\xi)^i/i!,$$

$$P(\eta \geq m) \approx \sum_{i=m}^{\infty} \exp\{-E(\xi)\}E(\xi)^i/i!. \qquad (17.7)$$

The required limiting procedure is quite restrictive and assumes a relatively "sparse" distribution of events relative to w. Glaz, Naus, Roos, and Wallenstein (1994) demonstrate that the above approximation for $P(\xi \geq m)$ behaves poorly in the range of values they considered (which are not necessarily close to the limiting procedure).

Glaz and Naus (1983) give an expression for Var(ξ). Huffer and Lin (1997a) find a simpler expression, given in (10.11).

It would be tempting to improve upon (17.7) utilizing a Poisson approximation for the distribution of η:

$$P(\eta \geq m) \approx \sum_{i=m}^{\infty} \exp\{-E(\eta)\}E(\eta)^i / i! . \tag{17.8}$$

However, the recursive nature of the definition in (17.5) precludes exact computation of the mean. In the next three sections, we will give three local definitions of declumping which allow the mean to be approximated: one closely mimicking the global, a Markovian one, and one related to the compound Poisson distribution.

17.2 Local Declumping which Mimics the Global One

Section 17.6 gives a simple method to approximate $E(\eta)$ based on a tail probability. It would appear preferable to estimate $E(\eta)$ directly, rather than what could be, in some applications, an exteme tail probability. Here, we approximate the expected number by replacing the recursive definition of a nonoverlapping cluster in (17.5) by a nonrecursive one put forward by Arratia, Goldstein, and Gordon (1990) in the context of discrete outcomes. Specifically, for $1 \leq j \leq n-r$, define the indicator variable for an observation starting a new clump (nonoverlapping cluster) as

$$I_j^*(w) = I_j(w) \prod_{i=1}^{r-1} [1 - I_{j-i}(w)]. \tag{17.9}$$

For the conditional case, the expected number of clumps using this definition is

$$\mu \equiv E\left[\sum_{j=1}^{N-r} I_j^*(w)\right] = \sum_{j=1}^{r-1} P[I_j^*(w) = 1] + (N - 2r + 1)P[I_j^*(w) = 1]. \tag{17.10}$$

Thus the suggested approximation is

$$P(\eta \geq m) \approx \sum_{i=m}^{\infty} e^{-\mu}\mu^i / i! . \tag{17.11}$$

For the conditional case, $P[I_j^*(w) = 1]$, denoted in Chapter 9 by α_1^*, is given by (17.1), while Berman and Eagelson (1985) have shown that $P[I_2^*(w) = 1]$, previously denoted as α_2^*, is given by

$$P[I_2^*(w) = 1] = \sum_{j=r}^{N} (-1)^{j-r} b(j; N, w). \tag{17.12}$$

Equation (9.36), derived in Glaz (1992), states that for $3 \le j \le r$:

$$P[I_j^*(w) = 1] = b(r; N, w) - b(r + 1; N, w)$$

$$+ \sum_{k=j}^{N-r} (-1)^{k-1} b(r + k; N, w) \prod_{i=1}^{j-2} \left[\frac{k(k-1)}{i(i+1)} - 1 \right]. \quad (17.13)$$

For the conditional case, μ is given by substituting the above equations into (17.10), and the approximation to $P(\eta = m)$ is given by (17.11). (Glaz, Naus, Roos, and Wallenstein (1994), come close to this suggestion, but suggest, but then reject, using this Poisson distribution to approximate the distribution of ξ rather than η.)

17.3   A Markovian Method of Declumping Leading to a Pólya–Aeppli Distribution

Su and Wallenstein (2000) use a Markovian method of declumping, in which a new clump starts if $I_j = 1$ and $I_{j-1} = 0$, leading to a definition of the number of nonoverlapping clusters as

$$C = I_1 + \sum_{j=2}^{N-r} (1 - I_{j-1}) I_j. \quad (17.14)$$

This *Markovian* definition of a clump could be viewed as an extension of the idea by Arratia, Goldstein, and Gordon (1990) who examine the probability of long head runs, in which a failure (tail) ends the clump.

From the definition of (17.14) it follows that

$$E(C) = P(I_1 = 1) + \sum_{j=2}^{N-r} P[I_{j-1} = 0, I_j = 1]$$

$$= P(I_1 = 1) + (N - r - 1) P(I_2^* = 1) \approx (N - r) P(I_2^* = 1).$$

Let U_j be the number of r-spacings less than w in the jth clump so that

$$\xi = \sum_{j=1}^{C} U_j.$$

(A more formal definition of U_j is given in Su and Wallenstein.) To approximate the distribution of ξ, Su and Wallenstein (2000) make the following assumptions:

(1) C has a Poisson distribution.

(2) The clump size $\{U_j, j = 1, 2, \ldots, C\}$ are independent and identically distributed (i.i.d.), independent of the number of clumps, C.

(3) $P\{A_j \mid A_{j-1}, A_{j-2}, \ldots, A_2, A_1\} = P\{A_j \mid A_{j-1}\}.$

They show that these assumptions imply that for $m = 1, 2, \ldots, N - r$:

$$P(\xi = m) \approx P(A_2 \mid A_1)^m \exp[-E(C)] \sum_{j=1}^{m} \binom{m-1}{j-1}$$

$$\times [E(C)P(A_2^c \mid A_1)/P(A_2 \mid A_1)]^j /j!. \qquad (17.15)$$

The distribution in (17.15) might, as in Johnson, Kotz, and Kemp (1992), be termed a "Poisson stopped geometric distribution." This is also known as a Pólya–Aeppli distribution (Pólya (1930)) which "arises in a model formed by supposing that objects arise in clusters, the numbers of clusters having a Poisson distribution, while the numbers of objects per cluster has a [shifted] geometric distribution" (Johnson, Kotz, and Kemp (1992, p. 378)).

It follows that

$$\mathrm{Var}(\xi) \approx E(C)[1 + P(A_2 \mid A_1)]/[1 - P(A_2 \mid A_1)]^2$$

$$\approx E(\xi)[1 + P(A_2 \mid A_1)]/[1 - P(A_2 \mid A_1)]. \qquad (17.16)$$

These expressions are the same for the conditional and unconditional cases except for different values of $P(A_1)$ and $P(A_2 \mid A_1)$, and replacing N by $E(N)$.

17.4 Compound Poisson Approach

Variants of the highly accurate approximation to be described in this section have been developed by Roos (1993a,b), Lin (1993), Glaz, Naus, Roos, and Wallenstein (1994), Huffer and Lin (1997a), and Su and Wallenstein (2000). As noted by Barbour, Holst, and Janson (1992) and Glaz, Naus, Roos, and Wallenstein (1994), there are two closely related methods to improve upon the simple Poisson approximation:

(i) those based on a declumping process; and

(ii) those based on a compound Poisson approach discussed in general by Barbour et al., and in detail for this application by Roos (1993a,b).

Huffer and Lin (1997a) acknowledge previous theoretical work that proved that the compound Poisson distribution is a limiting distribution for the distribution of ξ. However, they view the problem as approximating the distribution of ξ by that of

$$V = \sum i V_i, \qquad (17.17)$$

where V_i are independent variates with a Poisson distribution and $E(V_i) = \lambda_i$, so that $\sum \lambda_i < \infty$. From this definition it would follow that:

(i) The distribution of η would be the approximated by the sum of independent Poisson variates with mean $\sum E(V_i) = \sum \lambda_i$. Thus to approximate the distribution of η (and certainly that of $\sum V_i$), we would replace $E(\eta)$ in (17.8) with $E(\sum V_i)$.

(ii) The distribution of ξ can be approximated by a compound Poisson distribution (Glaz, Naus, Roos, and Wallenstein (1994)), that is,

$$P(\xi = m) \approx \sum \prod_{i=1}^{g-1} p(\beta_i, \lambda_i), \qquad (17.18)$$

where the summation is over all nonnegative integers β_i such that

$$\beta_1 + 2\beta_2 + \cdots + (g-1)\beta_{g-1} = m.$$

A particular useful consequence is

$$P(\xi = 0) = P(\eta = 0) \approx \exp\left(-\sum_i \lambda_i\right). \qquad (17.19)$$

Roos (1993a,b) and Glaz, Naus, Roos, and Wallenstein (1994) show that if $N \to \infty$ and $w \to 0$ in such a way that $E(\xi)$ remains fixed, then the maximum of the differences in probabilities in (17.18) is of order $1/N$. Note that these relationships are not as-yet well defined since the possibly infinite sequence of the λ's has not been defined.

The approximation based on (17.18) has a firmer methodological justification than some of the previously suggested approximations. However, the problem with this approximation is calculating the potentially infinite sequence of the λ's. A second technical problem is the calculation of λ_j, $j > r$ or $j > N$. The latter case is impossible, and the former introduces problems in the definition of η, since both intuition and the optimal definition precludes clumps with more than $k + 1 = r$ overlapping clusters. Fortunately, the methods developed for obtaining values of λ, solve both problems by setting $\lambda_j = 0$ for $j \geq r$.

Roos (1993a,b), and the citation by Glaz, Naus, Roos, and Wallenstein (1994), give an expression for the λ's, but this involves complicated probabilities, and no explicit expression of these is available. [It involves the probability that somewhere in a sequence of $2r$ dependent events, there will be g "successes," for example, $P(\sum_{j=i}^{2r} I_j) = g$.] Roos (1993a,b, Remark 3.6), suggests an approximation only involving probabilities concerning a sequence of r dependent events.

Glaz, Naus, Roos, and Wallenstein (1994) suggest a further approximation where the sequence of λ's is truncated at r, and $2 \leq j \leq r$:

$$\lambda_j = P(A_1)[E(N) - r][1 - \omega]^2 \omega^{j-1}, \qquad (17.20)$$

where $\omega = P(A_2 \mid A_1)$. The accuracy of the approximation is apparently enhanced by constraining the mean to be equal to $E(\xi)$ by setting

$$\lambda_1 = E(\xi) - \sum_{j=2}^{r} j\lambda_j = P(A_1)[E(N) - r][1 - 2\omega + \omega^2 - r\omega^r + (r+1)\omega^r].$$

(17.21)

Huffer and Lin (1997a) first note that the procedure based on (17.18) can be simplified by utilizing the identity

$$jP(\xi = j) = \sum_{i=1}^{j} (i\lambda_i)P(\xi = j - i).$$

(17.22)

They derive the λ's by equating the first g moments of ξ to those of V. Higher-ordered values of λ follow from a geometric series, or a linear programming approach. The expressions are quite complicated when $g \geq 3$, since the moments involve symbolic algebra and equating the moments is nontrivial. However, for $g = 2$, they obtain the expressions

$$\lambda_1 = E(\xi)(1 - u)^2,$$

and for $2 \leq i \leq r - 1$:

$$\lambda_i = \lambda_1 u^{i-1} = E(\xi)(1 - u)^2 u^{i-1},$$

(17.23)

where $u = [\text{Var}(\xi) - E(\xi)]/[\text{Var}(\xi) + E(\xi)]$, and where $\text{Var}(\xi)$ is derived by them and given in (10.11). When these expressions are substituted into (17.18) or (17.22), they yield the approximation termed CPG2.

17.5 The Dandekar-Modified Binomial as an Approximation to the Distribution of η

The Poisson approximations given previously all imply that $E(\eta) = \text{Var}(\eta)$. This could be unduly restrictive as simulations indicate that $E(\eta) > \text{Var}(\eta)$. Su, Wallenstein, and Bishop (2001), present an approximation using a modified binomial distribution derived by Dandekar (1955). Dandekar considered the distribution of M, the number of successes in t trials when the probability of a success in a single trial is π (constant), and the trials would be independent except for the proviso that if a trial produces a success, then the probability of success for the next $(s-1)$ trials is zero. He shows that for $m = 0, 1, 2, \ldots, [t/s]$:

$$P(M \leq m) = (1 - \pi)^{t-ms} \sum_{j=0}^{m} \binom{t - ms + j - 1}{j} \pi^j.$$

(17.24)

Based on the similarity of the two distributions, it is tempting to suggest an approximation for the distribution of η by modifying the three parameters: t, s, and π. It is most natural to set $s - 1 = r$ and $t = n - r$. The choice of π is open to more alternatives than the other choices. By analogy with the definition, we could use $\pi = P(I_r = 1 \mid I_{r-1} = 0, I_{r-2} = 0, \ldots, I_1 = 0)$, which can be expressed in terms of the probabilities given in (9.36). To avoid undue computational problems in (9.36) (that were noted by Glaz (1992)), we prefer to use a further Markovian approximation and replace π by $P(I_2 = 1 \mid I_1 = 0) = P(I_2^* = 1)/P(I_1 = 0)$.

Thus, applying (17.24) suggests the approximation

$$P\{\eta \leq m\} \approx [1 - \Pr(I_2 = 1 \mid I_1 - 0)]^{n-r-m(r+1)} \sum_{j=0}^{m}$$

$$\times \binom{n - r - m(r + 1) + j - 1}{j} [\Pr(I_2 = 1 \mid I_1 = 0)]^{j} (17.25)$$

A possible improvement on the approximation is to perform an iterative procedure and replace π by the value that yields $E(\eta) = \mu$, i.e., that π is the value that satisfies

$$\mu = \sum_{m=1}^{\infty} \left\{ 1 - (1 - \pi)^{n-r-m(r+1)} \sum_{j=0}^{m} \binom{n - r - m(r + 1) + j - 1}{j} \pi^j \right\}.$$

17.6   Another Approach Based on the Q_2/Q_3 Approximation

An approach to this problem in Chapter 3 assumes that the Poisson approximation is valid even fairly far out in the tails ($m = 0$) so that

$$1 - P(r + 1; N, w) = P(\eta = 0) \approx \exp(-E(\eta_r(w))),$$

and thus

$$E(\eta_r(w)) \approx -\ln[1 - P(r + 1; N, w)]. \tag{17.26}$$

We could now substitute any approximation for $P(r + 1; N, w)$, that is valid over the entire distribution (but not ones such as (2.3) that are only valid for small probabilities). In Chapter 3 we used the Q_2/Q_3 approximation, which would yield

$$E(\eta) \approx -(L - 2)\ln(Q_3/Q_2) - \ln(Q_2), \tag{17.27}$$

the last expression often being negligible.

17.7 Summary of Results and Comparison of Procedures

17.7.1 Overlapping Clusters

For the conditional case, the agreement between the probabilities, $P(\xi = m)$, and simulated values is described by Glaz, Naus, Roos, and Wallenstein (1994) (for $N = 100$ and $N = 500$, with $w = .01$ and $.10$), and by Huffer and Lin (1997a). Su and Wallenstein (2000) evaluate the approximation for the unconditional case. The formula based on the compound Poisson approximation (17.18), with the values of the λ's given by Glaz (17.20) or by Huffer and Lin (17.23) appear most accurate. (Huffer and Lin find that their approximation, CPG2, is better than the Glaz approximation for $r \leq 10$.) The approximation based on the Pólya–Aeppli distribution (17.15) gives an interesting insight, and is slightly simpler, but less accurate. The Poisson approximations cannot be recommended, as the variance is appreciably larger than the mean.

17.7.2 Nonoverlapping Clusters

For $N = 300$, Su, Wallenstein, and Bishop (2001) compare the different procedures with respect to estimating the probabilities per se. Despite the apparent failure of the Poisson assumption to hold, the Poisson approximation, substituting μ from (17.10) into (17.11), performs well. The modified binomial in (17.25) does about as well. A superior method is the one given at the end of the Section 17.5 using both the modified binomial and μ, but involves solving an implicit equation.

17.8 Exploratory Approach when r Cannot be Specified with Application to Detecting Clusters of Erythroid-Specific Transcription Factors

We will discuss, in Section 18.6, possible formal approaches for detecting clustering using the conventional "w-scan" statistic for the case where w, the distance between the $k+1 = r$ observations, is not specified a priori. In the example below, we give an alternative exploratory approach, based on a step-wise procedure.

We describe the use of overlapping r-scans to identify gene regulatory regions. These regulatory regions occur in the linear DNA molecule (specific sequences of purine (A or G) and pyrimidine (C or T) nucleotides), both proximal (nearby) and distal to gene transcriptional units. The proximal regulatory regions are termed promoters and the more distal regulatory regions, which can occur many kilobases away from genes or within the introns of genes, are termed enhancers or repressors. (Transcription factors are proteins that contain both DNA binding and protein–protein interaction domains that cooperate to create a multiprotein complex with RNA polymerase II that is competent to regulate transcription of a specific gene.) Tissue-specific control of genes frequently involves a limited set of sequence motifs for binding of transcription factors, some of which are expressed exclusively in the specific tissues. These DNA binding sites are frequently close enough together to result in protein–protein interactions between factors occupying adjacent binding sites. Since the DNA sequence motifs that specify the binding sites of transcription factors are typically only five to ten nucleotides, they occur in abundance throughout the genome by chance. While it is now possible to identify these sites with a high degree of confidence, using position weight matrices, it is not straightforward to determine which of such sites participate in the functional control of genes.

Su, Wallenstein, and Bishop (2001) propose to use the r-scan statistic to find clusters of transcription-factor binding sites that occur in higher density than expected for a uniform distribution, and thus to identify potential tissue-specific regulatory regions in genomic DNA sequences. Similar methods were previously used in a series of influential articles by Karlin and coauthors (Dembo and Karlin, 1992; Karlin and Brendel, 1992; Karlin and Macken, 1991) who found the asymptotic distribution of the "k greatest and k least lengths of sums of r-fragments," and used the statistics to assess inhomogeneities of DNA sequence data. The approach of Su et al. differs from those previously cited by focusing on nonoverlapping rather than overlapping clusters. They argue that to the extent that one is searching in a stepwise manner for clusters, identifying the same general regulatory region over and over again is of minimal interest, and thus efforts should be focused on nonoverlapping clusters.

Specifically, Su et al. apply the proposed method to the detection of significant clusters of erythroid-specific transcription factors (GATA-1, NF-E2, EKLF, and Sp1) within the human β-globin locus sequence with length $L = 73,308$ base pairs (bp). Figure 17.1 shows diagrammatically the locations of all $N = 403$ putative binding sites for transcription factors GATA-1, NF-E2, EKLF, and Sp1 in this sequence.

17.8.1   Calculations with Fixed r

Su et al. begin with seemingly arbitrarily setting $r = 6$. The shortest range containing seven putative binding sites is at 4618–4757 bp, encompassing 140/73,308 $= 0.19\%$ of the sequence ($w = .0019$); the next shortest nonoverlapping region goes from 1124 to 1302 bp encompassing 0.24%. The nonoverlapping six-scan statistic is used to calculate the probabilities of observing one or more six-spacings smaller than .0019, two or more smaller than .0024, etc.

To approximate $P[\eta_6(.0019) = 1]$, substitute $r = 6$ and $w = .0019$ in (17.1), (17.11), and (17.12) to find $P[I_1(.0019) = 1] = .000140$, $P[I_2^*(.0019) = 1] = .000113$, and $\mu = .04443$, so that by (17.11):

$$P[\eta_6(.0019) \geq 1] \approx 1 - e^{-.04443} = .0435.$$

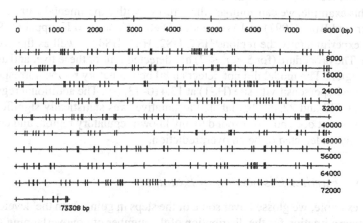

Figure 17.1. Locations of the 403 putative binding sites in human beta globin locus sequence. The 73308 bp is represented linearly as ten continuing horizontal lines. Each putative binding site is marked by a vertical line at the position where it occurs.

Alternatively we could have applied the modified binomial approximation in (17.25) to find $P[I_2^*(.0019) = 1 \mid I_1(.0019) = 0] = .000113$, so that

$$P[\eta_6(.0019) \geq 1] \approx 1 - (1 - .000113)^{397} = .0439.$$

To find the probability that two or more nonoverlapping six-spacings are less than .0024 note that, based on either approximation (17.11) or (17.25), $P[\eta_6(.00243) \geq 2] \approx .011$. Similarly, the probability that five or more nonoverlapping six-spacings are less than .0035 (259/L) (the smallest such distance observed) is .002. We continue this way until we stop since the sixth smallest six-spacing, of width $w = 0.52\%$, yields $P[\eta_6(.0052) = 6] = 0.235$. Thus we have found that under randomness, the probability is approximately .002 of observing five or more clusters of seven putative binding sites, each encompassing less than the fifth smallest observed six-spacing.

17.8.2 Calculations with Multiple Values of r Compared with Experimental Results

In actual application, r is not fixed a priori, and Su et al. repeat the procedure with different values of r. For both $r = 5$ and $r = 7$, they stop after the fifth step, and detect the same regions as for $r = 6$, although in a different order. For $r = 8$, they stop after detecting four of these regions, failing to detect the HS4 region. For $r = 4$, they stop after detecting eight possible regions; one of the additional ones caused by the algorithm now splitting HS3 into two parts. For $r = 3$, no significance was noted for any value of m we evaluated ($m < 10$), while setting $r = 9$, yielded only three of the five regions.

In this example, we can compare these results with experimental data. Crowley, Roeder, and Bina (1997) and Wingender, Dietze, Karas, and Knuppel (1996) detected experimentally the regions HS1, HS2, HS3, HS4, as well as the promoter region. The procedure (for $5 \le r \le 7$) has detected four of these five, and an additional region. The model did not detect an 80 bp regulatory region corresponding to DNAse hypersensitivity site (HS1) at 13,410–13,490. The additional region between 21,938 and 22,196 bp, labeled as putative, was statistically significant for $4 \le r \le 9$, but does not correspond to any known regulatory region, and could be previously undetected or be an overprediction.

17.8.3 Further Discussion of Example

In this example, we glossed over some of the steps in going from the development of an approximation for the distribution of the number of nonoverlapping ($r + 1$) clusters smaller than w, to the more exploratory detection of regulatory regions. First, and most obviously, the formal development assumes r known beforehand, whereas the application seeks out the value of r in an informal way based on the pattern of significance. Other investigators (e.g., Karlin and Brendel (1992), Karlin and Macken (1991), and Leung, Schachtel, and Yu (1994)) have also implicitly used at least somewhat similar stopping rules.

Su, Wallenstein, and Bishop (2001) were fortunate in yielding similar conclusions for a range of values of r. In other cases, the findings may be more inconclusive and there appears to be no omnibus test to summarize findings over r. (For omnibus tests for varying w, see Section 18.6.)

The development of a stopping rule similarly mixes biological expectations with the results of this analysis. We expect to need several regulatory regions (small r-spacings) to provide the flexibility of regulating a gene differently under different stages of development and varying metabolic needs. (To phrase this as a sports analogy: We are searching for a relay team with several (unspecified) fast runners rather than trying to find the fastest runner.) This motivation suggests that in the example discussed, one ignores the very early findings of nonsignificance for small m, but then once one begins to find statistical significance, the procedure terminates when the probability is "clearly" nonsignificant, perhaps $p > .15$.

18
Extensions of the Scan Statistic

18.1   The Double Scan Statistic

The previous chapters dealt primarily with unusual clusters of one type of event over time or space. In this section we deal with generalizations to the simultaneous clustering of multiple types of events. In the first generalization, two types of events occur over the same (discrete or continuous) time period. The period is scanned for a window of fixed length w, looking for unusual clusters that contain at least a certain number of each type of event. In the second generalization we look for unusual clustering of two types of letter patterns in a two-dimensional array.

Greenberg, Naus, Schneider, and Wartenberg (1991) were analyzing a dataset of different causes of death (homicide, suicide, accidents) among Americans aged 15–25 for a 7 year period. The data was broken down by day, type of death, race, gender, and by county. However, the dataset did not give identifiers that might link one death to another. They applied the scan statistic to test for unusual clustering of one type of cause of death. Do suicides cluster? Do homicides cluster? They were also interested in unusual clustering of homicide/suicides, or of accidents/suicides. This was the motivation for Naus and Wartenberg (1997) to develop a scan-type statistic based on clusters that contain at least one of each of two types of event occurring within the same w-day period.

Given that at least one of each of the two types of events occur within a w-day period, we say that a *two-type w-day cluster* has occurred. Over a long period of N days, a scientist may observe several such clusters. The scientist seeks to determine whether the observed number of clusters is unusually greater than what would be expected under certain chance models.

For the case $w = 1$, the number of two-type one-day clusters can be counted simply as the number of days in the N-day period that contain at least one of each of the two types of events. For $w > 1$, there are alternative ways to count the number of two-type w-day clusters. Naus and Wartenberg chose an approach that avoids multiple counting of closely overlapping clusters.

Define the event E_i to have occurred if anywhere within the w consecutive days $i, i + 1, \ldots, i + w - 1$ there are at least one of each of the two types of events. The event E_i indicates the occurrence of a two-type w-day cluster. Let $Z_i = 1$, if E_i occurred and none of $E_{i-1}, E_{i-2}, \ldots, E_{i-w+1}$ occur. Let $Z_i = 0$, otherwise; let

$$S_{w(2)} = \sum_{I=1}^{N-W+1} Z_i.$$

Naus and Wartenberg call $S_{w(2)}$ the *double scan statistic*. They note that

$$E(S_{w(2)}) = \sum_{i=1}^{N-w+1} P(Z_i = 1) = \sum_{i=1}^{w-1} P(Z_i = 1) + (N - 2w + 2)P(Z_w = 1).$$

$$(18.1)$$

To develop formula for variance of $S_{w(2)} = \mathrm{Var}(S_{w(2)})$, note that in terms of the 0–1 indicator variables Z_i:

$$\mathrm{Var}(S_{w(2)}) = \sum_{i=1}^{N-w+1} \mathrm{Var}(Z_i) + 2 \sum\sum_{i<j} \mathrm{Cov}(Z_i, Z_j), \qquad (18.2)$$

where

$$\mathrm{Var}(Z_i) = E\{(Z_i)^2\} - (E\{Z_i\})^2 = P_i(1 - P_i), \qquad (18.3)$$

and

$$\mathrm{Cov}(Z_i, Z_j) = E(Z_i Z_j) - E(Z_i)E(Z_j) = P_{ij} - P_i P_j, \qquad (18.4)$$

where $P_i = P(Z_i = 1)$ and $P_{ij} = P\{(Z_i = 1) \cap (Z_j = 1)\}$. Note that from the definition of Z_i, $P_{ij} = 0$ if $|i - j| < w$.

This method counts the number of times that an E_i occurs with no previously overlapping E_j's. When the events are relatively rare and distributed according to certain chance models, the number of such *declumped* clusters is approximately Poisson distributed. See Aldous (1989) and Barbour, Holst, and Janson (1992).

Results for the expectation and variance of $S_{w(2)}$ are derived for two chance models. In the *retrospective model*, there are exactly A of the N days where a type-one event occurs, and exactly B of the N days where a type-two event occurs. All $\binom{N}{A}$ ways of picking the A type-one days, and all $\binom{N}{B}$ ways of picking the B type-two days are equally likely, and the occurrence of the two types of days are independent. For this model the exact expectation and approximate variance of $S_{w(2)}$ are derived.

In the prospective model, let A_i denote the event that the ith day contains a type A event, and let B_i denote the event that the ith day contains a type B event. Let $\alpha_i = P(A_i)$, $\beta_i = P(B_i)$, and assume that all A_i and B_j are mutually independent. For this model the exact expectation is derived for general α_i and β_i, and the variance of $S_{w(2)}$ is derived for the simple case where $\alpha_i = \alpha$ and $\beta_i = \beta$ for all i.

Define

$$P_{A,J}(r,s) = \left\{ \prod_{i=J}^{r-s+J-1} (1 - \alpha_i) \right\} \left\{ \prod_{i=r-s+J}^{r-1+j} (\alpha_i) \right\}, \tag{18.5}$$

where for $s = 0$ the second product is 1. Let $P_{B,J}(r,s)$ be similarly defined with β's replacing α's. Let $Q_{A,J}(r,s)$ denote $1 - P_{A,J}(r,s)$.

Theorem 18.1 (Naus and Wartenburg, 1997). *Given the occurrence of events on the N different days are independently distributed, with probabilities α_i and β_i, respectively, for the two types of events on day i. Then $E(S_{w(2)})$ is given by (18.1), where*

$$P(Z_1 = 1) = Q_{A,1}(w,0)Q_{B,1}(w,0), \tag{18.6}$$

$$P(Z_2 = 1) = P_{A,1}(w+1,1)Q_{B,2}(w,0) + P_{B,1}(w+1,1)Q_{A,2}(w,0)$$
$$- P_{A,1}(w+1,1)P_{B,1}(w+1,1). \tag{18.7}$$

For the case $2 < k \le w$:

$$P(Z_k = 1) = P(d_{AB}) + P(d_{BA}) - P(d_{AB} \cap d_{BA})$$
$$+ \sum_{r=1}^{k-2} \{P(D_{AB,r}) + P(D_{BA,r})\}, \tag{18.8}$$

where

$$P(d_{AB}) = P_{A,1}(w+k-1,1)Q_{B,k}(w,0), \tag{18.9}$$

$$P(d_{AB} \cap d_{BA}) = P_{A,1}(w+k-1,1)P_{B,1}(w+k-1,1), \tag{18.10}$$

$$P(D_{AB,r}) = \alpha_r P_{A,r+1}(w+k-r-1,1)P_{B,1}(w+r-1,0)$$
$$\times Q_{B,w+r}(k-r-1,0), \tag{18.11}$$

and $P(d_{BA})$ and $P(D_{BA,r})$, are, respectively, just $P(d_{AB})$ and $P(D_{AB,r})$ with α and β switched.

For the case $w < k$, apply (18.8) for $k = w$, letting α_i take the value α_{k-d+i} for $i = 1, \ldots, 2w$, and similarly for β's. Given we have programmed (18.8) to compute $P(Z_w = 1)$ as a function of the first w α's and β's, we can use (18.8) iteratively to compute the remaining $P(Z_k = 1)$ for $k > w$.

The proof of Theorem 18.1 is given in detail in the Appendix of Naus and Wartenburg (1997). Equation (18.1) holds for the general case of varying probabilities α_i, β_i. The proof finds exact expressions for $P\{Z_i = 1\}$ for $i = 1, 2, \ldots , w$. We illustrate the approach for $i = 1, 2$. The event $\{Z_1 = 1\}$ is equivalent to there being at least one of each type of event within the first w trials, and the probability is given by the right-hand side of (18.6).

The event $\{Z_2 = 1\}$ occurs if either of the events C_{AB} or C_{BA} occur, where

$$C_{AB} = \left(\prod_{i=1}^{w} A_i^c\right) \cap A_{w+1} \cap \left(\prod_{i=2}^{w+1} (B_i)\right) \qquad (18.12)$$

and C_{BA} is similarly defined as C_{AB} with A's and B's switched. It follows that

$$C_{AB} \cap C_{BA} = \left(\prod_{i=1}^{w} A_i^c\right) \cap A_{w+1} \cap \left(\prod_{i=1}^{w} B_i^c\right) \cap B_{w+1}, \qquad (18.13)$$

and

$$P(C_{AB}) = P_{A,1}(w + 1, 1)Q_{B,2}(w, 0), \qquad (18.14)$$

$P(C_{BA})$ is just $P(C_{AB})$ with α's and β's switched:

$$P(C_{AB} \cap C_{BA}) = P_{A,1}(w + 1, 1)P_{B,1}(w + 1, 1). \qquad (18.15)$$

Compute $P(Z_2 = 1) = P(C_{AB}) + P(C_{BA}) - P(C_{AB} \cap C_{BA})$ to find (18.7).

Naus and Wartenberg also consider a mixed model where some of the two types of events are linked in time, but many are not, and illustrate how to evaluate the power of the double scan statistic against this alternative.

For $w > 1$, the double scan statistic $S_{w(2)}$ measures for a possibly delayed relation between two types of events, but no order is prespecified for the two events. For homicide/suicide clusters one would anticipate that the day of the homicide would be the same or earlier than the day of the suicide. This led Naus and Wartenberg to develop a *directional double scan statistic*, and illustrate its application. Define an E_i^* to have occurred if anywhere within the w consecutive days, $i, i + 1, \ldots , i + w - 1$, there are at least one of each of the two types of events with a type-A event on the same or previous day as a type-B event. The statistic counts the nonoverlapping E^*'s as before.

The discrete scan statistic can be generalized for the case of two types of events, to clusters where there are at least r type-A and s type-B events within a w-day period. For other applications, the statistics can be generalized to more than two types of events, and the distribution of the number of declumped clusters derived. Huntington (1976b) derived general results for the expected waiting time, until a cluster that contained at least one of each of the two types of events within w days of each other. Huntington generalized this to a cluster of at least k events within w days, that satisfy various constraints on the number of types of events.

18.2 Clustering of Two Types of Letter Patterns in a Two-Dimensional Array

Recently, a book hit the bestseller list simultaneously in several countries. The *Bible Code* by Drosnin (1997) scans the text of the *Bible* with a two-dimensional approach, and finds what appears to intuition to be unusual clustering. The controversies, claims, and counterclaims have led to intriguing web sites spinning claims of scientific intrigue. (See http://www.torahcodes.co.il and http:/cs.anu.edu.au/-bmd/dilugim.) We go back to an article by Witztum, Rips, and Rosenberg (1994) that looks at words appearing as equally spaced letters in a text. As Drosnin (1997) put it "Rips explained that each code is a case of adding every fourth or twelfth or fiftieth letter to form a word." The text is viewed as a continuous sequence of letters, and blanks are ignored. They call words, whose letters' position in the text form an arithmetic progression, *equidistant letter sequences* (ELS). They are interested in testing whether such ELS's contain *hidden information*, coded as related ELS words that are unusually close to each other.

If the positions of the letters of the ELS are $t, t + d, t + 2d, \ldots, t + (k - 1)d$, the *skip* is called d, t is the *start*, and k is the length of the word. For example, Drosnin uses the above quote to illustrate an embedded ELS message. Let $t = 1$, $d = 3$, and $k = 11$; "**R**ips **e**xplained th**a**t eac**h** co**d**e is **t**he **c**ase **o**f ad**d**ing **e**very..." contains the embedded ELS measage "Read the code."

The general problem is very complex in terms of selecting among many possibly related words and many different possible skips and starting positions. To reduce the possibilities, they focus on ELS's where the skip for that word is a minimum over all (or most of) the text. Drosnin gives a particularly dramatic example. The name Yitzkak Rabin (eight Hebrew letters) appears only once as an ELS in the 304,805 letters of the Torah (the five books of Moses). The skip is 4772 letters, making clear why a computer is needed to find such codes, and also illustrating the magnitude of multiple comparisons. The 304,805 letters were arranged into 64 rows, each row consisting of 4772 letters. (Technically each row is a circle and the rows are viewed as printed on a cylinder.) The name Yitzkak Rabin appears as eight consecutive letters in a column of the two-way grid. Given that this ELS was searched for in many ways, it is not necessarily surprising that it was found. What was dramatic was that the one place where it was found, it was intersected by the expression "The killer who will kill," 12 consecutive letters in the row of the original text. Drosnin claimed he had found this message before Rabin had been assassinated and had warned him by letter more than a year before the assassination. Drosnin notes "The odds against Rabin's full name appearing with the prediction of his assassination were at least 3000 to 1."

The calculation is presumably based on there being 304,805 starting positions for the 12 consecutive letters corresponding to "The killer who will kill" in the text; of these there are $12(8) = 96$ starting positions for this phrase where it intersects with the eight-letter name Yitzkak Rabin. 96/304,805 is about one in three thousand. This calculation does not take into account other similarly ominous expressions that might have intersected with the name. It doesn't take into account other orientations—such as diagonal—in which related ELS's can appear in the grid. It doesn't take into account the direction in which the word is written. In the same example, an ELS spelling out (backward) the first name of the killer was found within the same general area of the grid.

Witztum, Rips, and Rosenberg (1994) focus on a more narrowly defined experiment with an independently selected list of 34 great rabbis, with the related words being the names of the rabbis and their dates of death or birth. (There are actually multiple names and spellings of names, and describing dates, so even this simple example is quite complex.) They apply a randomization/simulation procedure to estimate the unusualness of the closeness of the related words. The procedure carries out a random assignment of the 34 names to the 34 dates and computes an average measure of closeness for that assignment. The procedure is replicated many times, and the unusualness of the average measure of closeness of the true set of 34 pairings of names with dates is guaged relative to the simulation distribution.

In the molecular biology examples of Chapter 6 we were looking at scanning aligned sequences looking for matching words, where each word consists of consecutive letters. Stephen Altschul (personal communication) had suggested looking at words that match allowing for a few skips between two letters. Such skips might arise due to insertion or deletion. In some cryptographic applications one might scan for common or related ELS words in multiple sequences, or in a two-way grid such as in the *Bible Code* examples.

Witztum, Rips, and Rosenberg (1994) use the simple illustration of two related words: The four-letter Hebrew word for hammer, and the three-letter Hebrew word for anvil. The first two letters of each word touch in the original text, and both words involve skips of certain sizes. Let us consider a simplified version of the combinatorial scan problem.

Consider an $R \times C$ grid of random letters. View the $R \times C$ letters as i.i.d. random variables from an $\mathcal{M}$-letter alphabet. Consider two given words—a type A word and a type B word. (In the simplest version of the problem we allow no skips between the letters of a word, and look at only horizontal or vertical words.) Now scan the $R \times C$ grid with a $w \times w$ subsquare whose sides are parallel to the sides of the grid. How likely is it to find the two words both contained within a $w \times w$ subsquare of the $R \times C$ square. What is the expected number of times we would observe a type A word and a type B word together in a $w \times w$ subsquare? This problem is related to a two-dimensional generalization of the double scan statistic of Naus and Wartenburg (1997).

Consider two given words, one of u letters, and one of v letters. If u and v are small relative to w, and w is small relative to R and C, a Poisson-type approximation may be reasonable. Assume that this is the case in what follows, and also assume that letters appear at random in positions on the grid. Suppose that the probability that the u letter word appears in a given position (and orientation) is P_A, and let P_B denote the respective probability for the v-letter word. In a given

$w \times w$ square, the u-letter word can appear in $4(w-u+1)w$ possible ways. (There are four combinations: horizontal and word starts at right or left; vertical and word starts at top or bottom.) The v-letter word can appear in $4(w-v+1)v$ possible ways. The number of times that the u-letter word appears in the $w \times w$ square is approximately Poisson distributed with expectation $\lambda(u) = 4(w-u+1)wP_A$. The number of times that the v-letter word appears in the $w \times w$ square is approximately Poisson distributed with expectation $\lambda(v) = 4(w-v+1)wP_B$. The probability that both words appear in the given $w \times w$ square is approximately

$$P_{AB}(w) = (1 - \exp\{-\lambda(u)\})(1 - \exp\{-\lambda(v)\}). \qquad (18.16)$$

This probability will be very small in many applications. However, this is misleading in that there is a large number of $(R - w + 1)(C - w + 1)$ possible (overlapping) positions for a $w \times w$ square within the $R \times C$ grid. The expected number of these $w \times w$ squares that contain both the u-letter and v-letter word is $(R - w + 1)(C - w + 1)P_{AB}(w)$, and the probability that at least one of these squares contains both words is approximately

$$1 - \exp\{-(R - w + 1)(C - w + 1)P_{AB}(w)\}. \qquad (18.17)$$

Approximation (18.17) could be improved by declumping, and more refined approximations developed. Simulations or bounds need to be conducted to evaluate the accuracy of the approximation under various circumstances. In cases where the probability (18.17) is small, one can use a Bonferroni-type upper bound to test for significance; the upper bound can be approximated in some cases by $(R - w + 1)(C - w + 1)P_{AB}(w)$.

For a simplistic example, consider 304,704 letters arranged in a 552×552 grid. Assume an equally likely 22-letter alphabet. How likely is it that two given five-letter words would appear together within a 10×10 square. (Assume no skips, words can be horizontal or vertical, and go up or down, or from the left or from the right.) Here

$$P_A = P_B = (1/22)^5, \qquad \lambda(5) = 4(6)10(P_A) = 240P_A = .000046569,$$
$$P_{AB}(5) = (1 - \exp\{-.000046569\})^2 = 2.16858E\text{-}9.$$

The probability that a 10×10 scanning square will somewhere simultaneously contain both five-letter words is from approximation (18.17), $1 - \exp\{-543(543)(2.16858E\text{-}9\} = .00064$. This appears quite unusual, but we don't know the accuracy of the approximation.

We can compute Bonferroni upper bound to the probability, and illustrate the approach for this example. For a given position of the 10×10 square, there are a maximum of 240(239) possible positions/orientations for the two pairs of five-letter words. (If the words do not share any letters in common, there are fewer possible positions.) The probability that the two five-letter words are in a specific (allowable) position/orientation is, for the assumptions of our example, $(1/22)^{10}$. The probability, $P_{AB}(10)$, that the two five-letter words appear in at least one of the 240(239) possible combinations of positions within the given 10×10 square is by the Bonferroni upper bound less than or equal to the sum of the probabilities for the different positions

$$P_{AB}(10) \leq 240(239)(1/22)^{10} = 2.1596E\text{-}9.$$

There are 543(543) possible positions for the 10×10 scanning square within the 552×552 grid. The probability that at least one of these 543(543) squares contains both five-letter words is by the Bonferroni upper bound less than or equal to the sum of the probabilities for the different positions for the squares. This is $\leq 543(543)P_{AB}(10)$, which in turn is $\leq 543(543)2.1596E\text{-}9 = .00064$. For the assumptions of this example, the upper bound supports the conclusion from the approximation that it is unlikely to find two five-letter words within a 10×10 subsquare of the 552×552 grid.

18.3   The Skip–Scan Statistic

Section 6.3 of Chapter 6 deals with matching words in DNA sequences. Researchers with newly sequenced segments search the data banks looking for similarities. Computer algorithms have been developed to scan two long DNA sequences, searching for subsequences or fragments that match perfectly or almost perfectly. In the process of comparing two long sequences, one would expect to find, purely by chance, some matching subsequences. To efficiently search, the researcher seeks to determine, for various chance models, what is an unusually large match.

In some applications, two sequences are aligned by global criteria, and the researcher looks for perfectly or almost perfectly matching *words* (subsequences) with a common location in the two aligned sequences. In comparing two aligned letters, one from each sequence, the researcher gives a score denoting the similarity of the two letters. For the $(0, 1)$ similarity scoring a run of m one's corresponds to perfectly matching m-letter word (in the same position) in the two sequences.

A perfect match of several consecutive letters in a short amino acid sequence can be unusual. One typically thinks in terms of looking at consecutive position matches. Stephen Altschul (personal communication) suggested the innovative idea of looking at words that are not consecutive letters. For example, instead of seeing whether there is a perfect match in positions $(1, 2, 3)$ or $(2, 3, 4)$ or $(3, 4, 5) \ldots$ (the regular discrete scan), one could look to see if there is a perfect match in positions $(1, 2, 4)$ or $(2, 3, 5)$ or $(3, 4, 6) \ldots$; we call this latter the *skip–scan*. If there is a *target* region where letters are more likely to match than in a *background* region, are we more likely to pick it up with the regular scan or with the skip–scan?

Let $X_1, X_2, \ldots, X_T$ be i.i.d. Bernoulli random variables with $P(X_i = 1) = p$, $P(X_i = 0) = 1 - p$. Let $S_3^* = \max\limits_{1 \leq i \leq T-2} \{X_i + X_{i+1} + X_{i+2}\}$ denote a regular discrete scan statistic; let $SS_3 = \max\limits_{1 \leq i \leq T-3} \{X_i + X_{i+1} + X_{i+3}\}$ denote a skip–scan

Table 18.1. Finding skip–scan probability, $P(SS_3 \geq 3)$ for $T = 12$, $m = 3$; $q = 1 - p$.

Number of ones	Number of sequences	Number of sequences where $SS_3 \geq 3$	Weight
12	1	1	p^{12}
11	12	12	$p^{11}q$
10	66	66	$p^{10}q^2$
9	220	220	p^9q^3
8	495	489	p^8q^4
7	792	702	p^7q^5
6	924	607	p^6q^6
5	792	303	p^5q^7
4	495	81	p^4q^8
3	220	9	p^3q^9
2	66	0	
1	12	0	
0	1	0	
Total	4096	2490	

statistic. Under the background (null), the two statistics have different probabilities of exceeding a level. For example, for $p = .1$, $P(S_3^* \geq 3 \mid T = 11) = .00819$, $P(S_3^* \geq 3 \mid T = 12) = .00909$, and $P(SS_3 \geq 3 \mid T = 12) = .00879$. Note that S_3^* for $T = 11$ and that SS_3 for $T = 12$, each involve the maximum of nine sums of three X_i's.

$P(SS_3 \geq 3 \mid T = 12)$ is computed as follows. For $T = 12$, there are only $2^{12} = 4096$ possible 0–1 sequences, and one can evaluate $P(SS_3 \geq 3)$ exactly. Table 18.1 breaks down the 4096 sequences in terms of the number of ones in the sequence, and gives for each the number of sequences where $SS_3 \geq 3$:

$$P(SS_3 \geq 3 \mid T = 12) = 1p^{12} + 12p^{11}q + 66p^{10}q^2 + 220p^9q^3$$
$$+ 489p^8q^4 + 702p^7q^5 + 607p^6q^6$$
$$+ 303p^5q^7 + 81p^4q^8 + 9p^3q^9. \qquad (18.18)$$

Similarly, one can show that

$$P(SS_3 \geq 3 \mid T = 8) = 1 - \{1p^6q^2 + 15p^5q^3 + 45p^4q^4 + 51p^3q^5$$
$$+ 28p^2q^6 + 8pq^7 + 1q^8\}. \qquad (18.19)$$

In terms of the Q_3/Q_2 approximation of Chapter 7, $1 - Q_2$ is given by the right-hand side of (18.19), and $1 - Q_3$ is given by the right-hand side of (18.18). For $p = .1$, $T = 50$, the Q_3/Q_2 approximation gives $P(S_3^* \geq 3 \mid T = 50) = .0425$, and $P(SS_3 \geq 3 \mid T = 50) = .0449$. (For the skip–scan, with $p = .1$, $Q_2 = .995086$, and $Q_3 = .99121$, based on 8 and 12 trials, respectively; the approximation is $1 - Q_2(Q_3/Q_2)^{(50/4)-2} = .0449$.) For $p = .2$ and $T = 200$, the approximation gives $P(S_3^* \geq 3) = .728$ and $P(SS_3 \geq 3) = .767$. Altshul's skip–scan has properties that may prove useful in a variety of applications, and it is of interest for further research.

18.4   Unusually Small Scans

In certain applications reseachers focus on unusually sparse regions of the data. Large regions on a petri dish where there are few bacterial colonies, or regions of space apparently absent certain sources of radiation, can spark scientific inquiries. Much of the research on scan statistics deals with unusually large clusters. This section discusses the research on scan statistics that measure unusual sparseness in certain parts of the data.

Given N points independently drawn from the uniform distribution on $[0, 1)$, recall that S_w denotes the largest number of points to be found in any subinterval of $[0, 1)$ of length w. The maximum cluster S_w is called the *scan statistic*, from the viewpoint that one scans time with a window of size w, and observes a large number of points. In a similar way, let D_w denote the smallest number of points to be found in any subinterval of $[0, 1)$ of length w.

In looking at unusually large clusters one could focus on S_w, the largest number of points in an interval of length w, or on W_k, the size of the smallest subinterval of $[0, 1)$ that contains k points. We noted previously that the distributions of the statistics S_w and W_k are related, $P(S_w \geq k) = P(W_k \leq w)$. In the same way, one could focus on D_w, the smallest number of points in an interval of length w, or on the related V_k, the size of the largest subinterval of $[0, 1)$ that contains k points. The distributions of the statistics D_w and V_k are related, $P(D_w \leq k) = P(V_k \geq w)$.

Formally, let $X_1, X_2, \dots, X_N$, be i.i.d. uniform random variables. Let $X_{(1)} \leq X_{(2)} \leq \dots \leq X_{(N)}$ denote the ordered values of the X's:

$$V_k = \max_{1 \leq i \leq N-k+1} \{X_{(i+k-1)} - X_{(i)}\} = \max_{1 \leq i \leq N-k+1} \left\{ \sum_{j=1}^{k-1} (X_{(j+i)} - X_{(j+i-1)}) \right\}.$$

The quantities $X_{(i+1)} - X_{(i)}$ are called the *spacings* between the ith and $(i + 1)$st point. The *r-scan statistic* W_{r+1} can be viewed as the minimum of a sum of r consecutive spacings. Similarly, the scan statistic V_{k+1} can be viewed as the maximum of the sum of k consecutive spacings. The interval V_{r+1} is called the *maximum rth-order gap*.

A variety of results have been derived for the related statistics D_w and V_k. Dembo and Karlin (1992) derive asymptotic results for the distribution of the order statistics of the rth order gaps, for i.i.d. distributed spacings $X_{(i+1)} - X_{(i)}$ (gaps between consecutive points) and some more general uniform mixing stationary processes. They use Poisson approximation with the Chen–Stein method to bound the error of the approximation. They simplify their results for the special cases of the maximum and minimum r-scans for i.i.d. uniform $[0, 1)$ spacings, and other distributions. The minimum rth-order scan is W_{r+1}; the maximum rth-order scan is V_{r+1}. For the case of $n (= N + 1)$ i.i.d. uniform $[0, 1)$ spacings, their corollaries (5.1) and (5.2) give

$$\lim_{n \to \infty} P\{W_{r+1} \geq y/N^{(r+1)/r}\} = \exp\{-y^r/r!\} \tag{18.20}$$

and

$$\lim_{n \to \infty} P\{V_{r+1} \leq [\log_e n + (r-1)\log_e \log_e n + y]/n\} = \exp\{e^{-y}/(r-1)!\}.$$
$$(18.21)$$

The asymptotic result (18.20) used as an approximation is equivalent to the Newell–Ikeda approximation for the distribution of the mimimum r-scan (see 3.1). As noted, this is a rough approximation for sufficiently small probabilities, but may not be reliable in other situations. The asymptotic convergence (as n gets large) is very slow.

For the case of N uniform distributed points on the line, Huntington (1978) derived the exact distribution of D_w and V_k. His result for the general scanning window w, is derived by the approach of Theorem 8.3. He divides the unit interval into $2R+1$ subintervals: $[0, b), [b, w), [w, w+b), [w+b, 2p), \ldots$, where R is the largest integer in $1/w$. Let m_i denote the number of points in the ith interval. His equation (3) gives

$$P(D_w > k) = N! \, b^M (w-b)^{N-M} \sum_\sigma \det |1/c_{rs}!| \det |1/d_{rs}!|, \quad (18.22)$$

$$c_{rs} = \sum_{i=2R-2s+2}^{2R-2r+2} m_i - (s-r)k, \qquad 1 \leq r \leq s \leq R,$$

$$= (r-s)k - \sum_{i=2R-2r+3}^{2R-2s+1} m_i, \qquad 1 \leq s < r \leq R,$$

and

$$d_{rs} = \sum_{i=2R-2s+3}^{2R-2r+3} m_i - (s-r)k, \qquad 1 \leq r \leq s \leq R,$$

$$= (r-s)k - \sum_{i=2R-2r+4}^{2R-2s+2} m_i, \qquad 1 \leq s < r \leq R,$$

where σ is the set of all partitions of N into $2R+1$ nonnegative integers, the m_i's, such that $m_i + m_{i+1} > k$ for $i = 1, \ldots, 2R$, and M is the sum of the m_i's for i odd. The result uses the convention of Theorem 8.3, that $1/x!$ is zero if $x > N$ or $x < 0$.

Huntington's equation (2) gives, for the special case $w = 1/L$, L an integer,

$$P(D_{1/L} > k) = N! \, L^{-N} \sum_\sigma \det |1/e_{rs}!|, \qquad (18.23)$$

where

$$e_{rs} = \sum_{i=L-s+1}^{L-r+1} n_i - (s-r)k, \qquad 1 \le r \le s \le L,$$

$$= (r-s)k - \sum_{i=L-r+2}^{L-s} n_i, \qquad 1 \le s < r \le L,$$

and where σ is the set of all partitions of N into L integers n_i each $> k$.

The Proof of (18.23). Divide the interval into L disjoint subintervals $[(i-1)/L, i/L)$ for $i = 1, 2, \ldots, L$. Let n_i denote the number, and $x_{1i}, x_{2i}, \ldots, x_{ni}$, the values of the points that fall into $[(i-1)L, i/L)$. Let $y_i(t)$ denote the number of x_{ij} that fall in the subinterval $[(i-1)L, \{(i-1)/L\}+t)$, where t is a given real number, $0 \le t \le 1/L$. Naus (1965a, 1966a) noted that

$$P(D_{1/L} > k) = \Pr\left\{\inf_{i,t}[n_i - y_i(t) + y_{i+1}(t)] > k\right\} \qquad (18.24)$$

$$= L^{-N} N! \sum_{\sigma} \Pr\left\{\inf_{i,t}[n_i - y_i(t) + y_{i+1}(t)] > k \mid \{n_i\}\right\} \Big/ \pi n_i!,$$

where the sum is over the set σ of all partitions of N into L positive integers each greater than k. Now view the L sets of x_{ij}'s as L samples, each rescaled to be over the interval $[0, 1/L)$. That is, set $x_{ij}^* = x_{ij} - (i-1)/L$. Note that $\inf_{i,t}[n_i - y_i(t) + y_{i+1}(t)] > k$ is equivalent to

$$y_1(t) < y_2(t) + (n_1 - k) < y_3(t) + (n_1 - k) + (n_2 - k)$$
$$< y_4(t) + (n_1 - k) + (n_2 - k) + (n_3 - k) < \cdots$$
$$< y_L(t) + (n_1 + n_2 + \cdots + n_{L-1}) - (L-1)k. \qquad (18.25)$$

Apply the Barton and Mallow corollary (8.20) to Karlin and McGregor's theorem following the approach of Section 8.5:

$$P\{A_1(m) + \alpha_1 > A_2(m) + \alpha_2 > \cdots > A_L(m) + \alpha_L;$$
$$m = 1, 2, \ldots, N \mid \{a_i, \alpha_i\}) = \det |a_r!/(a_r + \alpha_r - \alpha_s)!|.$$

In Barton and Mallow's corollary (8.20) substitute $y_{L-i+1}(t)$ for $A_i(m)$, n_{L-i+1} for a_i, and $\alpha_i = (n_1 + n_2 + \cdots + n_{L-i}) - (L-i)k$. Thus,

$$\alpha_r - \alpha_s = (n_{L-s+1} + \cdots + n_{L-r}) - (s-r)k, \qquad 1 \le r \le s \le L,$$
$$= -(n_{L-r+1} + \cdots + n_{L-s}) + (r-s)k, \qquad 1 \le s < r \le L. \quad (18.26)$$

Let e_{rs} denote $a_r + \alpha_r - \alpha_s = n_{L-r+1} + \alpha_r - \alpha_s$. Sum in the resulting equation to find

$$P\left(\inf_{i,t}\{n_i - y_i(t) + y_{i+1}(t)\} > k \mid \{n_i\}\right) \Big/ \prod_i n_i = \det |1/e_{rs}!|, \qquad (18.27)$$

where e_{rs} is defined in (18.23).

One can use the exact formulas (18.22) and (18.23) to derive simpler formulas for special cases. Huntington illustrates an approach to find $P(D_w > k)$ for $w > .5$. Chapters 8 and 10 illustrate the approach to derive exact formulas for the special cases $w = 1/2$ and $w = 1/3$. One can derive formulas similar to (18.22) and (18.23) for the unconditional Poisson case. Using (18.23), the Q_2/Q_3 approach of Section 7.5 can be used to derive an approximation for $P(D_w > k)$, in a similar way to the derivation of the highly accurate approximation for $P(S_w < k) = 1 - P^*(k; \lambda L, 1/L)$ given in (3.4)–(3.6).

Lin (1993) and Huffer and Lin (1997b) develop a general approach to find the distribution of the minimum or maximum of sums of adjacent spacings. They apply their approach to find the distribution of the scan statistic. Their approach uses a recursion to rewrite the joint distribution of linear combinations of spacings as the sum of simple explicit components. Their results give the piecewise polynomial expressions for the distribution of the scan statistics W_k and V_k. There is difficulty when k is small and n is large. They were able to go up to $N = 61$, but at that level only for k-values fairly close to $n/2$. The approach is described in detail in Section 8.10 of Chapter 8.

There is a dual relation between the maximum and minimum scan statistics for N points on the circle. If there exists a position of the scanning window of length w on the unit circle, where the window contains more than k points, then the complementary arc of length $q = 1 - w$ must contain less than $n - k + 1$ points. Given the distribution of the maximum scan on the circle for all w, one would have the distribution of the minimum scan as well. For the case $w \geq .5$, the distribution of the maximum scan is more complex for the circle than for the line. The distribution of the minimum scan for the circle for $w \leq .5$ is also complex.

The distribution of the minimum scan for the line and circle is related to multiple coverage problems. The simple coverage problem is as follows: Given N subarcs each of length w, dropped at random on the circumference of the unit circle, what is the probability that the arcs completely cover the circumference of the circle? More generally, one seeks the probability that the arcs completely cover the circumference of the circle m times. Kaplan (1977) gives bounds, and Glaz (1978) and Glaz and Naus (1979) give exact results for the probability of multiple coverage of the line and circle.

To relate the coverage with the scan problem, let the N points in the scan problem correspond to the midpoints of the subarcs in the coverage problem. If the N subarcs do not cover the circle m times, there must be some point on the circumference not so covered. This implies that the subinterval of length w centered at that point contains fewer than m of the N midpoints of the N subarcs; in this case, the minimum number of the N (mid)points in a scanning window of length w must be less than m.

The continuous minimum scan problems have discrete counterparts. Given a sequence of T Bernoulli trials, what is the probability that the smallest number of successes in any m consecutive trials is less than k? This is directly related to the distribution of the maximum number of failures in any m consecutive trials, discussed in Chapters 4 and 12. One can also look at minimum scan variations of the ratchet scan statistic of this chapter. A special case is the longest run of empty cells (LREC) test, introduced by Grimson, Aldrich, and Drane (1992). Mancuso (1998) studies the exact distribution of the LREC test, and investigates its power for sparse data.

18.5 The Ratchet Scan

In Chapter 2, Section 2.3, the ratchet scan was defined as the maximum number of events in m consecutive months and applied to monthly health records. The statistic was introduced by Wallenstein, Weinberg, and Gould (1989) for the circle, and described in greater detail for both the circle and line in a series of papers by Krauth (1992a,b, 1999).

There is a much more extensive literature on the case $m = 1$, which is termed the maximum multinomial. Krauth (1999) gives a good summary of work concerning this statistic and its relation to the scan statistic.

18.5.1   Definition of Ratchet Scan and Exact Distribution

The statistic has some elements of the continuous scan and some of the discrete scan statistic. Assume the interval is divided into L subintervals or cells. Let n_i be the number of observations in the ith cell, and let $Y_i(j)$ be the number of events in j consecutive cells, i.e.,

$$Y_i(j) = \sum_{g=i}^{(i+j-1) \bmod L} n_g.$$

For example, for calendar time, we might divide the time into months, and $Y_i(j)$ is the number of events in months $i, i+1, \ldots, i+j-1$.

Let $R(m)$, the ratchet scan statistic, be the maximum number of events in m consecutive months, that is,

$$R(m) = \max_{1 \le i \le h} Y_i(m), \tag{18.28}$$

where

$$h = L - m + 1 \quad \text{for the linear case,}$$
$$= L \quad \text{for the circular case.}$$

(In Chapter 2, we used the notation, R_w, where $w = m/L$, so that the statistics $R(m)$ and R_w can be used interchangeably.)

One would anticipate using the ratchet scan in cases where the optimal statistic is the usual scan but the precise data are not available. Thus the statistic would be a reasonable choice to detect a pulse which is a fraction $w = m/L$ of the total time frame.

Let π_i be the probability that an event is in the ith cell. In the simplest equiprobable case, we wish to find the distribution of $R(m)$ when these probabilities are all equal to a common value, $1/L$. (This would occur if the time unit under consideration is divided into exactly L equally spaced intervals.) Under the equiprobable case, the probabilities that the cell counts $n_1, n_2, \ldots, n_L$ take on some specific value is a multinomial with equal probabilities of $1/L$ so that

$$P[R(m) \geq k] = N! \, L^{-N} \sum \prod_{i=1}^{L} 1/n_i!,$$

where the sum is taken over all $n_1, n_2, \ldots, n_L$ that yield $\sum n_i = N$ and $R(m) \geq k$. For seasonal clustering and moderate sample sizes ($L = 12$, $m = 2$ or 3), Wallenstein, Weinberg, and Gould (1989) give the p-values in the range .001–.15 for $N = 8(1)25, 30, 35$.

More generally, we find the distribution when

$$\pi_i = \pi_i^0.$$

For example, to allow for the unequal size of calendar months let π_i be proportional to the number of days in a month, e.g., in a nonleap year for February, $\pi_2 = 28/365$. The cell counts $n_1, n_2, \ldots, n_L$ now have a general multinomial distribution, so that

$$P[R(m) \geq k] = N! \sum \prod_{i=1}^{L} (\pi_i^0)^{n_i}/n_i!,$$

where the sum is taken over all $n_1, n_2, \ldots, n_L$ that yield $\sum n_i = N$ and $R(m) \geq k$. The summation set rapidly increases with N, and the exact computations become difficult.

18.5.2 Approximate Distributions

We outline two approaches to approximating the distribution of the ratchet scan. In the following subsection, we use methods similar to those employed previously in this book and follow the outline of Krauth (1992a,b, 1999), in finding bounds on the probability. The second approach is based on the asymptotic normal approximation. A slight modification will be employed to handle the case when the π's are nearly but not exactly equal, as in calendar months.

18.5.3 Equal Size Intervals, Combinatorial-Type Bounds

Let

$$s_1 = \sum_{i=1}^{h-1} P[Y_i(m) \geq k]$$

and

$$s_2 = \sum_{i=1}^{h-1} \sum_{j=i+1}^{h} P[\{Y_i(m) \geq k\} \cap \{Y_j(m) \geq k\}],$$

where as above $h = L - m + 1$, or L, for the line and circle, respectively. By definition,

$$P[R(m) \geq k] = P\left[\bigcup_{i=1,\dots,h} \{Y_i(m) \geq k\}\right].$$

The Bonferroni inequalities, as introduced in Chapter 9, yield the bounds

$$s_1 - s_2 \leq P[R(m) \geq k] \leq s_1. \tag{18.29}$$

As follows from the material in Chapter 9, Krauth (1992a,b, 1999) notes that the Hunter upper bound is

$$P[R(m) \geq k] \leq s_1 - \max_{1 \leq j \leq h} \sum_i P[\{Y_i(m) \geq k\} \cap \{Y_j(m) \geq k\}], \tag{18.30}$$

where the sum is over $i = 1, \dots, h$, $i \neq j$. The Kwerel lower bound is

$$P[R(m) \geq k] \geq 2(as_1 - s_2)/[a(a + 1)], \tag{18.31}$$

where $a = 1 + 2[s_2/s_1]$ and $[x]$ is the greatest integer in x.

Evaluating $P[\{Y_i(m) \geq k\} \cap \{Y_j(m) \geq k\}]$ requires some care. When $|j - i| > m$, the points involved in the two events are distinct and the probability is a sum of trinomials. In other cases, the placement of a single point can influence both events, and greater care is needed. Krauth (1992a,b, 1999) simplifies these expressions for both the line and circle.

The simplest results apply in the equiprobable case. For example,

$$s_1 = hG_b(k, N, 1/L),$$

and as Krauth indicates, on the circle the upper bound is

$$s_1 - 2s_2/L.$$

The same general concepts hold for the more general case where the proportions are not equal. The reader is referred to the two papers by Krauth (1992a,b) that deal with the cases individually, or to the article in 1999 that deals with them together.

The discussion above described bounds. As noted in Chapter 10, we anticipate that usually the lower approximation will be closer to the exact probability than the upper bound. Thus if we were interested in an approximation, we would take the lower bound, or a weighted average in which the lower bound is weighted more heavily than the upper bound.

18.5.4   Multivariate Normal Asymptotic for Circular Ratchet Scan when $L = 12$

The most common area of application is for detecting seasonal clustering (see Chapter 2, Section 2.3) based on months of the year ($L = 12$), and examining clusters in consecutive months ($m = 2$), or seasons ($m = 3$). Wallenstein, Weinberg, and Gould (1989) develop asymptotic results for this application for $L = 12$. We will, at least conceptually, extend the approach to arbitrary L.

The derivation is based on the equiprobable case. To apply these methods we first obtain the moments. Note that

$$E[R_i(m)] = mN/L,$$
$$\text{Var}[R_i(m)] = Nm(12 - m)/L^2.$$

Next, note that the correlation matrix has identical values for fixed $|i - j|$. In particular, when $L = 12$: for $m = 1$ all correlations are $-1/11$; for $m = 2$ they are $-.2$ except when $|i - j| = 1$ or 11 in which case the correlation is $.4$; for $m = 3$ they are $-1/3$ except when $|i - j| = 1$ or 11 in which case the correlation is $5/9$, or if $|i - j| = 2$ or 10 in which case the correlation is $1/9$.

For $L = 12, m = 3$, the rank of the correlation matrix is 9. Let $(Z_1, \ldots, Z_9)$ be multivariate normal with mean 0, variance 1, and correlation structure as above. Let

$$Z_{10} = -Z_1 - Z_4 - Z_7, \quad Z_{11} = -Z_2 - Z_5 - Z_8 \quad \text{and} \quad Z_{12} = -Z_3 - Z_6 - Z_9.$$

Let $Z_\alpha^{(m)}$ be the α percentile of $\max(Z_1, \ldots, Z_{12})$. The $1 - \alpha$ percentile of $R(m)$ is then, by the central limit theorem, approximately

$$mN/L + \sqrt{N}\, Z_\alpha^{(m)} \sqrt{[m(12 - m)/L^2]}. \tag{18.32}$$

This is an interesting relationship, but unfortunately an analytic form for the values of $Z_\alpha^{(m)}$ is not available. (Were they to become available in the future, this approach would merit more interest.)

Thus, to apply this procedure, we must use simulation. Wallenstein, Weinberg, and Gould (1989) simulated values of $Z_\alpha^{(m)}$. For example, for the most common seasonal clustering application with $m = 3$, setting $\alpha = .05$ yields $Z_{.05}^{(3)} = 2.58$, so that, noting that $\sqrt{[m(12 - m)/L^2]} = \sqrt{36/144} = 0.433$, the critical .05 value for $R(3)$ is approximately

$$0.25N + 1.12\sqrt{N}. \tag{18.33}$$

The table below gives other simulated values for $Z_\alpha^{(m)}$ so that critical values can be approximated for $m = 1, 2,$ and 3:

α	$m = 1$	$m = 2$	$m = 3$
.50	1.66	1.58	1.52
.10	2.38	2.34	2.32
.05	2.63	2.62	2.58
.01		3.16	3.11
.005			3.32

Wallenstein, Weinberg, and Gould also gives plots which allow p-values to be readoff, and also give separate curves for $N = 25$, $N = 35$, and for $m = 1$, $N = 100$. In practice, they recommend a slight modification of the asymptotic results based on a correction for continuity in which 1.0 is subtracted from the numerator.

In reality, months are not equal in length. To adjust for the slight differences we use the exact mean and variance, but use the critical value which is based on equal months. Specifically, let w be the fraction of the calendar year encompassed by the m months under consideration. Thus for evaluating data from January, February, and March, $W = (31 + 28 + 31)/265 = .247$, while for February to April, $2 = (28 + 31 + 30)/365$. Then slightly extending (18.32), the $(1 - \alpha)$ critical value is

$$wN + Z_\alpha^{(m)}\sqrt{[Nw(1 - w)]}. \qquad (18.34)$$

18.6   Unknown Value of w

A defect of the scan statistic is the requirement to choose w beforehand. In many applications, there is no natural value for w. In these cases, one can view the procedure in the context of exploratory data analysis, or use a Bonferroni inequality based on two or three possible window sizes. The approaches in this section find the maximum of some function of $Y_t(w)$ over a range of values of w.

Kulldorff and Nagarwalla have, in several papers, evaluated the statistic based on a generalized likelihood ratio. They derive the generalized likelihood ratio for testing

$$H_0: f_0(t) = 1/T,$$

against the generalized pulse alternative

$$H_A: f_0(t) = c_1, \quad a < t < b,$$
$$f_0(t) = c_0, \quad \text{otherwise},$$

$c_1 > c_0$, a and b unknown, subject to the restriction $0 \le u \le b - a \le v \le T$. They show that the optimal test rejects H_0 for large values of

$$S' = \sup_{u \le w \le v} \sup_{w \le t \le 1-w} \mathcal{L}_N[Y_t(w), wN],$$

where

$$\mathcal{L}_N[O, E] = O \ln(O/E) + (N - O) \ln[(N - O)/(N - E)], \quad \text{if } O > E,$$
$$= 0, \qquad\qquad\qquad\qquad\qquad\qquad\qquad\qquad \text{otherwise.}$$

(Note that this is a second maximization beyond the single one in 15.5.) The authors indicate that the truncation ($0 < u \le w \le v < 1$) is both for power considerations, and also apparently for numerical stability, so that $\mathcal{L}_N[Y_t(w), wN]$ does not become infinite as w approaches zero or T.

This statistic had been applied, possibly with slight variants by Nagarwalla (1996), who applies the statistic to the one-dimensional problem considered here. Unlike the method above which keeps the statistic finite by truncating w, Nagarwalla truncates k. He uses simulation rather than an analytic result. Kulldorff, in a series of papers starting in 1995, applies the method of geographical clustering and generalizations in two and three dimensions. He also relies on simulations for these applications. Louv and Little (1986) give a somewhat similar result in a related context.

Let $h(w)$ be defined implicitly to be the value that satisfies the equation

$$\mathcal{L}_1[h(w), w] = c^2/2N.$$

Loader (1991) uses large deviation theory to find that as N goes to infinity as $c/\sqrt{N}$ remains constant

$$P(S' \ge c^2/2) \approx N^{3/2}\phi(c) \int_{w=u}^{v} \frac{1-w}{h'(w)} \left[h'(w) - \frac{1-h(w)}{1-w} \right]^2$$
$$\times \left[\frac{h(w)}{w} - \frac{1-h(w)}{1-w} \right] \frac{1}{\sqrt{[h(w)(1-h(w))]}} \, dw, \quad (18.35)$$

where $h'(w)$ is the derivative of w and $\phi(z)$ is the normal density. (If this equation would yield $h(w) \ge w$ or $w \ge \exp(-c^2/2N)$, then we set $h(w) = 1$.)

In addition, Loader gives a cruder but simpler approximation using the first term in a Taylor expansion

$$h(w) = w + c\sqrt{[w(1-w)/N]} + o(c/\sqrt{N}),$$

together with convergence arguments to yield

$$P(S' \ge c^2/2) \approx 0.25c^3\phi(c) \ln \left[\frac{v(1-u)}{u(1-v)} + \frac{1}{u} - \frac{1}{v} \right]. \quad (18.36)$$

The numerical comparison below, extracted from Loader, indicates that the asymptotic expression (18.36) does give order of magnitude agreement, but is not as accurate as (18.35), the expression based on large-deviation theory. (The example is for $u = .1$, $v = .9$, but the results presumably apply for the range of values used in practice.)

		$c = 3$	$c = 3.5$	$c = 4$
	18.36	.195	.061	.014
$N = 20$	18.35	.155	.043	.009
	Simulation	.165	.044	.010
$N = 100$	18.35	.158	.048	.011
	Simulation	.162	.049	.011
Sim(S.E.)		.004	.002	.001

18.6.1 Other Statistics

Cressie (1977b,c) relates the maximum of the unnormalized difference between the statistic $Y_t(w)$ and its mean value to a known statistic, specifically showing that

$$\mathcal{K}/\sqrt{N} \equiv \sup_t \sup_w [Y_t(w) - Nw]/\sqrt{N}$$

where $\mathcal{K}$ is the Kuiper (1960) statistic which is an analog of the Kolmogorov–Smirnov statistic on the circle. Loader (1999) gives an asymptotic distribution on the circle

$$P(\mathcal{K} \geq Nc) \approx \sqrt{Nc} \int_{u=c}^{1} \left[\frac{c}{1-u} \right]^2 \left[\frac{c}{u} - \rho(u) \right]$$
$$\times \exp[-N\mathcal{L}_1(c+u, u)]/\sqrt{[2\pi(u+c)(1-u-c)]} \, du,$$

where $\rho(u)$ is the solution of

$$\ln(1 + c/u) - c/u = \ln[1 - \rho(u)] + \rho(u).$$

Cressie also suggests use of the normalized statistic

$$\sup_t \sup_w [Y_t(w) - Nw]/\sqrt{[N(w(1 - 1w))]},$$

and gives a conjecture for its distribution. (Note that the denominator is $SE(Y_t(w))$.)

References

Adler, R.J. (1984). The supremum of a particular Gaussian field. *Annals of Probability* **12**, 436–444.

Adler, R.J. (1990). *An Introduction to Continuity, Extrema, and Related Topics for General Gaussian Processes*. IMS Lecture Notes–Monograph Series, Vol. 12, IMS, Hayward, CA.

Ahn, H. and Kuo, W. (1994). Applications of consecutive system reliability in selecting acceptance sampling strategies. In Godbole, A. and Papastravridis, S.G., eds., *Runs and Patterns in Probability*. Kluwer Academic Publishers, Netherlands, pp. 131–162.

Ajne, B. (1968). A simple test for uniformity of a circular distribution. *Biometrika* **55**, 343–354.

Aldous, D. (1989). *Probability Approximations via the Poisson Clumping Heuristic*. Springer-Verlag, New York.

Alexander, F.E. and Boyle, P., Eds. (1996). *Methods for Investigating Localized Clustering of Disease*. International Agency for Research on Cancer Scientific Publications, No. 135. World Health Organization, Lyon, France.

Alm, S.E. (1983). On the distribution of the scan statitic of a Poisson process. In Gut, A. and Helst, L., eds., *Probability and Mathematical Statistics*. Essays in honour of Carl-Gustave Esseen, Upsalla University Press, Upsalla, pp. 1–10.

Alm, S.E. (1997). On the distribution of scan statistics of two-dimensional Poisson processes. *Advances in Applied Probability* **29**, 1–18.

Alm, S.E. (1998). Approximation and simulation of the distribution of scan statistics for Poisson processes in higher dimensions. *Extremes* **1**, 111–126.

Alm, S.E. (1999). Approximations of the distributions of scan statistics of Poisson processes. In Glaz, J. and Balakrishnan, N., eds., *Scan Statistics and Applications*. Birkhäuser, Boston, pp. 113–139.

Anderson, N.H. (1992). Methods for the investigation of spatial clustering with epidemiological applications. Ph.D. Thesis, University of Glasgow.

Anderson, N.H. (1996). Methods for investigating localized clustering of disease. A scan statistic for detecting spatial clusters. In Alexander, F.E. and Boyle, P., eds., *Methods for Investigating Localized Clustering of Disease*. International Agency for Research on Cancer Scientific Publications, NO. 135. World Health Organization, Lyon, France, pp. 215–218.

Anderson, N.H. and Titterington, D.M. (1995). A comparison of two statistics for detecting clustering in one dimension. *Journal Statistical Computation and Simulation* **53**, 103–125.

Anderson, N.H. and Titterington, D.M. (1997). Some methods for investigating spatial clustering, with epidemiological applications. *Journal Royal Statistical Society, Series A* **160**, 87–105.

Anscombe, F.J., Godwin, H.J., and Plackett, R.L. (1947). Methods of deferred sentencing in testing. *Journal of Royal Statistical Society, Series B* **7**, 198–217.

Apostolico, A., Crochemore, M., Galil, Z., and Manbar, U., Eds. (1992). *Combinatorial Pattern Matching*. Lecture Notes in Computer Science, Vol. 644, Springer-Verlag, Berlin.

Appel, M.J.B. and Russo, R.P. (1997). The maximum vertex degree of a graph on uniform points in [0, 1](d). *Advances in Applied Probability* **29**, 567–581.

Arnold, B.C., Balakrishnan, N., and Nagaraja, H.N. (1992). *A First Course in Order Statistics*. Wiley, New York.

Arratia, R. and Gordon, L. (1989). Tutorial on large deviations for the binomial distribution. *Bulletin of Mathematical Biology* **51**, 125–131.

Arratia, R., Gordon, L., and Waterman, M.S. (1986). An extreme value theory for sequence matching, *Annals of Statistics* **14**, 971–993.

Arratia, R., Gordon, L., and Waterman, M.S. (1990). The Erdös–Rényi law in distribution for coin tossing and sequence matching. *Annals of Statistics* **18**, 539–570.

Arratia, R., Morris, P., and Waterman, M.S. (1988). Stochastic scrabble: A law of large numbers for sequence matching with scores. *Journal of Applied Probability* **25**, 106–119.

Arratia, R.A., Goldstein, L., and Gordon, L. (1989). Two moments suffice for Poisson approximations: The Chen–Stein method. *Annals of Probability* **17**, 9–25.

Arratia, R.A., Goldstein, L., and Gordon, L. (1990). Poisson approximation and the Chen–Stein method. *Statistical Science* **5**, 403–434.

Arratia, R.A. and Waterman, M.S. (1985a). Critical phenomena in sequence matching. *Annals of Probability* **13**, 1236–1249.

Arratia, R.A. and Waterman, M.S. (1985b). An Erdös–Rényi law with shifts. *Advances in Mathematics* **55**, 13–23.

Arratia, R.A. and Waterman, M.S. (1989). The Erdös–Rényi strong law for pattern matching with a given proportion of mismatches. *Annals of Probability* **17**, 1152–1169.

Arratia, R.A. and Waterman, M.S. (1994). A phase transition for the score in matching random sequences allowing deletions. *Annals of Applied Probability* **4**, 200–225.

Atwood, C. (1994). Tests of a homogeneous Poisson process against clustering and other alternatives. Ms. Idaho National Engineering Lab, EG&G, Idaho Inc., Idaho Falls, Idaho 83415. Paper presented at August, 1994, meeting of the American Statistical Association in Toronto, 1994.

Auer, P., Hornik, K., and Revesz, P. (1991). Some limits theorems for the homogeneous Poisson process. *Statistics and Probability Letters* **12**, 91–96.

Balakrishnan, N., Balasubramanian, K., and Viveros, R. (1993). On sampling inspection plans based on the theory of runs. *Mathematical Scientist* **18**, 113–126.

Barbour, A.D., Chen, L.H.Y., and Loh, W.L. (1992). Compound Poisson approximation for nonnegative random variables via Stein's method. *Annals of Probability* **20**, 1843–1866.

Barbour, A.D., Chryssaphinou, O., and Roos, M. (1996). Compound Poisson approximation in systems reliability. *Naval Research Logistics* **43**, 251–264.

Barbour, A.D., Holst, L., and Janson, S. (1992). *Poisson Approximation*. Oxford University Press, Oxford.

Barbour, A.D. and Mansson, M. (2000). Compound Poisson approximation and the clustering of random points. *Advances in Applied Probability* **32**, 19–38.

Barbujani, G. and Calzolari, E. (1984). Comparison of two statistical techniques for the surveillance of birth defects through a Monte Carlo simulation. *Statistics in Medicine* **3**, 239–247.

Barraclough, B.M. and White, S.J. (1978). Monthly variation of suicides and undetermined deaths compared. *British Journal of Psychiatry* **132**, 275–278.

Barton, D.E. and David, F.N. (1959). Combinatorial extreme value distributions. *Mathematika* **6**, 63–76.

Barton, D.E. and Mallows, C.L. (1965). Some aspects of the random sequence. *Annals of Mathematical Statistics* **36**, 236–260.

Bateman, G.I. (1948). On the power function of the longest run as a test for randomness in a sequence of alternatives. *Biometrika* **35**, 97–112.

Bauer, P. and Hackl, P. (1978). The use of MOSUMS for quality control. *Technometrics* **20**, 431–436.

Bauer, P. and Hackle, P. (1980). An extension of the MoSum technique for quality control. *Technometrics* **22**, 1–7.

Beirlant, J. and Einmahl, J.H.J. (1996). Maximal type test statistics based on conditional processes. *Journal of Statistical Planning Inferences* **53**, 1–19.

Beirlant, J. and Horvath, L. (1984). Approximation of m-overlapping spacings processes. *Scandinavian Journal of Statistics* **11**, 225–245.

Berg, W. (1945). Aggregates in one- and two-dimensional random distributions. *The London, Edinburgh, and Dublin Philosophical Magazine and Journal of Science* **36**, 319–336.

Berger, A.W. and Whitt, W. (1993). Asymptotics for open-loop window flow control. *Journal of Applied Mathematics and Stochastic Analysis*. In honor of Lajos Takac's 70th birthday.

Berman, M. and Eagleson, G.K. (1983). A Poisson limit theorem for incomplete symmetric statistics. *Journal of Applied Probability* **20**, 47–60.

Berman, M. and Eagleson, G.K. (1985). A useful upper bound for the tail probabilities of the scan statistic when the sample size is large. *Journal of the American Statistical Association* **84**, 560–566.

Besag, J. and Newell, J. (1991). The detection of clusters in rare disease. *Journal of the Royal Statistical Society, Series A* **154**, 143–155.

Binswanger, K. and Embrechts, P. (1994). Longest runs in coin tossing. *Insurance: Mathematics and Economics* **15**, 139–149.

Bogartz, R.S. (1965). The criterion method. Some analyses and remarks. *Psychology Bulletin* **64**, 1–14.

Bogush, Jr., A.J. (1972). Correlated clutter and resultant properties of binary signals. *IEEE Transactions on Aerospace and Electronic Systems* **9**, 208–213.

Boldin, M.B. (1993). On the distribution of run statistics in a linear regression scheme. *Theory of Probability and its Applications* **38**, 129–136.

Bolton, P., Pickles, A., Harrington, R., Macdonald, H., and Rutter, M. (1992). Season of birth: Issues, approaches and findings for autism. *Journal of Child Psychology and Psychiatry* **33**, 509–550.

Bonferroni, C.E. (1936). Teoria statistica delle classi e calcolo delle probabilita. *Publicazioni del R. Instituto Superiore di Scienze Econmiche e Commerciali de Firenze* **8**, 1–62.

Book, S.A. (1979). The stochastic geyser problem for sample quantiles. *Journal of Applied Probability* **16**, 445–448.

Boole, G. (1854). *The Laws of Thought*. Dover, New York (also a 1984 American reprint of a 1854 edition).

Boutsikas, M.V. and Koutras, M.V. (2000). Reliability approximations for Markov chain imbeddable systems. *Methodology and Computing in Applied Probability*, to appear.

Boyle, P., Walker, A.M., and Alexander, F.E. (1996). Historical aspects of leukemia clusters. In Alexander, F.E. and Boyle, P., eds., *Methods for Investigating Localized Clustering of Disease*. International Agency for Research on Cancer Scientific Publications, No. 135. World Health Organization, Lyon, France.

Bradley, J.V. (1968). *Distribution-Free Statistical Tests*. Prentice Hall, Englewood Cliffs, NJ.

Brendel, V. and Karlin, S. (1989). Association of charge clusters with functional domains of cellular transcription factors. *Proceedings of the National Academy of Sciences USA* **86**, 5698–5702.

Brenner, S.E., Chothia, C., and Hubbard, T. (1998). Assessing sequence comparison methods with reliable structurally identified distant evolutionary relationships. *Proceedings of the National Academy of Sciences USA* **95**, 6073–6078.

Brodsky, B.E. and Darkhovsky, B.S. (1993). *Nonparametric Methods in Change-Point Problems*. Reidel, Dordrecht Kluwer Academic, Boston.

Brookner, E. (1966). Recurrent events in a Markov chain. *Information and Control* **9**, 215–229.

Brown, M. and Ge, G. (1984). On the waiting time for the first occurrence of a pattern. In Abdel-Hameed, M.S., Cinlar, E., and Quinn, J., eds., *Reliability Theory and Models*. Academic Press, Orlando, FL.

Burnside, W. (1928). *Theory of Probability*. Cambridge University Press, Cambridge.

Burr, E.J. and Cane, G. (1961). Longest run of consecutive observations having a specified attribute. *Biometrika* **48**, 461–465.

Cai, J. (1994). Reliability of a large consecutive-k-out-of-R-from-N-F system with unequal component reliability. *IEEE Transactions on Reliability* **43**(1), 107–111.

Calzolari, E., Volpato, S., Bianchi, F., Cianciulli, D., Tenconi, R., Clementi, M., Calabro, A., Lungarotti, S., Mastroiacovo, P.P., Botto, L., Spagnola, A., and Milan, M. (1993). Omphalocele and gastroschisis: A collaborative study of five Italian congenital malformation registries. *Teratology* **47**, 47–55.

Cardon, L.R., Burge, C., Schachtel, G.A., Blaisdell, B.E., and Karlin, S. (1993). Comparative DNA sequence features in two long *Escherichia coli* contigs. *Nucleic Acids Research* **21**(6), 3875–3884.

Casella, G. and Berger, R.L. (1990). *Statistical Inference*. Duxbury Press, Belmont.

Casella, G. and Berger, R.L. (1994). Estimation with selected binomial information, or Do you really believe that Dave Winfield is batting 0.471? *Journal of the American Statistical Association* **89**, 1080–1090.

Centers for Disease Control (1990). Guidelines for investigating clusters of health events. *Morbidity and Mortality Weekly Reports (MMWR)* **39** (RR-11), 1–23.

Chan, H.P. (1998). Boundary crossing theory in change-point detection and its applications (fault detection). Ph.D. Thesis, Stanford University.

Chan, H.P. and Lai, T.L. (2000). Saddlepoint approximations for Markov random walks and nonlinear boundary crossing probabilities for scan statistics. Preprint.

Chao, M.T., Fu, J.C., and Koutras, M.V. (1995). Survey of reliability studies of consecutive-k-out-of-n: F and related systems. *IEEE Transactions on Reliability* **44**, 120–127.

Chen, C.F. (1996). Analysis of R-scan statistics for marker arrays in correlated sequences. Ph.D. Thesis, Stanford University, November, 1996, 92 pp.

Chen, C.F. and Karlin, S. (2000). Poisson approximations for conditional r scan lengths of multiple renewal processes and application in marker arrays in biomolecular sequences. *Journal of Applied Probability* **37**, 865–880.

Chen, J. (1998). Approximations and inequalities for discrete scan statistics. Ph.D. Dissertation, University of Connecticut, Storrs, CT.

Chen, J. and Glaz, J. (1996). Two-dimensional discrete scan statistics. *Statistics and Probability Letters* **31**, 59–68.

Chen, J. and Glaz, J. (1997). Approximations and inequalities for the distribution of a scan statistic for 0–1 Bernoulli trials. In Johnson, N.L. and Balakrishnan,

N., eds., *Advances in Theory and Practice of Statistics*. Wiley, New York, pp. 285–298.

Chen, J. and Glaz, J. (1998). Approximations for discrete scan statistics on the circle. Technical report.

Chen, J. and Glaz, J. (1999). Approximations for the distribution of the moments of discrete scan statistics. In Glaz, J. and Balakrishnan, N. eds. *Scan Statistics and Applications*. Birkhäuser, Boston, pp. 27–66.

Chen, J. and Glaz, J. (2000). Approximations for a conditional two-dimensional scan statistic. Technical Report.

Chen, J., Glaz, J., Naus, J., and Wallenstein, S. (2001). Bonferroni-type inequalities for conditional scan statistics. *Statistics and Probability Letters* **53**, 67–77.

Chen, L.H.Y. (1975). Poisson approximations for dependent trials. *Annals of Probability* **3**, 534–545.

Chen, R. (1978). A surveillance system for congenital malformations. *Journal of the American Statistical Association* **73**, 323–327.

Choi, Y.K. (1990). The Erdös–Rényi law for stationary Gaussian sequences. *Journal of Mathematics of Kyoto University* **30**, 559–573.

Chryssaphinou, O. and Papastavridis, S. (1988). A limit theorem for the number of occurrences of a pattern in a sequence pattern in a sequence of independent trials. *Journal of Applied Probability* **25**, 428–431.

Chryssaphinou, O. and Papastavridis, S. (1990). Limit distribution for a consecutive-*k*-out-of-*n*: *F* system. *Advances in Applied Probability* **22**, 491–493.

Chryssaphinou, O. and Papastavridis, S., and Tsapekas, T. (1993). On the number of overlapping success runs in a sequence of independent Bernoulli trials. *Applications of Fibonacci Numbers* **5**, 103–112.

Chu, J.T. (1957). Some uses of quasi-ranges. *Annals of Mathematical Statistics* **28**, 173–180.

Chung, K.L., Erdos, P., and Sirao, T. (1959). On the Lipschitz condition for Brownian motion. *Journal of the Mathematical Society of Japan* **11**, 263–274.

Chvatal, V. and Sankoff, D. (1975). Longest common subsequences of two random sequences. *Journal of Applied Probability* **12**, 306–315.

Cohen, P. (1994). Is duodenal ulcer a seasonal disease? Statistical considerations. *American Journal of Gastroenterology* **90**, 1189–1190.

Collins, J.H., Coulson, A.F.W., and Lyall, A. (1988). The significance of protein sequence similarities. *Computer Applications in Biological Sciences* **4**, 67–71.

Cone, A.F. and Dodge, H.F. (1963). A cumulative-results plan for small-sample inspection. Sandia Corp. Reprint, SCR-678, Alburquerque, NM.

Conover, W.J., Bement, T.R., and Iman, R.L. (1979). On a method of detecting clusters of possible uranium deposits. *Technometrics* **21**, 277–283.

Cressie, N. (1973). Testing for uniformity against a clustering alternative. Ph.D. Thesis, Department of Statistics, Princeton University.

Cressie, N. (1976). On the logarithms of high-order spacings. *Biometrika* **63**, 343–355.

Cressie, N. (1977a). On the minimum of higher-order gaps. *Australian Journal of Statistics* **19**, 132–143.

Cressie, N. (1977b). On some properties of the scan statistic on the circle and the line. *Journal of Applied Probability* 14, 272–283.

Cressie, N. (1977c). Clustering on the circle. *Bulletin of the International Statistical Institute* 47 (book 4), 124–127.

Cressie, N. (1978). Power results for tests based on high-order gaps. *Biometrika* 65, 214–218.

Cressie, N. (1979). An optimal statistic based on higher-order gaps. *Biometrika* 66, 619–627.

Cressie, N. (1980). The asymptotic distribution of the scan statistic under uniformity. *Annals of Probability* 8, 838–840.

Cressie, N. (1981). How useful are asymptotic results in extrema problems? *Bulletin of the International Statistical Institute* 49, 899–900.

Cressie, N. (1984). Using the scan statistic to test uniformity. *Colloquia Mathematica Societetis János Bolayai* 45, Goodness of Fit, Debrecen, Hungary, pp. 87–100.

Cressie, N. (1991). *Statistics for Spatial Data*. Wiley, New York.

Cressie, N. and Davis, R.W. (1981). The supremum distribution of another Gaussian process. *Journal of Applied Probability* 18, 121–138.

Crowley, E.M., Roeder, K., and Bina, M. (1997). A statistical model for locating regulatory regions in genomic DNA. *Journal of Molecular Biology* 268, 8–14.

Csaki, E., Foldes, A., and Komlos, J. (1987). Limit theorems for Erdös–Rényi-type problems. *Studia Scientiarum Mathematicarum Hungarica* 22, 321–332.

Csorgo, M. and Revesz, P. (1979). How small are the increments of a Wiener process? *Stochastic Processes and Their Applications* 8, 119–129.

Csorgo, M. and Revesz, P. (1981). *Strong Approximations in Probability and Statistics*. Academic Press, New York.

Csorgo, M. and Steinbach, J. (1981). Improved Erdös–Rényi and strong approximation laws for increments of partial sums. *Annals of Probability* 9, 988–996.

Curnow, R.N. and Kirkwood, T.B.L. (1989). Statistical analysis of deoxyribonucleic acid sequence data—A review. *Journal of the Royal Statistical Society, Series A* 152, 199–220.

Dandekar, V. (1955). Certain modified forms of binomial and Poisson distributions. *Sankhya: the Indian Journal of Statistics* 15, 237–250.

Darling, R.W.R. and Waterman, M.S. (1985). Matching rectangles in d dimensions: Algorithms and laws of large numbers. *Advances in Mathematics* 55, 1–12.

Darling, R.W.R. and Waterman, M.S. (1986). Extreme value distribution for the largest cube in a random lattice. *SIAM Journal on Applied Mathematics* 46, 118–132.

Dat, N. van (1982). Tests for time–space clustering of disease. Ph.D. Thesis, University of North Carolina at Chapel Hill, 106pp.

David, F.N. (1947). A power function for tests for randomness in a sequence of alternatives. *Biometrika* 34, 335–339.

David, H.A. and Kinyon, L.C. (1983). The probability that out of n events at least r ($\geq n - 2$), occur within the time span t. In Sen, P.K., ed., *Contributions to*

Statistics: Essays in Honour of Norman L. Johnson. North-Holland, Amsterdam, pp. 107–113.

David, H.A. and Newell, D.J. (1965). The identification of annual peak periods for a disease. *Biometrics* **21**, 645–650.

David, H.T. (1958). A three sample Kolmogorov–Smirnov test. *Annals of Mathematical Statistics* **29**, 842–851.

Dawson, D.A. and Sankoff, D. (1967). An inequality for probabilities. *Proceedings of American Mathematical Society* **18**, 504-507.

Dayhoff, J.E. (1984). Distinguished words in data sequences: Analysis and applications to neural coding and other fields. *Bulletin of Mathematical Biology* **46**, 529–543.

Deheuvels, P. (1985a). On the Erdös–Rényi theorem for random fields and sequences of its relationships with the theory of runs and spacings. *Zeitschrift Wahrscheinlicheitstheorie* **70** 91–115.

Deheuvels, P. (1986b). Spacings and applications. *Probability and Statistical Decision Theory* A (Bad Tatzmannsdorf, 1983), pp. 1–30.

Deheuvels, P. (1997). Strong laws for local quantile processes. *Annals of Probability* **25**, 2007–2054.

Deheuvels, P. and Devroye, L. (1983). Limit laws related to the Erdös–Rényi theorem. Technical Report #6, LSTA, Universite Paris VI.

Deheuvels, P., Erdos, P., Grill, K., and Revesz, P. (1987). Many heads in a short block. *Math. Statist. Prob. Theory* (M.L. Puri et al., eds.) A, pp. 53–67.

Deheuvels, P. and Steinbach, J. (1986). Exact convergence rate of Erdös–Rényi strong law for moving quantiles. *Journal of Applied Probability* **23**, 355–369.

Deheuvels, P. and Steinbach, J. (1987). Exact convergence rates in strong approximation laws for large increments of partial sums. *Probability Theory and Related Fields* **76**, 369–393.

Deken, J. (1983). Probabilistic behavior of the longest common subsequence length. In Sankoff, D. and Kruskal, J.B., eds., *Time Warps, String Edits, and Macromolecules: The Theory and Practice of Sequence Comparisons.* Addison-Wesley, Reading, MA, pp. 359–362.

Dembo, A. and Karlin, S. (1992). Poisson approximations for r-scan processes. *Annals of Applied Probability* **2**, 329–357.

de Moivre, A. (1738). *The Doctrine of Chances.* 3rd ed., Chelsea Publishing Co., New York, 1967.

Dersch, E. and Steinbach, J. (1987). On improved versions of generalized Erdös–Rényi laws and large deviation asymptotics. In Sendler, W., ed., *Contributions of Stochastics: In Honour of the 75th Birthday of Walther Eberl, Sr.* Physica-Verlag, Heidelberg, Springer-Verlag, New York, pp. 38–49.

Diaconis, P. and Mosteller, F. (1989). Methods for studying coincidences. *Journal of the American Statistical Association* **84**, 853–861.

Dinneen, G.P. and Reed, I.S. (1956). An analysis of signal detection and location by digital methods. *IRE Transactions on Information Theory* **IT-2**, 29–39.

Doheer, M.G., Carpenter, T.E., Wilson, W.D., and Gardner, I.A. (1999). Evaluation of temporal and spatial clustering of horses with Corynebacterium pseudoturberculosis infection. *American Journal of Veterinary Research* **60**(3), 284–291.

Domb, C. (1947). The problem of random intervals on a line. *Proceedings of the Cambridge Philosophical Society* **43**, 329–341.

Domb, C. (1950). Some probability distributions connected with recording apparatus II. *Proceedings of the Cambridge Philosophical Society* **46**, 429–435.

Domb, C. (1972). A note on the series expansion method for clustering problems. *Biometrika* **59**, 209–211.

Drosnin, M. (1997). *The Bible Code*. Simon & Schuster, New York.

Du, D.Z. (1986). Optimal consecutive-2-out-of-*n* system. *Mathematics Operation Research* **11**, 187–191.

Du, D.Z. and Hwang, F.K. (1988). A direct algorithm for computing reliability of a consecutive-*k* cycle. *IEEE Transactions in Reliability* **37**, 70–72.

Dunkel, O. (1925). Solutions of a probability difference equation. *American Mathematical Monthly* **32**, 354–370.

Ebneshahrashoob, M. and Sobel, M. (1990). Sooner and later waiting time problems for Bernoulli trials: Frequency and run quotas. *Statistics and Probability Letters* **9**, 5–11.

Ederer, F., Myers, M.H., and Mantel, N. (1964). A statistical problem in space and time. Do leukemia cases come in clusters? *Biometrics* **20**, 626–636.

Edmonds, L. and James, L.M. (1993). Temporal trends in birth prevalence of selected congenital malformations in the Birth Defects Monitoring Program/Commission on Professional and Hospital Activities, 1979–1989. *Teratology* **48**, 647–649.

Edwards, J.H. (1961). The recognition and estimation of cyclic trends. *Annals of Human Genetics* **25**, 83–86.

Eggleton, P. and Kermack, W.O. (1944). A problem in the random distribution of particles. *Proceedings of the Royal Society of Edinburgh, Series A* **62**, 103–115.

Ekbom, A., Zack, M., Adami, H.O., and Helmick, C. (1991). Is there clustering of inflammatory bowel disease at birth? *American Journal of Epidemiology* **134**, 876–886.

Elteren, Van P.H. and Gerritis, H.J.M. (1961). Ein wachtprobleem voorkomende bij drempelwaardemetingen aan het oof. *Statistica Neerlandica* **15**, 385–401 (English summary).

Engelberg, O. (1964a). (see also Percus). Exact and limiting distribution of the number of lead positions in an unconditional ballot problem. *Journal of Applied Probability* **1**, 168–172.

Engelberg, O. (1964b). Generalization of the ballot problem. *Zeitschrift für Wahrscheinlichkeitstheorie und Verwandte Gebiete* **3**, 271–275.

Erdös, P. and Rényi, A. (1970). On a new law of large numbers. *Journal d'Analyse Mathematique* **23**, 103–111.

Erdös, P. and Revesz, P. (1975). On the length of the longest head-run. *Topics in Information Theory, Colloquia Mathematica Societatis János Bolyai* **16**, 219–228. Keszthely, Hungary.

Erdös, P. and Revesz, P. (1987). Problems and results on random walks. In P. Bauer, F. Konecny, and W. Wertz, eds., *Mathematical Statistics and Probability Theory, Proc. 6th Pannonian Symposium on Mathematical Statistics, Bad Tatzmanndorf, Austria*, Sept. 14–20, 1986, Vol. B. Reidel, Dordrecht, pp. 59–65.

Esary, J.D., Proschan, F., and Walkup, D. (1967). Association of random variables with applications. *Annals of Mathematical Statistics* **38**, 1466–1474.

Everett, J. (1953). State probabilities in congestion problems characterized by constant holding times. *Operations Research* **1**, 279–285.

Farrington, C.P., Andrews, N.J., Beale, A.A., and Catchpole, M.A. (1996). A statistical algorithm for the early detection of outbreaks of infections disease. *Journal of the Royal Statistical Association, Series A* **159**, 547–563.

Feinberg, S.E. and Kaye, D.H. (1991). Legal and statistical aspects of some mysterious clusters. *Journal of the Royal Statistical Association, Series A* **154**, 61–74.

Feller, W. (1957, 1958, 1967, 1968). *An Introduction to Probability Theory and its Applications*. Vol. I, 2nd ed., Wiley, New York.

Fisher, R.A. (1959). *Statistical Methods and Scientific Inference*. Hafner, New York.

Flatto, L. (1973). A limit theorem for random coverings of a circle. *Israel Journal of Mathematics* **15**, 167–184.

Foldes, A. (1979). The limit distribution of the length of the longest head run. *Periodica Mathematica Hungarica* **10**, 301–310.

Fousler, D. and Karlin, S. (1987). Maximal success runs for semi-Markov processes. *Stochastic Processes and their Applications* **24**, 203–224.

Freedman, D. (1974). The Poisson approximation for dependent events. *Annals of Probability* **2**, 256–269.

Frieze, A.M., Preparata, F.P., and Upfal, E. (1999). Optimal reconstruction of a sequence from its probes. *Journal of Computational Biology* **6**, 361–368.

Frosini, B.V. (1981). Distribution of the smallest interval that contains a given cluster of points. *Statistica* **41**, 255–280.

Fu, J.C. (1986). Reliability of consecutive-k-out-of-n-F system with $(k-1)$ step Markov dependence. *IEEE Transactions on Reliability* **35**, 602–606.

Fu, J.C. (2000). Distribution of scan and related statistics for a sequence of Bernoulli trials. Manuscript Department of Statistics, The University of Manitoba, Winnipeg, Manitoba, Canada.

Fu, J.C. and Hu, B. (1987). On reliability of large consecutive-k-out-of-n-F system with $(k-1)$ step Markov dependence. *IEEE Transactions on Reliability* **36**, 75–77.

Fu, J.C. and Koutras, M.V. (1994a). Poisson approximations for two-dimensional patterns. *Annals of the Institute of Statistical Mathematics* **46**, 179–192.

Fu, J.C. and Koutras, M.V. (1994b). Distribution theory of runs: A Markov chain approach. *Journal of the American Statistical Association* **89**, 1050–1058.

Fu, J.C., Lou, W.Y., and Chen, S.C. (1999). On the probability of pattern matching in nonaligned DNA sequences: A finite Markov chain embedding approach. In

Glaz, J. and Balakrishnan, N., eds., *Scan Statistics and Applications*. Birkhäuser, Boston, pp. 287–302.

Fu, Y. and Curnow, R.N. (1990). Locating a changed segment in a sequence of Bernoulli variables. *Biometrika* **77**, 295–304.

Furth, R. (1920). Schwankungserscheinungen un der Physik. Braunschweig: *Sammlung Vieweg*, 1–17.

Galambos, J. and Simonelli, I. (1996). *Bonferroni-Type Inequalities with Applications*. Springer-Verlag, New York.

Galati, G. and Studer, F.A. (1982). Angular accuracy of the binary moving window detector. *IEEE Transactions on Aerospace and Electronic Systems* **18** 416–422.

Gates, D.J. (1985). Asymptotics of two integrals from optimization theory and geometric probability. *Advances in Applied Probability* **17**, 908–910.

Gates, D.J. and Westcott, M. (1984). On the distribution of scan statistics. *Journal of the American Statistical Association* **79**, 423–429.

Gates, D.J. and Westcott, M. (1985). Accurate and asymptotic results for distributions of scan statistics. *Journal of Applied Probability* **22**, 531–542.

Giglyavskii, A.A. and Kraskovskii, A.E. (1988). *Disorder Detection for Random Sequences in Radiotechnical Problems*. Leningrad State University, Leningrad (Russian).

Gilbert, E.N. and Pollack, H.O. (1957). Coincidences in Poisson patterns. *Bell System Technical Journal* **39**, 1005–1033.

Glaz, J. (1978). Multiple coverage and clusters on the line. Ph.D. Thesis, Rutgers University.

Glaz, J. (1979a). Expected waiting time for the visual response. *Biological Cybernetics* **35**, 39–41.

Glaz, J. (1979b). The number of dense arrangements. *Journal of Combinatorial Theory, Series A* **27**, 367–370.

Glaz, J. (1981). Clustering of events in a stochastic process. *Journal of Applied Probability* **18**, 268–275.

Glaz, J. (1983). Moving window detection for discrete scan. *IEEE Transactions on Information Theory* **IT-29**(3), 457–462.

Glaz, J. (1989). Approximations and bounds for the distribution of the scan statistic. *Journal of the American Statistical Association* **84**, 560–569.

Glaz, J. (1990). A comparison of Bonferroni-type and product-type inequalities in the presence of dependence. In H.W. Block, A.R. Sampson, and T.H. Savits, eds., *Topics in Statistical Dependence*, IMS Lecture Notes–Monograph Series, Vol. 16. IMS, Hayward, CA, pp. 223–235.

Glaz, J. (1992). Approximations for tail probabilities and moments of the scan statistic. *Computational Statistics and Data Analysis* **14**, 213–227.

Glaz, J. (1993a). *Extreme Order Statistics for a Sequence of Dependent Random Variables. Stochastic Inequalities*. IMS Lecture Notes–Monograph Series, Vol. 22. IMS, Hayward, CA, pp. 100–115.

Glaz, J. (1993b). Approxiations for tail probabilities and moments of the scan statistic. *Statistics in Medicine* **12**, 1845–1852.

Glaz, J. (1996). Discrete scan statistics with applications to minefields detection. *Proceedings of Conference SPIE*, Orlando, Florida, *SPIE*, **2765**, 420–429.

Glaz, J. and Balakrishnan, N. (1999a). Introduction to scan statistics. In Glaz, J. and Balakrishnan, N., eds., *Scan Statistics and Applications*. Birkhäuser, Boston, pp. 3–24.

Glaz, J. and Balakrishnan, N. (1999b). *Scan Statistics and Applications*. Birkhäuser, Boston.

Glaz, J., Hormel, P., and Johnson, B. (1986). Moving window detection for 0–1 Markov trials. *Symposium on Interface of Computer Science and Statistics*, pp. 571–576.

Glaz, J. and Johnson, B. (1986). Approximating boundary crossing probabilities with applications to sequential tests. *Sequential Analysis* **5**, 37–72.

Glaz, J. and Johnson, B. (1988). Bounary crossing for moving sums. *Journal of Applied Probability* **25**, 81–88.

Glaz, J. and Naus, J. (1979). Multiple coverage of the line. *Annals of Probability* **7**, 900–906.

Glaz, J. and Naus, J. (1983). Multiple clusters on the line. *Communications in Statistics—Theory and Methods* **12**, 1961–1986.

Glaz, J. and Naus, J. (1986). Approximating probabilities of first passage in a particular Gaussian process. *Communications in Statistics—Theory and Methods, Section A* **15**, 1709–1722.

Glaz, J. and Naus, J. (1991). Tight bounds and approximations for scan statistic probabilities for discrete data. *Annals of Applied Probability* **1**, 306–318.

Glaz, J., Naus, J., Roos, M., and Wallenstein, S. (1994). Poisson approximations for the distribution and moments of ordered m-spacings. *Journal of Applied Probability* **31A**, 271–281.

Godbole, A.P. (1990). Specific formulae for some success run distributions. *Statistics and Probability Letters* **10**, 119–124.

Godbole, A.P. (1991). Poisson approximations for runs and patterns of rare events. *Advances in Applied Probability* **23**, 851–865.

Godbole, A.P. (1993). Approximate reliabilities of m-consecutive-k-out-of-n failure systems. *Statistical Sinica* **3**, 321–327.

Godbole, A.P. and Papastavridis, S.G. (1994). *Runs and Patterns in Probability*. Kluwer Academic, Amsterdam.

Godbole, A.P., Potter, L.K., and Sklar, J. (1998). Improved upper bounds for the reliability of d-dimensional consecutive-k-out-of-n: FS systems. *Naval Research Logistics* **45**, 219–230.

Goldman, A.J. and Bender, B.K. (1962). The first run preceded by a quota. *Journal of Research National Bureau of Standards* Sect. **B**, 77–89.

Goldstein, L. and Waterman, M.S. (1992). Poisson, compound Poisson and process approximations for testing statistical significance in sequence comparisons. *Bulletin of Mathematical Biology* **54**, 785–812.

Gonzalez-Barrios, J.M. (1996). The volume of the smallest parallelepiped including m random points. *Statistics and Probability Letters* **30**, 139–145.

Goodwin, J.M. and Giese, E.W. (1965). Reliability of spare part support for a complex system with repair. *Operations Research* **13**, 413–423.

Gordon, L., Schilling, M.F., and Waterman, M.S. (1986). An extreme value theory for long head runs. *Probability Theory and Related Fields* **72**, 279–288.

Gould, M.S., Petrie, K., Kleinman, M.N., and Wallenstein, S. (1994). Clustering of attempted suicide—New Zealand national data. *International Journal of Epidemiology* **23**, 2285–2289.

Gould, M.S., Wallenstein, S., and Davidson, L. (1989). Suicide clusters: A critical review. *Suicide and Life Threatening Behavior* **19**, 17–29.

Gould, M.S., Wallenstein, and Kleinman, M.G. (1990). Time–space clustering of teenage suicide. *American Journal of Epidemiology* **31**, 71–78.

Gould, M.S., Wallenstein, S., Kleinman, M.G., O'Carroll, P., and Mercy, J. (1990). Suicide clusters: An examination of age specific effects. *American Journal of Public Health* **80**, 211–213.

Gower, B. (1987). Planets and probability: Daniel Bernouilli on the inclination of the planetary orbits. *Studies in History and Philosophy of Science* **18**, 441–454.

Grant, D.A. (1947). Additional tables of the probability of "runs" of correct responses in learning and problem-solving. *Psychological Bulletin* **44**, 276–279.

Greenberg, I. (1970a). The first occurrence of N successes in M trials. *Technometrics* **12**, 627–634.

Greenberg, I. (1970b). On sums of random variables defined on a two-state Markov chain. *Journal of Applied Probability* **13**, 604–607.

Greenberg, M., Naus, J., Schneider, D., and Wartenberg, D. (1991). Temporal clustering of homicide and suicide among 15–24 year old white and black Americans. *Ethnicity and Disease* **1**, 342–350.

Griffith, W.S. (1986). On consecutive-k-out-of-n failure systems and their generalizations. In Basu, A.P., ed., *Reliability and Quality Control*. Elsevier, Amsterdam, pp. 157–166.

Griffith, W.S. (1994). Runs and patterns with applications to reliability. In Godbole, A.P. and Papastavridis, S.G., eds., *Runs and Patterns in Probability*. Kluwer Academic, Amsterdam, pp. 173–181.

Grimson, R.C., Aldrich, T.E., and Drane, J.W. (1992). Clustering in sparse data and an analysis of Rhabdomyosarcoma incidence. *Statistics in Medicine* **11**, 761–768.

Grind, Van de, W.A., Koenderink, J.J., Heyde, Van der, G.L., Landman, H., and Bowman, M.A. (1971). Adapting coincidence scalers and neural modeling studies of vision. *Kybernetik* **8**, 85–105.

Grind, Van de, W.A., Schalm, T. Van, and Bowman, M.A. (1968). A coincidence model of the processing of quantum signals by the human retina. *Kybernetik* **4**, 141–146.

Guibas, L.J. and Odlyzko, A.M. (1980). Long repetitive patterns in random sequences. *Zeitschrift für Wahrscheinlichkeitstheorie Verwandte Gebiete* **53**, 241–262.

Guttorp, P. and Lokhart, R.A. (1989). On the asymptotic distribution of high-order spacings statistics. *Canadian Journal of Statistics* **17**, 419–426.

Haiman, G. (1987). Etudes des extremes d'une suite stationnaire m-dependante avec une application relative aux accroissements du processus de Wiener. *(Paris University) Annales de l'Institut Henri Poincaré* **23**, 425–458.

Hald, A. (1990). *A History of Probability and Statistics and their Applications before 1750*. Wiley, New York.

Hall, P. (1984). Limit theorems for sums of general functions of m-spacings. *Mathematical Proceedings of the Cambridge Philosophical Society* **96**, 517–532.

Hall, P. (1986). On powerful distributional tests based on sample spacings. *Journal of Multivariate Analysis* **19**, 201–224.

Hamilton, J.F., Lawton, W.H., and Trabka, E.A. (1972). Some spatial and temporal point processes in photographic science. In Lewis, P.A.W., ed., *Stochastic Point Processes: Statistical Analysis, Theory and Applications*. Wiley Interscience, New York, 1972, pp. 817–867.

Hewitt, D., Milner, J., Csima, A., and Pakula, A. (1971). On Edwards' criterion of seasonality and a non-parametric alternative. *British Journal of Preventive and Social Medicine* **25**, 174–176.

Hirano, K. and Aki, S. (1993). On number of occurrences of success runs of specified length in a two-state Markov chain. *Statistica Sinica* **3**, 313–320.

Hjalmers, U., Kulldorff, M., Gustafsson, G., and Nagarwalla, N. (1996). Childhood leukemia in Sweden using GIS and a spatial scan statistic for cluster detection. *Statistics in Medicine* **15**, 707–715.

Hoh, J. and Ott, J. (2000). Scan statistics to scan markers for suspectibility genes. *Proceedings of the National Academy of Sciences USA* **97**, 9615–9617.

Holst, L. (1980). The multiple covering of a circle with random arcs. *Journal of Applied Probability* **17**, 284–290.

Holst, L. and Janson, S. (1990). Poisson approximation using the Stein–Chen method and coupling the number of exceedances of Gaussian random variables. *Annals of Probability* **18**, 713–723.

Hoover, D.R. (1989). Bounds on expectations of order statistics for dependent samples. *Statistics and Probability Letters* **8**, 261–264.

Hoover, D.R. (1990). Subset complement addition upper bounds—An improved inclusion–exclusion method. *Journal of Statistical Planning and Inference* **24**, 195–202.

Hoppe, F.M. and Seneta, E. (1990). A Bonferroni-type identity and permutation bounds. *International Statistical Review* **58**, 253–261.

Hourani, L.L., Warrack, A.G., and Cohen, P.R. (1997). Suicide in the U.S. Marine Corps. 1990–1996. U.S. Naval Health Center Report #97-32, San Diego, CA, Sept. 1997, pp. 1–20.

Hryhorczuk, D.O., Frateschi, L.J., Lipscomb, J.W., and Zhang, R. (1992). Use of the scan statistic to detect temporal clustering of poisonings. *Journal of Toxicology, Clinical Toxicology* **30**, 459–465.

Huffer, F.W. (1982). The moments and distributions of some quantities arising from random arcs on the circle. Ph.D. Dissertation, Department of Statistics, Stanford University, Stanford, CA.

Huffer, F.W. (1988). Divided differences and the joint distribution of linear combinations of spacings. *Journal of Applied Probability* **25**, 346–354.

Huffer, F.W. and Lin, C.-T. (1997a). Approximating the distribution of the scan statistic using moments of the number of clumps. *Journal of American Statistical Association* **92**, 1466–1475.

Huffer, F.W. and Lin, C.-T. (1997b). Computing the exact distribution of the extremes of sums of consecutive spacings. *Computational Statistics and Data Analysis* **26**, 117–132.

Huffer, F.W. and Lin, C.-T. (1999a). An approach to computations involving spacings with applications to the scan statistic. In Glaz, J. and Balakrishan, N., eds., *Scan Statistics and Applications*. Birkhäuser, Boston, pp. 141–163.

Huffer, F.W. and Lin, C.-T. (1999b). Using moments to approximate the distribution of the scan statistics. In Glaz, J. and Balakrishan, N., eds., *Scan Statistics and Applications*. Birkhäuser, Boston, pp. 165–190.

Hunter, D. (1976). An upper bound for the probability of a union. *Journal of Applied Probability* **13**, 597–603.

Huntington, R.J. (1974a). Distributions and expectations for clusters in continuous and discrete cases, with applications. Ph.D. Thesis, Rutgers University.

Huntington, R.J. (1974b). Distributions for clusters in continuous and discrete cases. *Northeast Science Review* **4** (W.H. Long and M. Chatterjii, eds.), 153–161.

Huntington, R.J. (1976a). Mean recurrence times for k successes within m trials. *Journal of Applied Probability* **13**, 604–607.

Huntington, R.J. (1976b). Expected waiting time till a constrained quota. Technical report, AT&T.

Huntington, R.J. (1978). Distribution of the minimum number of points in a scanning interval on the line. *Stochastic Processes and their Applications* **7**, 73–77.

Huntington, R.J. and Naus, J.I. (1975). A simpler expression for Kth nearest neighbor coincidence probabilities. *Annals of Probability* **3**, 894–896.

Husler, J. (1982). Random coverage of the circle and asymptotic distributions. *Journal of Applied Probability* **19**, 578–587.

Husler, J. (1987). Minimal spacings of non-uniform densities. *Stochastic Processes and their Applications* **25**, 73–81.

Hwang, F.K. (1974). A discrete clustering problem. Manuscript, Bell Laboratories, Murray Hill.

Hwang, F.K. (1977). A generalization of the Karlin–McGregor theorem on coincidence probabilities and an application to clustering. *Annals of Probability* **5**, 814–817.

Hwang, F.K. (1982). Fast solutions for consecutive-k-out-of-n: F systems. *IEEE Transactions on Reliability* **R-31**(5), 447–448.

Hwang, F.K. and Wright, P.E. (1995). An $O(k^3 \log |n/k|)$ algorithm for the consecutive-k-out-of-n: F system. *IEEE Transactions on Reliability* **R-44**, 128–131.

Hwang, F.K. and Wright, P.E. (1997). An $O(n/\log n)$ algorithm for the generalized birthday problem. *Computational Statistics and Data Analysis* **23**, 443–451.

Ikeda, S. (1965). On Bouman–Velden–Yamamoto's asymptotic evaluation formula for the probability of visual response in a certain experimental research in quantum biophysics of vision. *Annals of the Institute of Statistical Mathematics* **17**, 295–310.

Jacquez, G.M., Ed. (1993). *Proceedings of the Workshop on Statistics and Computing in Disease Clustering.* Port Washington, New York, 1992. *Statistics in Medicine* **12**, 1751–1968.

Jacquez, G.M., Grimson, R., Waller, L.A., and Wartenberg, D. (1996). The analysis of disease clusters, Part II: Introduction to techniques. *Infection Control and Hospital Epidemiology* **17**, 385–397.

Jain, M. and Ghimire, R.P. (1997). Reliability of k-in-r-out-of-N G system subject to random and common cause failure. *Performance Evaluation* **29**, 213–218.

Janson, S. (1984). Bounds on the distributions of extremal values of a scanning process. *Stochastic Processes and their Applications* **18**, 313–328.

Jiang, G.X., Cheng, Q., Link, H., and de Pedro-Cuesta, J. (1997). Epidemiological features of Guillain–Barre syndrome in Sweden, 1978–1993. *Journal of Neurology, Neurosurgery and Psychiatry* **62**, 447–453.

Johnson, N.L., Kotz, S., and Kemp, A.W. (1992). *Univariate Discrete Distributions*, 2nd ed. Wiley, New York.

Kaplan, N. (1977). Two applications of a Poisson approximation for dependent events. *Annals of Probability* **5**, 787–794.

Karlin, S. (1988). Coincident probabilities and applications in combinatorics. *Journal of Applied Probability*, 25th Year Anniversary Volume, pp. 185–200.

Karlin, S. (1994). Statistical studies of biomolecular sequences: Score-based methods. *Phil. Transactions of the Royal Society of London, Series B* **344**, 391–402.

Karlin, S. (1995). Statistical significance of sequence patterns in proteins. *Current Opinion in Structural Biology* **5**, 360–371.

Karlin, S. and Altschul, F. (1990). Methods for assessing the statistical significance of molecular sequence features by using general scoring schemes. *Proceedings of the National Academy of Science USA* **87**, 2264–2268.

Karlin, S. Blaisdell, B., Mocarski, E., and Brendel, V. (1989). A method to identify distinctive charge configurations in protein sequences, with application to human Herpes virus polypeptides. *Journal of Molecular Biology* **205**, 165–177.

Karlin, S., Blaisdell, B.E., Sapolsky, R.J., Cardon, L., and Burge, C. (1993). Assessments of DNA inhomogeneities in yeast chromosome III. *Nucleic Acids Research* **21**(3), 703–711.

Karlin, S. and Brendel, V. (1992). Chance and statistical significance in protein and DNA sequence analysis. *Science* **257**, 39–49.

Karlin, S. and Cardon, L.R. (1994). Computational DNA sequence analysis. *Annual Review of Microbiology* **48**, 619–654.

Karlin, S. and Dembo, A. (1992). Limit distributions of maximal segmental score among Markov-dependent partial sums. *Advances in Applied Probability* **24**, 113–140.

Karlin, S., Dembo, A., and Kawabata, T. (1990). Statistical composition of high scoring segments from molecular sequences. *Annals of Statistics* **18**, 571–581.

Karlin, S. and Ghandour, G. (1985). Multiple-alphabet amino acid sequence comparisons of the immunoglobulin *k*-chain constant domain. *Proceedings of the National Academy of Science USA* (Genetics) **82**, 8597–8601.

Karlin, S., Ghandour, G., and Foulser, D.E. (1985). DNA sequence comparisons of the human, mouse, and rabbit immunoglobulin kappa gene. *Molecular Biology and Evolution* **2**, 35–52.

Karlin, S. and Leung, M.Y. (1991). Some limit theorems on distributional patterns of balls in urns. *Annals of Applied Probability* **1**, 513–538.

Karlin, S. and MacDonald, M., and Schaechtel, G. (1993). Exact formulas for multitype run statistics in a random ordering. *SIAM Journal of Discrete Mathematics* **6**, 70–86.

Karlin, S. and Macken, C. (1991). Some statistical problems in the assessment of inhomogeneities of DNA sequence data. *Journal of the American Statistical Association* **86**, 27–35.

Karlin, S. and McGregor, G. (1959). Coincidence probabilities. *Pacific Journal of Mathematics* **9**, 1141–1164.

Karlin, S. and Ost, F. (1985). Maximal segmental match length among random sequences from a finite alphabet. In LeCam, L.M. and Olshen, R.A., eds., *Proceedings of the Berkeley Conference in Honor of Jerzy Neyman and Jack Kiefer*, Vol. 1. Wadsworth, Belmont, CA, pp. 225–243.

Karlin, S. and Ost, F. (1987). Counts of long aligned word matches among random letter sequences. *Advances in Applied Probability* **19**, 293–351.

Karlin, S. and Ost, F. (1988). Maximal length of common words among random letter sequences. *Annals of Probability* **16**, 535–563.

Karwe, V.V. (1993). The distribution of the supremum of integer moving average processes with application to the maximum net charge in DNA sequences. Ph.D. Thesis, Rutgers University.

Karwe, V.V. and Naus, J. (1997). New recursive methods for scan statistic probabilities. *Computational Statistics and Data Analysis* **23**, 389 404.

Kase, L.M. (1996). Why community cancer clusters are often ignored. *Scientific American*, September, pp. 85–86.

Katiyar, S.K., Visvesvara, G.S., and Edlind, T.D. (1995). Comparisons of ribosomal RNA sequences from amitochondrial protozoa: Implications for processing *m*RNA binding and paromomycin susceptibility. *Gene* **152**, 27–33.

Kay, L.A.W. (1997). Properties of the Ederer–Myers–Mantel statistic and ordered equiprobable multinomial vectors. Ph.D. Thesis, University of Kentucky, 112 pages.

Kerstan, J. (1964). Verallgemeinerung eines Satzes von Prochorov und Le Cam. *Zeitschrift für Wahrscheinlichkeitstheorie Verwandte Gebiete* **2**, 173–179.

Kevan, S.M. (1980). Perspectives on season of suicide: A review. *Social Science and Medicine* **14D**, 369–378.

Khashimov, Sh.A. (1987). Asymptotic properties of functions of spacings. *Theory of Proability and its Applications* **34**, 298–306.

Khatri,C.G. and Mitra, S.K. (1969). Some identities and approximations concering positive and negative multinomial distributions. In Krishnaiah, P.R., ed., *Multivariate Analysis* II. Academic Press, New York, pp. 241–260.

Kim, B.S. and Kim, G.H. (1993). A review on the development of a scan statistic and its applications. *Korean Journal of Applied Statistics* 6, 125–143.

King, W., Darlington, G.A., Kreiger, N., and Fehringer, G. (1993). Response of a cancer registry to reports of disease clusters. *European Journal of Cancer* 29a, 1414–1418.

Kirkwood, T.B.L. (1989). Methods for comparing DNA sequences. Special Topics Section, *Biometric Bulletin*, pp. 20–21.

Knox, G. and Lancashire, R. (1982). Detection of minimal epidemics. *Statistics in Medicine* 1, 186–189.

Koen, C. (1991). A computer program package for the statistical analysis of spatial point processes in a square. *Biometric Journal* 33, 493–503.

Koestler, A. (1972). *The Roots of Coincidence*. Vantage Books, New York.

Kokic, P.N. (1987). On tests of uniformity for randomly distributed arcs on the circle. *Australian Journal of Statistics* 29, 179–187.

Komlos, J. and Tusnady, G. (1975). On sequences of pure heads. *Annals of Probability* 3, 608–617.

Kopocinski, B. (1991). On the distribution of the longest success-run in Bernoulli trials. *Matematyka Stosowana (Applied Mathematics) Polski Towarzystwo Mat (Polish Mathematical Society)* 34, 3–13.

Kounias, S. and Sfakianakis, M. (1991). The reliability of a linear system and its connection with the generalized birthday problem. *Statistica Applicata* 3, 531–543.

Koutras, M.V. (1994). Distribution theory of runs: A Markov chain approach. *Journal of the American Statistical Association* 89, 1050–1058.

Koutras, M.V. (1996). On a Markov chain approach for the study of reliability structures. *Journal of Applied Probability* 33, 357–367.

Koutras, M.V. (1997). Consecutive k-r-out-of-n DFM systems. *Microelectronics and Reliability* 37, 597–603.

Koutras, M.V. and Alexandrou, V.A. (1995). Runs, scans, and urn model distributions: A unified Markov chain approach. *Annals of Institute of Statistical Mathematics* 47, 743–766.

Koutras, M.V. and Balakrishnan, N. (1999). A start-up demonstration test using a simple scan-based statistic. In Glaz, J. and Balakrishnan, N., eds., *Scan Statistics and Applications*. Birkhäuser, Boston, pp. 251–267.

Koutras, M.V., Papadopoulos, G.K., and Papastavridis, S.G. (1993). Reliability of two-dimensional consecutive-k-out-of-n: F system. *IEEE Transactions on Reliability* 42, 658–661.

Koutras, M.V., Papadopoulos, G.K., and Papastavridis, S.G. (1995). Runs on a circle. *Journal of Applied Probability* 32, 396–404.

Koutras, M.V. and Papastavridis, S.G. (1993). On the number of runs and related statistics. *Statistica Sinica* 3, 277–294.

Kozelka, R. (1980). Approximate upper percentage points for extreme values in multinomial sampling. *Annals of Mathematical Statistics* **27**, 507–512.

Krauth, J. (1988). An improved upper bound for the tail probability of the scan statistic for testing non-random clustering. Classification and related methods of data analysis. *Proc. 1st Conference International Federation Classif. Soc., Technical University of Aachen, F.R.G.* North-Holland, Amsterdam, pp. 237–244.

Krauth, J. (1991). Lower bounds for the tail probabilities of the scan statistic. In Bock, H.H. and Ihm, P., eds., *Classification, Data Analysis, and Knowledge Organization: Models and Methods with Applications.* Springer-Verlag, New York, pp. 61–67.

Krauth, J. (1992a). Bounds for the upper-tail probabilities of the circular ratchet scan statistic. *Biometrics* **48**, 1177–1185.

Krauth, J. (1992b). Bounds for the upper-tail probabilities of the linear ratchet scan statistic. In Schader, M., ed., *Analyzing and Modeling Data and Knowledge.* Springer-Verlag, Berlin, pp. 51–61.

Krauth, J. (1996). Bounds for *p*-values of combinatorial tests for clustering in epidemiology. In Bock, H.H. and Polasek, W., eds., *Analysis and Information Systems.* Springer-Verlag, Berlin, pp. 64–72.

Krauth, J. (1998). Upper bounds for the *p*-values of a scan statistic with a variable window. *Studies in Classification, Data Analysis, and Knowledge Organization.* Springer-Verlag, New York, pp. 155–163.

Krauth, J. (1999). Ratchet scan and disjoint statistics. In Glaz, J. and Balakrishnan, N., eds., *Scan Statistics and Applications.* Birkhäuser, Boston.

Kruskal, J.B. (1956). On the shortest spanning subtree of a graph and the traveling salesman problem. *Proceedings of the American Mathematical Society* **39**, 2154–2158.

Kruskal, W. and Mosteller, F. (1979). Representative sampling III: The current statistical literature. *International Statistical Review* **47**, 245–265.

Kuiper, N. (1960). Tests concerning random points on a circle. *Nederlandse Akademie van Wetenschappen Proceedings, Series A* **63**, 38 47.

Kulldorff, M. (1997). A spatial scan statistic. *Communications in Statistics, A — Theory and Methods* **26**, 1481–1496.

Kulldorff, M. (1998). Letters to the Editors. *Journal of the Royal Statistical Society, Series A* **161**, 273.

Kulldorff, M. (1999). Spatial scan statistics: Models, calculations and applications. In Glaz, J. and Balakrishnan, N., eds., *Scan Statistics and Applications.* Birkhäuser, Boston, pp. 303–322.

Kulldorff, M., Atlas, W.F., Feurer, E.J., and Miller, B.A. (1998). Evaluating cluster alarms: A space–time scan statistic and brain cancer in Los Alamos, New Mexico. *American Journal of Public Health* **88**, 1377–1380.

Kulldorff, M., Feurer, E.J., Miller, B.A., and Freedman, L.S. (1997). Breast cancer clusters in the Northeast United States: A geographical analysis. *American Journal of Epidemiology* **146**, 161–170.

Kulldorff, M. and Nagarwalla, N. (1995). Spatial disease clusters: Detection and inference. *Statistics in Medicine.* **14**, 799–810.

Kulldorff, M., Rand, K., Gherman, G., Williams, G., and DeFrancesco, D. (1988). SaTScan versin 2.1.3. Software for the spatial and space–time scan statistics. National Cancer Institute, Bethesda, MD.
(http://dcp.nci.nih.gov/BB/SaTScan.html.

Kulldorff, M. and Williams, G. (1997). *SaTScan v. 1.0, Software for the Space and Space–Time Scan Statistics.* Bethesda, MD: National Cancer Institute.

Kuo, M. and Rao, J.S. (1979). Tests based on higher-order spacings. Manuscript, University of California, Santa Barbara. 42nd Session of ISI collection of contributed papers, 9.

Kwerel, S.M. (1975). Most stringent bounds on aggregated probabilities of partially specified dependent probability systems. *Journal of the American Statistical Association* **70**, 472–479.

Lai, T.L. (1973). Gaussian processes, moving averages, and quick detection problems. *Annals of Probability* **1**, 825–837.

Lai, T.L. (1995). Sequential change point detection in quality control and dynamical systems. *Journal of the Royal Statistical Society, Series B* **57**, 613–658.

Lai, T.L. and Shan, J.Z. (1999). Efficient recursive algorithms for detection of abrupt changes in signals and control systems. *IEEE Transactions on Automatic Control* **44**, 952–966.

Laszlo, Z. and Mihalyko, E.O. (1992a). Probability approximation for reliability of pipeline networks. Manuscript, Department of Mathematics and Computer Sciences, University of Veszprem, Hungary. 8200 Veszprem, Egyetem U. 10.

Laszlo, Z. and Mihalyko, E.O. (1992b). On the increasement of Poisson processes. Manuscript, to appear in *Annales Scientifiques de l'Université de Budapest*, Section Computatorica.

Leadbetter, M.R., Lindgren, G., and Rootzen, H. (1983). *Extemes and Related Properties of Random Sequences and Processes.* Springer-Verlag, New York.

Leontovich, A.M. (1992). On the optimality of the Dayhoff matrix for computing the similarity scoring between fragments of biological sequences. In Gindikin, S., ed., *Mathematical Methods of Analysis of Biopolymer Sequences.* DIMACS Series in Discrete Mathematics and Theoretical Computer Science. American Mathematical Society, Providence, RI, Vol. 8, pp. 1–9.

Leslie, R.T. (1967). Recurrent composite events. *Journal of Applied Probability* **4**, 34–61.

Leslie, R.T. (1969). Recurrence times of clusters of Poisson points. *Journal of Applied Probability* **6**, 372–388.

Leung, M.-Y. (1989). Probabilistic models and computational algorithms for some problems from molecular sequence analysis. Ph.D. Thesis, Stanford University, 76 pages.

Leung, M.-Y. (1993). Application of the scan statistics in identifying non-random clusters of markers in genomic DNA sequences. Abstract *IMS Bulletin* **22**, 46 (Bloomington, Indiana, meeting).

Leung, M.-Y., Blaisdell, B.E., Burge, C., and Karlin, S. (1991). An efficient algorithm for identifying matches with errors in multiple long molecular sequences. *Journal of Molecular Biology* **221**, 1367–1378.

Leung, M.-Y., Marsh, G.M., and Speed, T.P. (1996). Over- and under-representation of short DNA words in Herpes virus genomes. *Journal of Computational Biology* **3**, 345–360.

Leung, M.-Y., Schachtel, G.A., and Yu, H.S. (1994). Scan statistics and DNA sequence analysis: The search for an origin of replication in a virus. *Nonlinear World* **1**, 445–471.

Leung, M.-Y. and Yamashita, T.E. (1999). Application of the scan statistic in DNA sequence analysis. In Glaz, J. and Balakrishnan, N., eds., *Scan Statistics and Applications*. Birkhäuser, Boston,

Levin, B. and Kline, J. (1985). The CUSUM test of homogeneity with an application in spontaneous abortion epidemiology. *Statistics in Medicine* **4**, 469–488.

Lin, C.-T. (1993). The computation of probabilities which involve spacings, with applications to the scan statistic. Ph.D. Thesis, The Florida State University, Tallahassee, FL.

Lin, C.-T. (1999). Scan statistics and multiple scan statistics. In Glaz, J. and Balakrishnan, N., eds., *Scan Statistics and Applications*. Birkhäuser, Boston, pp. 203–223.

Ling, K.D. (1988). On binomial distributions of order k. *Statistics and Probability Letters* **6**, 247–250.

Liu, K.H. (1987). A new probability estimation of the longest run and its application. *Kexue Tongbao* (English Edition) **32**, 729–731.

Loader, C. (1990a). Large deviation approximations to distribution of scan statistic. AT&T Bell Laboratorie Technical Memorandum 11214-900914-12TM.

Loader, C. (1990b). Scan statistics for Bernoulli random variates. AT&T Bell Laboratorie Technical Memorandum 11214-901025-15TM.

Loader, C. (1991). Large deviation approximations to distribution of scan statistics. *Advances Applied Probability* **23**, 751–771.

Lou, W.Y. (1996). On runs and longest run tests: A method of finite Markov chain embedding. *Journal of the American Statistical Association* **91**, 1595–1601.

Lou, W.Y. (1997). An application of the method of finite Markov chains into runs tests. *Statistics and Probability Letters* **31**, 155–161.

Louv, W.C. and Little, R.C. (1986). Combining one-sided binomial tests. *Journal of the American Statistical Association* **81**, 550–554.

Mack, C. (1948). An exact formula for $Q_k(n)$, the probable number of k-aggregates in a random distribution of n points. *London, Edinburgh, and Dublin Philosophical Magazine and Journal of Science* **39**, 778–790.

Mack. C. (1950). The expected number of aggregates in a random distribution of n points. *Proceedings of the Cambridge Philosophical Society* **46**, 285–292.

Mactavish, J.K. (1998). An inquiry into the phenomenology of meaningful coincidences (synchronicity). Ph.D. Thesis, The Fielding Institute, 203 pp.

Makri, F.S. and Phillippou, A.N. (1994). Binomial distributions of order k on the circle. In Godbole, A.P. and Papastavridis, S.G., eds., *Runs and Patterns in Probability*. Kluwer Academic, Amsterdam, pp. 65–81.

Malinowski, J. and Preuss, W. (1996). A recursive algorithm evaluating the exact reliability of a circular consecutive-k-within-m-out-of-n F system. *Microelectron Reliability* **36**(10), 1389–1394.

Mancuso, J.P. (1998). Exact null distributions of runs statistics for occupancy models with applications to disease cluster analysis. Ph.D. Thesis, State University of New York at Stony Brook.

Mansson, M. (1994). Covering uniformly distributed points by convex scanning sets. Preprint 1994:17/ISSN 0347-2809, Department of Mathematics, Chalmers University of Technology, Goteborg, Sweden.

Mansson, M. (1995). Intersections of uniformly distributed translations of convex sets in two and three dimensions. Preprint NO 1995:11/ISSN 0347-2809, Department of Mathematics, Chalmers University of Technology, Goteborg, Sweden.

Mansson, M. (1996). On clustering of random points in the plane and in space. Thesis, ISBN 91-7197-290-0/ISSN 0346-718X, Department of Mathematics, Chalmers University of Technology, Goteborg, Sweden.

Mansson, M. (1999a). Poisson approximation in connection with clustering of random points. *Annals of Applied Probability* **9**(2), 465–492.

Mansson, M. (1999b). On Poisson approximation for continuous multiple scan statistics in two dimensions. In Glaz, J. and Balakrishnan, N., eds., *Scan Statistics and Applications*. Birkhäuser, Boston.

Mantel, N., Kryscio, R.J., and Myers, M.H. (1976). Tables and formulas for extended use of the Ederer–Myers–Mantel disease-clustering procedure. *American Journal of Epidemiology* **104**, 576–584.

Marrero, O. (1983). The performance of several statistical tests for seasonality in monthly data. *Journal of Statistical Computation and Simulation* **17**, 275–296.

Mason, D.M., Shorack, G.R., and Wellner, J.A. (1982). Strong limit theorems for oscillation moduli of the uniform empirical process. Manuscript (also correspondence dated 3/12/82 from Wellner, with inequality for scan statistic in uniform case).

Matthews, R. and Stones, F. (1998). Coincidences: The truth is out there. *Teaching Statistics* **20**, 17.

McClure, D.E. (1976). Extreme uniform spacings. Notes I and II. *Report No. 44 in Pattern Analysis*, Brown University, Providence, RI.

Melzak, Z.A. (1962). Scattering from random linear arrays with closest approach. *Quarterly of Applied Mathematics* **20**, 151–159.

Melzak, Z.A. (1967). A combinatorial coincidence problem. *Bulletin of the American Mathematics Society* **73**, 955–957.

Melzak, Z.A. (1968). On a class of configuration and coincidence problems. *Bell Systems Technical Journal* **47**, 1105–1129.

Melzak, Z.A. (1979), Multi-indexing and multiple clustering. *Mathematical Proceedings of the Cambridge Philosophical Society* **86**, 313–337.

Menon, M.V. (1964). Clusters in a Poisson process [abstract]. *Annals of Mathematical Statistics* **35**, 1395. Also unpublished manuscript, IBM Research Laboratories, San Jose, CA.

Mevorach, Y. and Pollak, M. (1991). A small sample size comparison of the CUSUM and Shirayev–Roberts approaches to change-point detection. *American Journal of Mathematical and Management Science* **11**, 277–298.

Michell, J. (1767). An inquiry into the probable parallax and magnitude of the fixed stars from the quantity of light which they afford us, and the particular circumstances of their situation. *Philosophical Transactions* **57**, 234–264.

Mirkin, B. and Roberts, F. (1993). Consensus functions and patterns in molecular sequences. *Bulletin of Mathematical Biology* **55**, 695–713.

Mizuki, M. (1996). The number of generalized runs in a Markov chain sequence of a fixed length. Ph.D. Thesis, Harvard University.

Mood, A.M. (1940). The distribution theory of runs. *Annals of Mathematical Statistics* **11**, 367–392.

Morant G.M. (1920). On random occurrences in space and time when followed by a closed interval. *Biometrika* **13**, 309–337.

Moreno, C., Ardanaz, E., Olivera, J.E., Castilla, J., and de Pedro-Cuesta, J. (1994). A temporal–spatial cluster of sudden infant death syndrome in Navarre, Spain. *European Journal of Epidemiology* **10**, 129–134.

Mori, T. (1993). The a.s. limit distribution of the longest head run. *Canadian Journal of Mathematics* **45**, 1245–1262.

Mori, T. (1994). On long runs of heads and tails. *Statistics and Probability Letters* **19**, 85–89.

Morris, J.K., Alberman, E., and Mutton, D. (1998). Is there evidence of clustering in Downs syndrome. *International Journal of Epidemiology* **27**, 495–498.

Moser, W.O.S. and Abramson, M. (1969). Enumeration of combinations with restricted differences and cospan. *Journal of Combinatorial Theory* **7**, 162–170.

Mosteller, F. (1941). Note on an application of runs to quality control charts. *Annals of Mathematical Statistics* **12**, 228–232.

Mosteller, F. (1965). *Fifty Challenging Problems in Probability*. Addison-Wesley, Reading, MA.

Mott, R.F., Kirkwood, T.B.L., and Curnow, R.M. (1989). A test for the statistical significance of DNA sequence similarities for application in databank searches. *Computer Applications in the Biosciences: CABIOS* **5**, 123–131.

Mott, R.F., Kirkwood, T.B.L., and Curnow, R.M. (1990). An accurate approximation to the distribution of the length of the longest matching word between two random DNA sequences. *Bulletin of Mathematical Biology* **52**, 773–784.

Murray, M.R. and Baker, D.E. (1991). MWINDOW: An interactive FORTRAN-77 program for calculating moving window statistics (STMA V33 0372). *Computers and Geosciences* **17**, 423–430.

Muslli, M. (2000). Useful inequalities for the longest run distribution. *Statistics and Probability Letters* **46**, 239–249.

Nagarwalla, N. (1996). A scan statistic with a variable window. *Statistics in Medicine* **15**, 845–850.

Naiman, D.Q. and Carey, P. (1998). Computing scan statistic *p*-values using importance sampling, with applications to genetics and medical image analysis. Technical report. Department of Mathematics, The Johns Hopkins University, Baltimore, MD.

Naus, J.I. (1963). Clustering of random points in line and plane. Ph.D. Thesis, Harvard University.

Naus, J.I. (1965a). The distribution of the size of the maximum cluster of points on a line. *Journal of the American Statistical Association* **60**, 532–538.

Naus, J.I. (1965b). A power comparison of two tests of non-random clustering. *Technometrics* **8**, 493–517.

Naus, J.I. (1968). An extension of the birthday problem. *The American Statistician* **22**, 27–29.

Naus, J.I. (1974). Probabilities for a generalized birthday problem. *Journal of the American Statistical Association* **69**, 810–815.

Naus, J.I. (1979). An indexed bibliography of clusters, clumps, and coincidences. *International Statistical Review* **47**, 47–78.

Naus, J.I. (1982). Approximations for distributions of scan statistics. *Journal of the American Statistical Association* **77**, 177–183.

Naus, J.I. (1988). Scan statistics. In Johnson, N.L. and Kotz, S., eds., *Encyclopedia of Statistical Sciences*, vol. 8. Wiley, New York, pp. 281–284.

Naus, J.I. (1999). Scanning multiple sequences. In Glaz, J. and Balakrishnan, N., eds., *Scan Statistics and Applications*. Birkhäuser, Boston.

Naus, J.I. and Sheng, K.N. (1996). Screening for unusual matched segments in multiple protein sequences. *Communications in Statistics, Simulation and Computation* **25**, 937–952.

Naus, J.I. and Sheng, K.N. (1997). Matching among multiple random sequences. *Bulletin of Mathematical Biology* **59**, 483–496.

Naus, J.I. and Wartenberg, D. (1997). A double scan statistic for clusters of two types of events. *Journal of the American Statistical Association* **92**, 1105–1113.

Neff, N. (1978). Piecewise polynomials for the probability of clustering on the unit interval. Unpublished Ph.D. dissertation, Rutgers University.

Neff, N. and Naus, J. (1980). *Selected Tables in Mathematical Statistics*, Vol. VI: *The Distribution of the Size of the Maximum Cluster of Points on a Line*. American Mathematical Society, Providence, RI.

Nelson, J.B. (1978). Minimal order models for false alarm calculations on sliding windows. *IEEE Transactions on Aerospace and Electronic Systems* **14**, 351–363.

Nemetz, T. and Kusolitsch, N. (1982). On the longest run of coincidences. *Zeitschrift für Wahrscheinlichkeitstheorie und Verwandte Gebiete* **61**, 59–73.

Neuhauser, C. (1994). A Poisson approximation for sequence comparisons with insertions and deletions. *Annals of Statistics* **22**, 1603–1629.

Neuhauser, C. (1996). A phase transition for the distribution of matching blocks. *Combinatorics, Probability and Computing* **5**, 139–159.

Newell, G.F. (1958). Some statistical problems encountered in a theory of pinning and breakaway of dislocations. *Quarterly of Applied Mathematics* **16**, 155–168.

Newell, G.F. (1963). Distribution for the smallest distance between any pair of Kth nearest-neighbor random points on a line. In Rosenblatt, M., ed., *Time Series Analysis, Proceedings of a Conference Held at Brown University*. Wiley, New York, pp. 89–103.

Newell G.F. (1964). Asymptotic extremes for n-dependent random variables. *Annals of Mathematical Statistics* **35**, 1322–1325.

Nikitin, Y.Y.   (1984). Large deviations of Durbin's statistic for testing uniformity on the square. *Studies in Mathematical Statistics* **VI**, 165–167.

Novak, S.Y. (1992). Longest runs in a sequence of m-dependent random variables. *Probability Theory of Related Fields* **91**, 268–291.

Novak, S.Y. (1998). On the Erdös–Rényi maximum of partial sums. *Theory of Probability and its Applications* **42**, 254–270.

Nunnikhoven, T.S. (1992). A birthday problem solution of nonuniform birth frequencies. *The American Statistician* **46**, 270–274.

Olmstead, P. (1958). Runs determined in a sample by an arbitrary cut. *Bell System Technical Journal* **37**, 55–82.

Openshaw, S. (1996). Using a geographical analysis machine to detect the presence of spatial clustering and the location of clusters in synthetic data. In Alexander, F.E. and Boyle, P., eds., *Methods for Investigating Localized Clustering of Disease*. International Agency for Research on Cancer Scientific Publications, No. 135. World Health Organization, Lyon, France.

Openshaw, S., Charlton, M., and Craft, A. (1988). Searching for leukemia clusters using a Geographical Analysis Machine. *Papers of the Regional Science Association* **64**, 95–106.

Openshaw, S., Charlton, M., Wymer, C., and Craft, A. (1987). A Mark I Geographical Analysis Machine for the automated analysis of point data sets. *International Journal of Geographical Information Systems* **1**, 335–358.

Orear, J. and Cassel, D. (1971). Aplication of statistical inference to physics. In Godambe, V.P. and Sprott, D., eds., *Foundations of Statistical Inference, Proceedings of the Symposium on the Foundations of Statistical Inference Prepared Under the Auspices of the Rene Descartes Foundation and Held at the Department of Statistics, University of Waterloo, from March 31 to April 9, 1970*. Holt, Reinhart & Winston, Toronto, Canada, pp. 280–289.

Orford, K.J. (2000). The analysis of cosmic ray data. *Journal of Physics G— Nuclear and Particle Physics* **26**(4), R1–R26.

Ozols, V. (1956). Generalization of the theorem of Gnedenko–Korolyuk to three samples in the case of two one-sided boundaries. *Latvijas PSR Zintānu Akadēmijes Vestis* **10**(111), 141–152.

Page, E.S. (1955). Control charts with warning lines. *Biometrika* **42**, 243–257.

Pai, G., Valle, D., Thomas, G., and Rosenblum, K. (1978). Cluster of trisomy 13 live births. *Lancet* (i), 613.

Panayirci, E. and Dubes, R.C. (1983). A test for multidimensional clustering tendency. *Pattern Recognition* **16**, 433–444.

Paneth, N., Kiely, M., Hegyi, T., and Hiatt, I.M. (1984). Investigation of a temporal cluster of left-sided congenital heart disease. *Journal of Epidemiology and Community Health* **38**(4), 340–344.

Papastavridis, S.G. (1988). A Weibull limit for the reliability of a consecutive k-within-m-out-of-n system. *Advances in Applied Probability* **20**, 690–692.

Papastavridis, S.G. and Koutras, M.V. (1993). Bounds for reliability of consecutive k-within-m-out-of-n: F system. *IEEE Transactions on Reliability* **42**, 156–160.

Papastavridis, S.G. and Koutras, M.V. (1994). Consecutive-k-out-of-n systems. In Misra, K.B., ed., *New Trends in System Reliability Evaluation*. Elsevier, Amsterdam, pp. 228–248.

Papastavridis, S.G. and Sfakianakis, M.E. (1991). Optimal arrangements and importance of the components in a consecutive-k-out-of-r-from-n: F system. *IEEE Transactions on Reliability* **R-40**, 277–279.

Pare, J., Carpenter, T.E., and Thurmond, M.C. (1996). Analysis of spatial and temporal clustering of horses with Salmonella Krefeld in an intensive care unit of a veterinary hospital. *Journal of the American Veterinarian Medicine Association* **209**, 558–560.

Parzen, E. (1960). *Modern Probability Theory and its Applications*. Wiley, New York.

Patefield, W.M. (1981). An efficient method of generating $R \times C$ tables with given row and column totals. *Applied Statistics* **30**, 91–97.

Pearson, E.S. (1963). Comparison of tests for randomness of points on a line. *Biometrika* **50**, 315–325.

Percus, O.E. (1990). Why use Chen–Stein for sequence comparison? Manuscript, Courant Institute.

Percus, O.E. and Percus, J.K. (1994). String matching for the novice. *American Mathematical Monthly* **101**, 944–947.

Pfaltz, J.L. (1983). Convex clusters in discrete m-dimensional space. *Journal of Computation* **12**, 746–750.

Phillippou, A.N. and Makri, F.S. (1986). Successes, runs and longest runs. *Statistics and Probability Letters* **4**, 101–105.

Pinkel, D. and Nefzger, D. (1959). Some epidemiological features of childhood leukemia. *Cancer* **12**, 351–358.

Piterbarg, V.I. (1992). On the distribution of the maximum similarity score for fragments of two random sequences. In Gindikin, S., ed., *Mathematical Methods of Analysis of Biopolymer Sequences*. DIMACS Series in Discrete Mathematics and Theoretical Computer Science, Vol. 8. American Mathematical Society, Providence, RI.

Polya, G. (1930). Sur quelques points de la theorie des probabilites. *Annales de l'Institut Henri Poincaré* **1**, 117–161.

Prekopa, A. (1988). Boole–Bonferroni inequalities and linear programming. *Operations Research* **36**, 145–162.

Priebe, C.E., Olson, T., and Healy, Jr., D.M. (1997). A spatial scan statistic for stochastic scan partitions. *Journal of the American Statistical Association* **92**, 1476–1484.

Psillakis, Z.M. (1995). A simulation algorithm for computing failure probability of a consecutive-k-out-of-R-from-N-F system. *IEEE Transactions on Reliability* **44**(3), 523–531.

Pyke, R. (1965). Spacings. *Journal of the Royal Statistical Society, Series B* **27**, 395–449.

Pyke, R. (1972). Spacings revisited. *Proceedings of the Sixth Berkeley Symposium on Mathematical Statistics and Probability* **1**, 417–427.

Qualls, C. and Watanabe, H. (1972). Asymptotic properties of Gaussian processes. *Annals of Mathematical Statistics* **43**, 580–596.

Quetelet, A. (1835). *Sur L'Homme*. William & Robert Chambers, Edinburgh.

Rabinowitz, D. (1984). Detecting clusters in disease incidence. In Carlstein, E., Muller, H.G., and Siegmund, D., eds., *Change-Point Problems*. Institute of Mathematical Statistics, Hayward, CA.

Rabinowitz, L. and Naus, J.I. (1975). The expectation and variance of the number of components in random linear graphs. *Annals of Probability* **3**, 159–161.

Rayens, M.K. and Kryscio, R.J. (1993). Properties of Tango's index for detecting clustering in time. *Statistics in Medicine* **12**, 1813–1827.

Revesz, P. (1982). On the increments of Wiener and related processes. *Annals of Probability* **10**, 613–622.

Revesz, P. (1984). How random is random? *Probability and Mathematical Statistics* **4**, 109–116.

Riordan, J. (1984). *An Introduction to Combinatorial Analysis*. Wiley, New York.

Roberts, S.W. (1958a). Properties of control chart zone tests. *Bell System Technical Journal* **37**, 83–114.

Roberts, S.W. (1958b). Duration of an m-player game of chance that ends when a player achieves k successes within n consecutive trials. Technical Report Bell Laboratorie, MM58-5214-1.

Roos, M. (1993a). Stein–Chen method for compound Poisson approximation. Ph.D. Dissertation, University of Zurich, Zurich, Switzerland.

Roos, M. (19993b). Compound Poisson approximations for the numbers of extreme spacings. *Advances in Applied Probability* **25**, 847–874.

Roos, M. (1994). Stein's method for compound Poisson approximation. *Annals of Applied Probability* **4**, 1177–1187.

Rosenfeld, A. (1978). Clusters in digital pictures. *Information and Control* **39**, 19–34.

Rothenberg, R.B., Steinberg, K.K., and Thacker, S.B. (1990). The public health importance of clusters: A note from the Centers for Disease Control. *American Journal of Epidemiology* **132** (Supplement 1), S3–5.

Rothman, E. (1967). Tests for clusters in a Poisson process. *Annals of Mathematical Statistics* **38**, 967.

Rothman, E. (1969a). Tests for uniformity against regularly spaced alternatives. Technical Report Number 119, Johns Hopkins University, Baltimore, MD.

Rothman, E. (1969b). Properties and applications of test statistics invariant under rotation of a circle. Ph.D. Thesis, Johns Hopkins University, Baltimore, MD.

Rothman, E. (1972). Tests for uniformity of a circular distribution. *Sankhyā Series A* **34**, 23–32.

Rothman, K.J. (1990). A sobering start for the cluster busters' conference. *American Journal of Epidemiology* **132** (Supplement 1), S6–13.

Runnels, L.K., Thompson, R., and Runnels, P. (1968). Near perfect runs as a learning criterion. *Journal of Mathematical Psychology* **5**, 362–368.

Russo, R.P. (1988). Strong laws for quantiles corresponding to moving blocks of random variables. *Annals of Probability* **16**, 162–171.

Sahu, S.K., Bendel, R.B., and Sison, C.P. (1993). Effect of relative risk and cluster configuration on the power of the one-dimensional scan statistic. *Statistics in Medicine* **12**, 1853–1865.

Salvia, A.A. and Lasher, W.C. (1990). Two-dimensional consecutive-k-out-of-n: F models. *IEEE Transactions on Reliability* **39**, 382.

Samarova, S.S. (1981). On the length of the longest head-run for a Markov chain with two states. *Theory of Probability and its Applications* **26**, 498–509.

Samuel-Cahn, E. (1983). Simple approximations to the expected waiting time for a cluster of any given size, for point processes. *Advances in Applied Probability* **15**, 21–38.

Sankoff, D. and Kruskal, J.B. (Eds.) (1983). *Time Warps, String Edits, and Macromolecules: The Theory and Practice of Sequence Comparisons*. Addison-Wesley, Reading, MA.

Saperstein, B. (1969). Some generalizations of the birthday problem and related problems with applications. Ph.D. Thesis, New York University.

Saperstein, B. (1972). The generalized birthday problem. *Journal of the American Statistical Association* **67**, 425–428.

Saperstein, B. (1973). On the occurrence of n successes within N Bernoulli trials. *Technometrics* **15**, 809–818.

Saperstein, B. (1974). Unrestricted solution of the generalized birthday problem. Manuscript.

Saperstein, B. (1975). Note on a clustering problem. *Journal of Applied Probability* **12**, 629–632.

Saperstein, B. (1976). The analysis of attribute moving averages: MIL-STD-105D reduced inspection plans. *Sixth Conference Stochastic Processes and Applications*, Tel Aviv.

Scheaffer, R., Mendenhall, W., and Ott, L. (1996). *Elementary Survey Sampling*, 5th ed. Duxbury Press, Boston.

Schilling, M.F. (1990). The longest run of heads. *The College Mathematics Journal* **3**, 196–207.

Schroedinger, E. (1944). Rate of N-fold accidental coincidences. *Nature* **153**, 592–593.

Schuster, E.F. (1991). Distribution theory of runs via exchangeable random variables. *Statistics and Probability Letters* **11**, 379–386.

Schuster, E.F. (1994). Exchangeability and recursion in the conditional distribution theory of numbers and lengths of runs. In Godbole, A.P. and Papastavridis, S.G., eds., *Runs and Patterns in Probability*. Kluwer Academic, Amsterdam, pp. 91–118.

Schuster, E.F. (1996). The conditional distribution of the longest run in a sample from a multi-letter alphabet. *Communications in Statistics, Simulation and Computation* **25**, 215–224.

Schuster, E.F. and Gu, X. (1997). On the conditional and unconditional distribution of the number of runs in a sample from a multisymbol alphabet. *Communications in Statistics, Simulation and Computation* **26**, 423–442.

Schwager, S.J. (1983). Run probabilities in sequences of Markov-dependent trials. *Journal of the American Statistical Association* **78**, 168–175.

Schwager, S.J. (1984). Bonferroni sometimes loses. *American Statistician* **3**, 192–197.

Seneta, E. (1988). Degree, iteration and permutation in improving Bonferroni-type bounds. *Australian Journal of Statistics* **30A**, 27–38.

Serfling, R.J. (1975). A general Poisson approximation theorem. *Annals of Probability* **3**, 726–731.

Sfakianakis, M.E. (1991). Reliability of the k out-of-r consecutive-out-of-n: F systems. Ph.D. Thesis, University of Athens.

Sheng, K.-N. and Naus, J. (1994). Pattern matching between two non-aligned random sequences. *Bulletin of Mathematical Biology* **56**, 1143–1162.

Sheng, K.-N. and Naus, J. (1996). Matching fixed rectangles in two dimensions. *Statistics and Probability Letters* **26**, 83–90.

Sheperd, J., Creasey, J.W., and Fisher, N.I. (1981). Statistical analysis of spacings between geological discontinuities in coal mines, with applications to short-range forecasting of mining conditions. *Australian Coal Geology* **3**, 71–80.

Shepp, L. (1971). First passage time for a particular Gaussian process. *Annals of Mathematical Statistics* **42**, 946–951.

Shmueli, G. and Cohen, A. (2000). Run-related probability functions applied to sampling inspection. *Technometrics* (to appear).

Siegel, A.F., Roach, J.C., and Van Den Engh, G. (1998). Expectation and variance of true and false fragment matches in DNA restriction mapping. *Journal of Computational Biology* **5**, 101–111.

Siegmund, D. (1988). Tail probabilities for the maxima of some random fields. *Annals of Probability* **16**, 487–501.

Siegmund, D. (1992). Tail approximations for maxima of random fields. *Probability Theory: Proceedings of the Singapore Probability Conference*. Springer-Verlag, New York, pp. 147–158.

Siegmund, D. and Ventrakaman, E. (1995). Using the generalized likelihood ratio statistics for sequential detection of a change point. *Annals of Statistics* **23**, 255–271.

Siegmund, D. and Yakir, B. (2000a). Tail probabilities for the null distribution of scanning statistics. *Bernoulli* **6**, 191–213.

Siegmund, D. and Yakir, B. (2000b). Approximate *p*-values for local sequence alignments. Preprint.

Silberstein, L. (1945). The probable number of aggregates in random distributions of points. *London, Edinburgh, and Dublin Philosophical Magazine and Journal of Science* **36**, 319–336.

Singer, R.S., Case, J.T., Carpenter, T.E., Walker, R.L., and Hirsh, D.C. (1998). Assessment of spatial and temporal clustering of ampicillin- and tetracycline-resistant strains of *Pasteurella multocida* and *P. haemolytical* isolated from cattle in California. *Journal of the American Veterinary Medical Association* **212**(7), 1001–1005.

Smeeton, N. and Wilkinson, G. (1988). The identification of clustering in parasuicide. *British Journal of Psychiatry* **153**, 218–221.

Sobel, E. and Martinez, H.M. (1986). A multiple sequence alignment program. *Nucleic Acids Research* **14**, 363–374.

Sobel, M., Uppuluri, V.R.R., and Frankowski, K. (1985). *Dirichlet Integrals of Type II and Their Applications: Selected Tables in Mathematical Statistics*, vol. IX. American Mathematical Society, Providence, RI., 480 pp.

Solov'ev, A.D. (1966). A combinatorial identity and its application to the problem concerning the first occurrence of a rare event. *Theory of Probability and Its Applications* **11**, 276–282.

Steele, J.M. (1982). Long common subsequences and the proximity of two random strings. *SIAM Journal of Applied Mathematics* **42**, 731–737.

Stefanov, V.T. (1999a). On the occurrence of composite events and clusters of points. *Journal of Applied Probability* **36**, 1012–1018.

Stefanov, V.T. (1999b). Markov renewal processes and exponential families. In Taussen, T. and Liwuios, N., eds., *Semi-Markov Models and Applications*. Kluwer Academic, Amsterdam.

Stefanov, V.T. and Pakes, A.G. (1997). Explicit distributional results in pattern formation. *Annals of Applied Probability* **7**, 666–678.

Stefanov, V.T. and Pakes, A.G. (1999). Explicit distribution results in pattern formation II. *Australian and New Zealand Journal of Statistics* **41**(1), 79–90.

Stein, C. (1972). A bound for the error in the normal approximations to the distribution of a sum of dependent random variables. *Proceedings of the Sixth Berkeley Symposium on Mathematical Statistical Probability* **2**, 583–602.

Stevens, W.L. (1939). Solution to a geometrical problem in probability. *Annals of Eugenics* **9**, 315–320.

Stewart, I. (1998). What a coincidence. *Scientific American* (Mathematical Recreations) June, pp. 95–96.

Stroup, D.F., Williamson, G.D., and Herndon, J.L. (1989). Detection of aberrations in the occurrence of notifiable disease surveillance data. *Statistics in Medicine* **8**, 323–329.

Stroup, N.E., Edmonds, L., and Obrien, T.R. (1990). Renal agenesis and dysgenesis: Are they increasing? *Teratology* **42**, 383–395.

Su, X. (1999). Scan statistics and DNA sequence analysis: The search for tissue-specific regulatory regions. Ph.D. Thesis, Mount Sinai Bioinformatics Group.

Su, X. and Wallenstein, S. (2000). New approximations for the distribution of the r-scan statistic. *Statistics and Probability Letters* **46**, 411–419.

Su, X., Wallenstein, S., and Bishop, D. (2001). Non-overlapping clusters: Approximate distribution and application to molecular biology. *Biometrics* **57**, 420–426.

Suman, K.A. (1994). The longest run of any letter in a randomly generated word. In Godbole, A.P. and Papastavridis, S.G., eds., *Runs and Patterns in Probability*. Kluwer Academic, Amsterdam, pp. 119–130.

Swanepoel, J.W.H. and De Beer, C.F. (1990). A powerful test for uniformity to detect highly peaked alternative densities. *Communications in Statistics — Theory Methods* **19**, 2781–2798.

Takacs, L. (1951). Coincidence phenomena in case of happenings with arbitrary distribution law of duration. *Acta Mathematica Hungarica* **2**, 275–298.

Takacs, L. (1953). Coincidence problems arising in the theory of counters. *Publications of the Mathematical Institute of the Hungarian Academy of Science*, (Hungarian) *Magyar Tud. Akad. Alkalm. Mat. Int. Kozl.* **2**, 153–163.

Takacs, L. (1958). On a coincidence problem concerning telephone traffic. *Acta Mathematica Hungarica* **9**, 45–81.

Takacs, L. (1961). On a coincidence problem concerning particle counters. *Annals of Mathematics and Statistics* **32**, 739–756.

Takacs, L. (1980). The problem of coincidence. *Archive for History of Exact Sciences* **21**, 229–244.

Takacs, L. (1995). On a test for uniformity of a circular distribution. *Mathematical Methods of Statistics* **5**, 77–98.

Takacs, L. (1997). On the ballot theorems. In Balakrishnan, N., ed., *Advances in Combinatoric Methods and Applications to Probability and Statistics*. Birkhäuser, Basel, pp. 97–114.

Ten Hoopen, M. and Reuver, H.A. (1963). On a waiting time problem in physiology. *Statistica Neerlandica* **19**, 27–34.

Ten Hoopen, M. and Reuver, H.A. (1965). An n-fold coincidence problem in physiology. *Journal of Theoretical Biology* **9**, 117–123.

Todd, P.H. (1981). Direct minimal-order Markov model for sliding-window detection probabilities. *IEEE Proceedings* **128**, 152–154.

Tomescu, I. (1986). Hypertrees and Bonferroni inequalities. *Journal of Combinatorial Theory, Series B* **41**, 209–217.

Troxell, J.R. (1972). An investigation of suspension systems for small scale inspections. Ph.D. Thesis, Department of Statistics, Rutgers University, New Brunswick, NJ.

Troxell, J.R. (1980). Suspension systems for small sample inspections. *Technometrics* **22**, 517–533.

Trusov, A.G. (1979). Estimation of the optical signal arrival time under conditions of photon counting in free space. *Proc. IEEE Radio–Optics* **19**, 137–139.

Tu, I.-P. (1997). Theory and applications of scan statistics. Ph.D. Thesis, Stanford University, Stanford, CA, 111 pp.

Turnbull, B.W., Iwano, E.J., Burnett, W.S., Howe, H.L., and Clark, L.C. (1990). Monitoring for clusters of disease: Application to leukemia incidence in upstate New York. *American Journal of Epidemiology* **132**, S136–S143.

Uspensky, J.V. (1937). *Introduction to Mathematical Probability*. McGraw-Hill, New York, pp. 77–84.

Velandia, M., Fridkin, S.K., Cardenas, V., Boshell, J., Ramirez, G., Bland, L., Iglesias, A., and Jarvis, W. (1995). Transmission in HIV in dialysis centre. *Lancet* **345**, 1417–1422.

Viel, J.-F., Arveus, P., Baveral, J., and Cahn, J.-Y. (2000). Soft-tissue sarcoma and non-Hodgkin's lymphoma clusters around a municipal solid waste incinerator with high dioxin emission levels. *American Journal of Epidemiology* **152**, 13–19.

Viveros, R. and Balakrishnan, N. (1993). Statistical inference from startup demonstration test data. *Journal of Quality Technology* **25**, 119–130.

Votaw, D.F. (1946). The probability distribution of the measure of a random linear set. *Annals of Mathematical Statistics* **17**, 240–244.

Wallenstein, S. (1971). Coincidence probabilities used in nearest-neighbor problems on the line and circle. Ph.D. Thesis, Department of Statistics, Rutgers University, New Brunswick, NJ.

Wallenstein, S. (1980a). A test for detection of clustering over time. *American Journal of Epidemiology* **11**, 367–372.

Wallenstein, S. (1980b). Distributions of some one-sided k-sample Smirnov-type statistics. *Journal of the American Statistical Association* **75**, 441–446.

Wallenstein, S. (1999). Applying ballot problem results to compute probabilities required for a generalization of the scan statistics. In Glaz, J. and Balakrishnan, N., eds., *Scan Statistics and Applications*. Birkhäuser, Boston.

Wallenstein, S., Gould, M.S., and Kleinman, M. (1989). Use of the scan statistic to detect time–space clustering. *American Journal of Epidemiology* **130**, 1057–1064.

Wallenstein, S. and Naus, J. (1973). Probabilities for the kth nearest neighbor problem on the line. *Annals of Probability* **1**, 188–190.

Wallenstein, S. and Naus, J. (1974). Probabilities for the size of largest clusters and smallest intervals. *Journal of the American Statistical Association* **69**, 690–697.

Wallenstein, S., Naus, J., and Glaz, J. (1993). Power of the scan statistic for detection of clustering. *Statistics in Medicine* **12**, 1–15.

Wallenstein, S., Naus, J., and Glaz, J. (1994). Power of the scan statistic in detecting a changed segment in a Bernoulli sequence. *Biometrika* **81**, 595–601.

Wallenstein, S., Weinberg, C.R., and Gould, M. (1989). Testing for a pulse in seasonal event data. *Biometrics* **45**, 817–830.

Wallqvist, A., Fununishi, Y., Murphy, L.R., Fadel, A., and Levy, R. (1999). Protein sequence matching using secondary structure similarities: Comparison with amino acid sequence alignments and application to fold recognition in genome databases. Department of Chemistry, Rutgers University.

Walter, S.D. and Elwood, J.M. (1975). A test for seasonality of events with a variable population at risk. *British Journal of Preventive and Social Medicine* **29**, 18–21.

Warburton, D., Kline, J., Stein, Z., and Susser, M. (1977). Trisomy cluster in New York. *Lancet* (ii), 201 (July 23).

Ward, M.P. and Carpenter, T.E. (2000). Techniques for analysis of disease clustering in space and in time in veterinary epidemiology. *Preventive Veterinary Medicine* **45**(3–4), 257-284.

Waterman, M.S. (1986). Multiple sequence alignment by consensus. *Nucleic Acids Research* **14**, 9095–9102.

Waterman, M.S. Ed. (1989). *Mathematical Methods for DNA Sequences*. CRC Press, Boca Raton, FL.

Waterman, M.S. (1995). *Introduction to Computational Biology*. Chapman & Hall, New York.

Waterman, M.S., Arratia, R., and Galas, D.J. (1984). Pattern recognition in several sequences: Consensus and alignment. *Bulletin of Mathematical Biology* **46**, 515–527.

Waterman, M.S., Gordon, L., and Arratia, R. (1987). Phase transitions in sequence matches and nucleic acid structure. *Proceedings of the National Academy of Sciences USA* **84**, 1239–1243.

Watson, G. (1967). Another test for the uniformity of a circular distribution. *Biometrika* **54**, 675–677.

Weinberg, R. (1980). A test for clustering on the circle. Ph.D. Thesis, University of Washington, Seattle, WA.

Weinstock, M. (1981). A generalized scan statistic for the detection of clusters. *International Journal of Epidemiology* **10**, 289–293.

Weiss, L. (1959). The limiting joint distribution of the largest and the smallest sample spacings. *Annals of Mathematical Statistics* **30**, 590–593.

Weiss, W. (1982). Epidemic curve of respiratory cancer due to chloromethyl ethers. *Journal of National Cancer Institute* **69**, 1265–1270.

Whitworth, W.A. (1901). *Choice and Chance*. Hafner, New York.

Wingender, E., Dietze, P., Karas, H., and Knuppel, R. (1996). TRANSFAC: A database on transcription factors and their DNA binding sites. *Nucleic Acids Research* **24**, 238–241.

Witztum, D., Rips, E., and Rosenberg, Y. (1994). Equidistant letter sequences in the book of Genesis. *Statistical Science* **9**, 429–438.

Wolf, E.H. (1968). Test for randomness on the line and a related k-sample test for homogeneity. Ph.D. Thesis, Rutgers University.

Wolf, E. and Naus, J.I. (1973). Tables of critical values for a k-sample Kolmogorov–Smirnov test statistic. *Journal of the American Statistical Association* **68**, 994–997.

Worsley, K.J. (1982). An improved Bonferroni inequality and applications. *Biometrika* **69**, 297–302.

Wu, J.S. and Chen, R.J. (1994). Reliability of consecutive-weighted K out of N: F system. In Godbole, A.P. and Papastavridis, S.G., eds., *Runs and Patterns in Probability*. Kluwer Academic, Amsterdam, pp. 205–211.

Yamamoto, H. and Miyakawa, M. (1995). Reliability of a linear connected-(r, s)-out-of-(m, n): F lattice system. *IEEE Transactions on Reliability* **44**, 333–336.

Zakai, M. and Ziv, J. (1969). On the threshold effect in radar range estimation. *IEEE Transactions on Information Theory* **IT-15**, 167–170.

Zhang, H. (1999). The spatial scan statistic and its application. Master of Arts Thesis, Truman State University.

Zubkov, A.M. and Mihailov, V.G. (1974). Limit distributions of random variables that are connected with long duplications in a sequence of independent trials. *Theory of Probability and its Applications* **19**, 172–179.

Zuo, M.J. (1993). Reliability and design of a two-dimensional consecutive k-out-of-n system. *IEEE Transactions on Reliability* **42**, 488–490.

Index

acceptance sampling, 49, 51
airplane crashes, 5, 30
amitochondrial protozoa, 90
ARL (average run length), 49, 52
astronomy, 6, 274

Bible Code, 9, 317
ballot problems, 101, 103, 121, 139,
    192, 261, 271
Bernoulli process, 6, 38, 44, 87, 203,
    205, 210, 212, 221, 241,
    275, 325
birthdays, 9, 15, 56, 137, 201
blowfly strike, 4
Bonferroni inequalities, 68, 104, 141,
    145, 158, 164, 205, 207,
    226, 230, 276, 279, 287,
    292, 328, 330
Boole's inequality, 104
bounds, 141, 147, 155, 156, 163, 164,
    176, 178, 183, 186, 189,
    205, 210, 225, 232, 236,
    240, 249, 300, 319, 328

cancer, 14, 64, 85, 262

brain, 4, 65
breast, 4, 65
cell occupancy, 118, 128, 131, 161,
    170, 182, 248, 250
charges in DNA, 236
Chen–Stein method, 322
chess, 57
circular scan statistics, 18, 41, 137,
    158, 210, 329
clumping, 281
coal mine discontinuities, 18
coincidences, 8, 56
combinatorial approach, 101, 115, 116,
    123, 126, 138, 318, 327
compound Poisson approximations,
    38, 77, 108, 111, 168, 169,
    215, 218, 241, 282, 287,
    291, 305
computer science, 170, 182, 239, 256,
    274, 296
control chart, 51
correlated sequences, 95
cosmic ray source, 70
Crohn's disease, 15
crossovers, 96

CUSUM, 51
cytomegalovirus, 83

DAM sites, 82, 235
Dandekar-modified binomial, 307
declumping, 110, 165, 291, 305, 314, 319
descendant sequences, 95
discrete scan, 5, 77, 88, 201, 221, 243, 245, 261, 273, 283, 287, 316, 320
disease surveillance, 36, 137, 261
DNA, 3, 81, 82, 84, 94, 95, 137, 235, 309
double scans, 95, 313, 318
Down's Syndrome, 4
dyad, 84, 90

E. coli, 90, 137
E. coli, 82
ecology, 274
embedding in Markov chain, 224, 225, 262, 283
Epstein–Barr virus, 83, 85
Erdös–Rényi laws, 46, 59, 233

failure systems, 43, 165, 201, 210, 240
flaws in crystals, 18
food poisonings, 36
fragment sequencing, 94, 320

galaxy super-clustering, 79
generalized likelihood ratio, 245, 263, 274, 330
generating function, 233
genome, 8, 82, 94, 310
global declumping, 303
Guillain–Barre syndrome, 4, 33

higher-order gaps, 113, 307
HIV, 4, 13
homicide–suicide clusters, 32, 313
Huffer–Lin approach, 133
Hunter inequalities, 144, 145, 178, 205, 328

hypergeometric distribution, 203, 207, 219, 295

identical by descent, 95
image analysis, 274
inflammatory bowel disease, 4, 15

Janson bounds, 198, 229

k-in-m-in-N failure systems, 54
Karlin–McGregor theorem, 103, 121, 125, 189, 203, 248, 271, 324
Kolmogorov–Smirnov statistic, 120, 332

laryngeal cancer, 4, 66
lattice, 69, 76, 111
learning, 53
leukemia, 4, 15, 65
linkage, 95
local declumping, 165
longest success run, 58, 222, 232, 240, 326
LREC test, 326

Markov-type approximations, 161, 167, 174, 213, 249, 258, 265, 275, 286, 289
matching
    almost perfect, 86, 88, 89, 91, 222, 320
    in DNA, 85, 90, 222, 320
    multiple, 86, 89, 91
maximum rth-order gap, 322
maximum likelihood estimates, 72
method of moments, 154, 161, 162, 166, 168, 170
minefields, 72, 78, 274
moments, 21, 37, 59, 166, 199, 239, 241, 307, 329
MOSUM, 51
multiple scan statistic, 85, 155, 286
muons, source of, 70, 71

nonoverlapping clusters, 36, 40, 164, 185, 302, 303, 309, 316
nonuniform, 244, 261
number of clusters, 39, 170, 301

open-loop flow control, 33
optimal test, 262, 263, 266, 330
order statistic, 99, 147, 152, 154, 164, 322
origin of replication, 84
overlapping clusters, 40, 65, 101, 249, 306, 309, 314, 319

palindrome clusters, 3, 83
parasuicide, 12
pattern recognition, 82, 84, 274, 317
photography, 13
piecewise polynomials, 123, 126, 131
pipeline networks, 33
poisoning, carbon monoxide, 26
Poisson approximations, 67, 77, 90, 92, 108, 110, 163, 168, 214, 218, 281, 287, 290, 303, 309, 318, 322
Poisson process, 27, 38, 72, 95, 121, 185, 190, 197, 222, 229, 241, 243, 297
police deaths, 32
population size estimation, 71
power, 7, 243, 247, 251, 258
product-type approximation, 161, 175, 182, 212, 214, 218, 275, 277, 287, 288
prospective case, 56
pulse alternatives, 244, 247, 255, 263, 330

Q_2/Q_3 approximation, 164
Q_2/Q_3 approximation, 107
Q_2/Q_3 approximation, 175, 182, 183, 196, 249, 255, 256, 265, 308, 321
quality control, 43
quasi-ranges, 113
quota, 5, 44, 54, 56, 87, 201, 202, 233, 241

random walks, 101, 121, 198
ratchet scan, 20, 66, 71, 84, 90, 326
recursion formula, 144, 179, 207, 222, 236, 239, 276, 325
reflection principle, 101, 102, 118, 119, 138
reliability, 54, 79, 274
remote sensing, 274
representativeness of samples, 16
retrospective case, 25, 56, 201, 314
runs, 58, 87, 168, 233, 304, 320

salmonella, 36
sample size, 120, 179
Saperstein's recursion, 202, 236, 237, 239, 278
seasonality, 19, 20, 35, 261, 267, 269, 329
shape of scan window, 65
skip–scan statistic, 320
small scans, 322
spacings, 113, 133, 147, 162, 233, 245, 301, 310, 322, 325
spare part, stocking, 32
sparse data, 302, 322, 326
sports, 52, 312
star cluster, 67
streaks, 52
success run, 47, 58, 89, 201
Sudden Infant Death Syndrome, 4
suicide, 4, 13
    adolescent, 19, 20
    copy-cat, 22

telephone systems, 26
two dimensions, 61, 66, 70, 78, 79, 273, 297, 331
two-type clusters, 313

uniform distribution, 11, 100, 101, 113, 118, 137, 141, 147, 152, 158, 185, 192, 244, 299, 310, 322, 323
upcrossings, 197, 298
uranium deposits, 62

visual perception, 31

waiting time, 38, 49, 60, 186, 199,
        221, 226, 241, 316
web sites, 12, 73, 317
Weinstock's approach, 262

window
    fixed, 3, 71, 87, 96, 262, 313
    size unknown, 249
    variable, 96, 263

zone control charts, 48

Springer Series in Statistics

(continued from p. ii)

Kotz/Johnson (Eds.): Breakthroughs in Statistics Volume I.
Kotz/Johnson (Eds.): Breakthroughs in Statistics Volume II.
Kotz/Johnson (Eds.): Breakthroughs in Statistics Volume III.
Küchler/Sørensen: Exponential Families of Stochastic Processes.
Le Cam: Asymptotic Methods in Statistical Decision Theory.
Le Cam/Yang: Asymptotics in Statistics: Some Basic Concepts, 2nd edition.
Liu: Monte Carlo Strategies in Scientific Computing.
Longford: Models for Uncertainty in Educational Testing.
Mielke, Jr./Berry: Permutation Methods: A Distance Function Approach.
Miller, Jr.: Simultaneous Statistical Inference, 2nd edition.
Mosteller/Wallace: Applied Bayesian and Classical Inference: The Case of the
    Federalist Papers.
Parzen/Tanabe/Kitagawa: Selected Papers of Hirotugu Akaike.
Politis/Romano/Wolf: Subsampling.
Ramsay/Silverman: Functional Data Analysis.
Rao/Toutenburg: Linear Models: Least Squares and Alternatives.
Read/Cressie: Goodness-of-Fit Statistics for Discrete Multivariate Data.
Reinsel: Elements of Multivariate Time Series Analysis, 2nd edition.
Reiss: A Course on Point Processes.
Reiss: Approximate Distributions of Order Statistics: With Applications
    to Non-parametric Statistics.
Rieder: Robust Asymptotic Statistics.
Rosenbaum: Observational Studies.
Rosenblatt: Gaussian and Non-Gaussian Linear Time Series and Random Fields.
Särndal/Swensson/Wretman: Model Assisted Survey Sampling.
Schervish: Theory of Statistics.
Shao/Tu: The Jackknife and Bootstrap.
Siegmund: Sequential Analysis: Tests and Confidence Intervals.
Simonoff: Smoothing Methods in Statistics.
Singpurwalla and Wilson: Statistical Methods in Software Engineering:
    Reliability and Risk.
Small: The Statistical Theory of Shape.
Sprott: Statistical Inference in Science.
Stein: Interpolation of Spatial Data: Some Theory for Kriging.
Taniguchi/Kakizawa: Asymptotic Theory of Statistical Inference for Time Series.
Tanner: Tools for Statistical Inference: Methods for the Exploration of Posterior
    Distributions and Likelihood Functions, 3rd edition.
Tong: The Multivariate Normal Distribution.
van der Vaart/Wellner: Weak Convergence and Empirical Processes: With
    Applications to Statistics.
Verbeke/Molenberghs: Linear Mixed Models for Longitudinal Data.
Weerahandi: Exact Statistical Methods for Data Analysis.
West/Harrison: Bayesian Forecasting and Dynamic Models, 2nd edition.

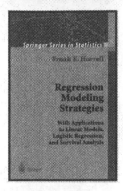
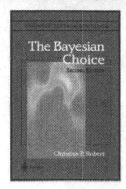
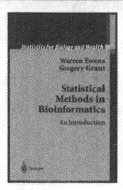
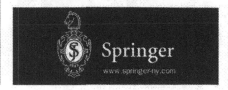

Errata

Scan Statistics

Joseph Glaz, Joseph Naus, and Sylvan Wallenstein

Page 3, 2 lines from bottom: "April 4" should be "April 14."

Page 67, 3 lines from bottom: "$E(X)$ = 1499, p=" should be "$E(X)$ = 1499 p =."

After the final galleys were returned by the authors to the publisher for final printing, the printer used a pdf file for the entire book except for the three pages where figures appeared (69, 102 & 117). The wrong version of these three pages was used. The following errors resulted:

Page 69. The first two lines of the footnote repeat the two lines on the bottom of page 68.

Page 70: The first line on the top of the page was left out and is as follows:
"motivated by astronomers' search of the "celestial sphere for a point source of..."

Page 101: The last line is repeated on page 102.

Page 117: Figure 8.1. "*****" should be "****."

The authors will post other errors found at the following URL:

http://merlot.stat.uconn.edu/~joe/